PSYCHIATRIC NURSING IN THE HOSPITAL AND THE COMMUNITY

PSYCHIATRIC
IN THE
AND THE

Ann Wolbert Burgess, R.N., D.N.Sc.

Associate Professor and Coordinator
Graduate Program in Community Health Nursing
Boston College, Chestnut Hill
Massachusetts

Aaron Lazare, M.D.

Associate Professor of Psychiatry at the Massachusetts General Hospital,
Harvard Medical School
Director of Outpatient Psychiatry
Massachusetts General Hospital

SECOND EDITION

NURSING
HOSPITAL
COMMUNITY

Prentice-Hall, Inc., Englewood Cliffs, New Jersey

Library of Congress Cataloging in Publication Data

BURGESS, ANN WOLBERT, (date)
  Psychiatric nursing in the hospital and the community.

  Includes bibliographies and index.
  1. Psychiatric nursing. I. Lazare, Aaron, joint
author. II. Title. [DNLM: 1. Community mental
health services. 2. Psychiatric nursing. WY160 B955p]
RC440.B89 1976   610.73'68   75-35946
ISBN 0-13-731901-0

second edition
Psychiatric Nursing in the Hospital and the Community
Ann Wolbert Burgess | Aaron Lazare

10 9 8 7 6 5 4 3 2 1

Printed in the United States of America

PRENTICE-HALL INTERNATIONAL, INC., LONDON
PRENTICE-HALL OF AUSTRALIA PTY. LIMITED, SYDNEY
PRENTICE-HALL OF CANADA, LTD., TORONTO
PRENTICE-HALL OF INDIA PRIVATE LIMITED, NEW DELHI
PRENTICE-HALL OF JAPAN, INC., TOKYO
PRENTICE-HALL OF SOUTHEAST ASIA PTE. LTD., SINGAPORE

*We dedicate this book
to the memory of our mothers:*
Anna Kehrli Wolbert
Anne Lazare

CONTRIBUTING AUTHORS

MARIANNE TIPMORE CANNON, R.N., M.S.

Marianne Cannon is a child psychiatric nurse clinician at the Newton-Wellesley Hospital, Newton, Massachusetts. She works with children and their families and consults with departments within the hospital and community agencies. She is a nurse-educator and has worked in a psychiatric crisis in-patient hospital unit, a day treatment center for adults, and an in-patient center for children.

JOHN A. RENNER, JR., M.D.

John Renner is Director of the Alcohol Clinic and Drug Treatment Program at Massachusetts General Hospital. He is an Instructor in Psychiatry at Harvard Medical School. Dr. Renner brings administrative, clinical, and theoretical expertise to these issues.

CONTENTS

THREE
CONCEPTUAL FRAMEWORK FOR PRACTICE

FOUR
THE CLINICAL SYNDROMES

FIVE
THE COMMUNITY

FOREWORD

If this book surprises some teachers of psychiatric nursing, it is because it is not a cookbook presentation with multiple recipes for the quick and sure approach to the mentally ill. It is also not a Rand McNally guide to the intricacies of the diagnostic nomenclature with the entire clinical entities neatly mapped out. It presents, rather, an exciting way to think and to be concerned about those human beings who are suffering and at times dying from emotional illness. The text stimulates us to become involved, yet helps us to remain objective. It calls upon us not only to understand but demands an empathetic acceptance of the patient with all his hurts no matter how frightened we may be. Its major purpose is clear: to motivate nurses as human beings to acknowledge and respond to another human in a way that is therapeutic. It demonstrates a catalytic approach where the nurse catalysts are intimately involved yet ultimately themselves and not part of the pathological process.

Although the focus is the student in the psychiatric setting, the principles are clearly applicable to all areas of nursing and indeed often to situations outside of the profession.

The authors have devoted attention to stalls in the therapeutic process. How often in the past have students felt they alone were the only ones who experienced no movement in their relationships? How reassuring to learn otherwise. The text strips away the facade of detached omnipotence behind which the nurse, in the past, could safely hide. It identifies the pitfalls in relationships that are universal and tells us how to heal ourselves after traumatic encounters.

Ann Burgess and Aaron Lazare have told it as it is.

GERTRUDE E. FLYNN, R.N., D.N.SC.
Chairperson, Department of Nursing
Bloomsburg State College
Bloomsburg, Pennsylvania

PREFACE

This book addresses itself to students and practitioners of psychiatric nursing and community mental health nursing and to all other disciplines that provide mental health services. The central focus of this book is on the *human dimension* in psychiatric nursing. Patients matter as people. They must be seen as individuals who are suffering in their behaviors, in their thoughts, and especially in their feelings. Mental illness represents the patients' attempts to cope with overwhelming experiences. It is their way of making the best out of a bad situation.

By the human dimension, we also mean that nurses matter as people. Their discomfort with patients represents not a treatment failure but a diagnostic clue that there is a subtle and complicated clinical situation to be understood. The nurses' feelings must be attended to by themselves, their colleagues, and their supervisors if they are to fully develop their skills as clinicians.

The past five years have seen an increase in the need for the delivery of mental health services to individual citizens, the family, and the community. In order to meet the requests for services, psychiatric nursing has expanded its practice in scope and direction. This second edition attempts to elaborate on and enhance the focus on the human dimension in psychiatric nursing with four objectives in mind:

1. To update the theoretical framework of existing clinical syndromes that will add to the knowledge base for the nurse;
2. To present current research findings in contemporary social problems and issues with which nurses deal daily in the community;
3. To present new clinical techniques useful in client situations for nurses to add to their nursing practice;
4. To respond to the critical comments and suggestions recommended by instructors and students who have used the first edition of this text.

Part One includes two chapters that apply the humanistic perspective to both student and patient. We first make nurses aware of the subjective experiences of their predecessors in order for them to appreicate that their anxiety is understandable. The subjective experiences of the patient are then presented to keep in sight from the very beginning that the patient is a real, live person with extraordinary capacities to sense what is going on around him.

Part Two, "Theoretical Framework," includes three new chapters as a response to the requests for theoretical depth. Current advances that have been made in ego psychology and contemporary formulations of psychodynamic concepts are included. In addition, the illustration of a four-year course of treatment of an adolescent male by the authors is presented to show the application of concepts to practice.

Part Three is a conceptual framework for practice. The nursing process includes the steps of assessment, planning, negotiating, intervening, and evaluating nurse-patient interaction. Standards of psychiatric-mental health nursing practice are included within the appropriate chapters. We attempt to conceptualize the therapeutic process in a way that enables the nurses to "get close," allowing their individual human styles to do their job. Formulations and intellectualizations—which separate the nurse from the patient—are avoided. Subsequent chapters include techniques of interviewing that facilitate the humanistic process and a description of stall factors that might impede the process. The psychiatric interventions are described according to the four models of patient care.

Part Four, "The Clinical Syndromes," applies what has been learned thus far to the various syndromes that are encountered in clinical practice. Some believe that diagnostic categories are not relevant to the practice of psychiatric nursing. They advocate the teaching of nursing care of behavior patterns. Although there are limitations to the diagnostic categories, we believe that the historically derived syndromes do lend themselves to study of the human dimension. In addition, there can be no interdisciplinary collaboration between nursing and other professions without knowledge of these syndromes. We attempt to conceptualize each syndrome as a complex of feelings, thoughts, and behaviors, all of which represent ways of coping with human miseries. In this way, clinical pathology may be treated independent of diagnosis. New chapters added to this section are "Problems of Children and Adolescents," written by a child psychiatric nurse, Marianne Tipmore Cannon, and a chapter entitled "Liaison Psychiatric Nursing."

Part Five, "The Community," helps the nurse move from the hospital to the community. We begin by discussing recently acquired knowledge in the understanding of social factors in mental illness and include the history of the community mental health movement, the impact of the feminist movement, and patients' rights in the field. We describe two specific approaches in community work: crisis intervention and the treatment of unresolved grief. We conclude this section with a discussion of some community problems, which include chapters on alcoholism and drug abuse written by a psychiatrist, John A. Renner, Jr., and a chapter on the elderly in the community.

Part Six, "Perspectives," describes the expanding and increasing responsibilities of the nurse in the delivery of adequate mental health services. The broadened dimension of nursing care moving out to a social context has implications that lead to a whole new orientation of training and skill for the nurse.

This book addresses itself to the increasing clinical responsibilities of psychiatric nurses, who, in many situations, have become primary caretakers. Often they are the first ones to see a patient, and sometimes they are the only ones. This makes it necessary for psychiatric nurses to become general practitioners of psychiatric care, possessing a broad range of information that will enable them to determine what specialists, if any, need to be called upon.

In summary, we wish to emphasize in this text an often understated aspect of patients — that is, their *humanness*. Somehow this dimension seems to have been overlooked, with the consequence that patients are seen as diagnostic entities rather than as people with feelings, concerns, and problems. Only by raising the human dimension of patienthood to its proper perspective will optimal treatment be possible in the delivery of health care services.

Many individuals have aided us in our efforts to portray and present the human dimension. We take this opportunity to express our appreication and gratitude to our teachers, our students, our patients, our colleagues, and our families, who have been instrumental in teaching us much more than they perhaps will ever realize.

Special recognition is given to Elvin Semrad, Professor of Psychiatry at Harvard Medical School and Director of Psychiatry at the Massachusetts Mental Health Center, Boston, Massachusetts, who taught both authors the humanistic approach to the psychiatric patient.

Nursing students played an important part in the evolution of the book and recognition is accorded to the Class of 1971 of the Lasell Junior College Nursing Program, Auburndale, Massachusetts, whose efforts provided in large part the content for Chapter 1.

We wish to thank Sister Cecile Couture, Margaret Smith Hamilton, Anna Melone Pollack, Eleanor Rosenwald, Gloria Edlehauser Shapiro, Carolyn J. Thomas, Dawn Huber Warrington, and Edward Wellin for their assistance in contributing to the clinical examples cited in the book.

A distinct comment is in order for the resourceful and effective manuscript review program managed and directed by our editor, Harry A. McQuillen and his assistant, Barbara Nissen-Bartlett of Prentice-Hall, Inc. The careful and precise editorial production of the editions by Margaret G. McNeily were most helpful to the final details of the project.

The painstaking reading and scrupulous editorial attention that were paid to each line of the manuscript were provided by John N. Wolbert. A very special acknowledgement is made of his untiring assistance, patience, and enthusiasm with the manuscript in all its stages.

Our warmest thanks go to our children, Elizabeth, Benton, Clayton, and Sarah Burgess; and Jacqueline, Samuel, Sarah, Thomas, Hien, Robert, and David Lazare, who reluctantly but usually good naturedly loaned us the time to work on the manuscript.

We are deeply appreciative of the unfailing support and encouragement of Allen G. Burgess and Louise C. Lazare, who provided those therapeutic qualities of optimism, sensitivity, involvement, caring, patience, and persistence — thus providing the momentum necessary to maintain the "lift" for the flight of this book.

A.W.B.
A.L.

Boston, Massachusetts

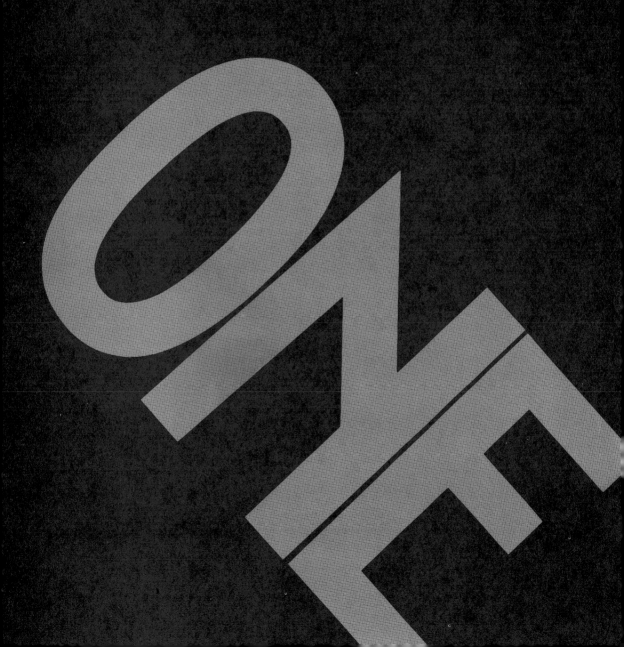

The introduction helps the reader to develop an attitude of involvement with the human dimension. By this, it is meant to develop insights to see patients as they really are regardless of the particular setting in which they are found.

The first two chapters are as follows:

Chapter 1 Student Reactions to Psychiatric Nursing

Being aware of the thoughts, feelings, and actions of the student in the beginning of the psychiatric nursing experience facilitates understanding of the learner's human dimension.

Chapter 2 Through the Eyes of the Patient

Knowledge of the thoughts, feelings, and actions of the patient facilitates understanding of his human dimension.

STUDENT REACTIONS TO PSYCHIATRIC NURSING

1

One's initial experience in a new setting can trigger a broad spectrum of human responses. Consider the following statement.

"... terror, that was what I felt. My legs literally wobbled as I walked down the corridor. I couldn't even remember the name of the person I was looking for . . .then I looked and saw her . . . sitting at the table with a knife in her hand. She was sitting there peeling apples . . . I just wished she would hurry up and run out of apples or finish the pie or that three o'clock would come. I was afraid to say anything; afraid to talk . . . what if she asked me a question . . . what would I say . . . I thought the id in my mind would come out and say something."

The feelings described above are those of a nursing student on her first day on a psychiatric ward. She is concerned that her fears are unique to her and that they symbolize her inability to function effectively as a psychiatric nurse. This student's reaction in anticipating her first psychiatric contact is, in fact, quite normal.

It is our belief that there is a wide range of normal feelings, worries, and concerns that the student experiences at the start of the psychiatric nursing experience. We regard these feelings as *role appropriate* since they are understandable and appropriate to the situation. They are to be distinguished from *subjective* feelings that are unique reactions having their origins in the student's past. For instance, a student may be repulsed by an alcoholic male, not because of his condition but because of painful recollections of an alcoholic relative. The student is responding subjectively to him on the basis of past personal experiences.

In this chapter we will describe a wide range of normal questions, worries, and fears experienced by the beginner in psychiatric nursing. The authors gathered this material during meetings with two groups of nursing students who had just completed their second visit to a psychiatric ward. The students were asked how they felt before the first visit and after their second visit.

We will discuss more fully the difference between the role appropriate and subjective feelings and reactions of the nurse.

Feeling anxious before the first interview

1. I have a friend who is in a psychiatric hospital—locked up and bars on the windows. He was just having problems with drugs. I thought the hospital would be like that one. . . .

2. I went in blank, not knowing what to expect. You hear stories about keys and locked doors. I feared what to talk to my patient about. Mental hospitals are so stereotyped; set up on a hill. . . .

3. I was looking forward to this experience 'till the first class and then I began to wonder how I was going to react to my patient. Was really shaking on the bus going over. I didn't know what I'd find there. My patient really talked to me and told me how scared she was and I forgot how scared I was listening to her.

4. In every phase of nursing I'm ready to jump in and love it. Each new experience is something different and I'm looking forward to it. But the psychiatric hospital wasn't a situation I automatically jumped into. The whole six-week vacation before this experience I thought about how I'd feel at ease when I came here. But this is another part of nursing and I want to do good in all parts of nursing. But psychiatric nursing scares you and it bothers you. Just knowing you have to go into the hospital and talk with a patient. I'm the type who talks a lot and when I got to my patient's door, I couldn't even say her name hardly. When her roommate said she wasn't there, I was so relieved. But then I knew I would have another day to wait and the other students had already talked to their patients. . . . I just hope I get along with this patient and that I don't chatter a lot.

In anticipating the first interview the student commonly feels scared and inadequate to the task. As it is with many new ventures, we have fantasies about the very worst happening. These fantasies can come from past experience (see statement 1), from stories or stereotypes (see statement 2), or from the depths of our imaginations. It would be most unusual for the student to feel calm and assured before her first interview.

Feeling useless and appearing like a beginner

5. I was excited this summer thinking of coming to the psychiatric hospital, because I think the mind is very important—maybe even more so than the body in terms of feeling well. I had visions of really helping the patients—really trying and being able to do something. But when I got there, I had the feeling that I'm not that intelligent as a doctor and maybe I won't really be able to get into this as I want. I began to worry that I'd be failing at this; that I wouldn't have enough knowledge to help this person.

6. I wondered what good I could be to someone; I have no knowledge of psychological problems.

7. I remember being told in Fundamentals if a patient asked us if this was our first time doing a dressing, to look rather indignant. I was trying to think how could I look like this wasn't the first time I had even been in a place like this . . . how could I look like this was something I had done before.

The major theme of statements 5 and 6 is the lack of enough knowledge to be helpful to the patient. If students do not know how to help, then they are in the awkward situation of looking like beginners (see statement 7).

The students' feelings and concerns are normal and understandable.

They are beginners. They do not know what to do and must learn to deal with the uncertainty of a first experience.

In another sense, students in psychiatric nursing are never beginners. They have spent years talking with and listening to people. Many non-patients (friends and relatives) have at times turned to them for psychological help in time of trouble. The students certainly have a great deal to learn about listening and talking, but they already have a good start.

Will the patient talk?

Many students voiced concern over whether or not the patient would talk.

8. When the patient saw me, she got right on the phone and stayed there for 30 minutes. She wouldn't even talk to me.

9. I was afraid the patient wouldn't talk and she is talking real good and I feel extremely lucky.

10. My patient doesn't talk. She said it's because she doesn't trust anyone. It seems everyone else's patient is talking to them and I feel it must be me.

It certainly is easier for the beginning student who is understandably anxious if the patient is verbal. If the patient speaks little or is mute, the student feels compelled to speak although she is unsure of whether or not this will be helpful to the patient. The student must remember, however, that it is the patient's problem—not the student's—that he is not verbal. The student should not begin by assuming that she is failing. Instead, she should ask herself what it is about the patient's past experience and present illness that leads him to his current state of mental functioning. What the student can do to help may then become more apparent.

It may be appropriate to ask the patient why he is silent. It may be useful to sit with the patient in silence. It may even be therapeutic to leave the patient. Which course of action makes most sense will depend on the assessment of the individual patient.

Wanting to know the patient's history before the interview

Whether it is necessary or useful to have background information about the patient prior to the first interview depends on a joint decision between instructor and student. Sentiments reflecting both points of view are described below.

11. What confuses me is that the patient knows what he is there for and we walk in and say we are students. They know we're to ask them about their illness and they know what they are there for, but we are out in the cold because we know little about them.

12. I would like to have the patient's family background and environmental background. We were just told the bare essentials like age, sex, religion, diagnosis, and that was it; we had to go and talk to our patients. I'd like to know what got her so upset. When my patient told me about her family, it was all very new and I didn't know how to react. I had no idea what in the

environment had upset her so much and therefore I had trouble saying anything . . . . With a physical disease or an operation, if you know what they have, you know how to deal with them.

13. I don't agree. You can read a chart and prejudge them. We're here to listen and understand them and help them communicate. If you know the background, what's the sense of talking to them. You're trying to find out what's troubling them and if you already know, they can probably sense this . . . and with emotional illness, it isn't so clear-cut. It's not like she has this symptom and this is the way she'll act.

If it is thought best to learn by not having the history prior to the interview, the student need not be concerned. The patient does not necessarily expect that she will have read the chart. He might even resent the student's knowing more about him than he was willing to reveal himself.

It may be that the student's desire to know the historical details before meeting the patient reflects understandable anxiety over making contact with the patient. Knowing the history may allow the student to feel more in control of the situation and therefore less anxious.

Some unpleasant reactions to the first interview

The patient rejects the student

14. The patient I had rejected having any student nurse. Prior to seeing her, I had tried to build my self-confidence up. I walked in and told her who I was and she said she didn't want anything to do with a student nurse. I could feel my self-confidence slipping away. I tried to think that she doesn't know us and it must be from past experiences. She kept saying that she had no intention of being talked to by a student nurse.

15. My patient was hiding from me. She'd make all kinds of excuses not to see me, like she had to put her makeup on or go to lunch or something. I looked one whole hour for her; all I'm doing is chasing her. She makes me feel like a jerk.

16. My patient immediately told me she only told her doctor her problem and she had no intention of telling me. She just talked about superficial things.

The patient's rejection of the student nurse during the initial interview is not uncommon. In statement 14 the student made the astute observation that the patient did not know anything about the students. Therefore, the patient must be reacting to her own past experience. One can only speculate what that experience might have been. Perhaps a previous student was not helpful. More likely the patient has recently "lost" a student through graduation or the completion of training. The patient still misses the student, is angry about the termination, and refuses to establish a new relationship. (If the new student learns that this is why the patient is resisting the new relationship, a supervisor should offer some techniques for establishing a working relationship with the patient.)

There are many other reasons why a patient rejects the student. The patient may prefer to keep all personal material between herself and her doctor. The patient may have a child who is close in age to the student and she cannot tell her new "child" certain personal problems. The patient may be angry at her physician and the anger is then displaced onto the next person who enters the room, the student nurse.

The student becomes depressed

17. I had a patient who has been depressed for years. It was hard to set a goal with her. I wanted to bring her out of her depression, but I knew I couldn't. She told me everything she had done in life was a failure; she didn't like herself; she wanted me to take her down to the railroad tracks. . . . It's depressing.

18. This experience is depressing me beyond words. I was sitting listening to the social worker talk to us and I almost fell asleep. And I know I'm not tired. I knew I had to go up and talk to my patient after the class. While I was seeing her, I couldn't wait to get out of there. There is something to do with my having to talk with her.

Although there are many reasons why the student may feel depressed, one of the most common reasons is the student's feeling of helplessness, a normal reaction, especially for the beginner. This feeling diminishes considerably once the student becomes better acquainted with the tools of psychiatric nursing. Independent of the experience of the nurse, the patient who is depressed often communicates his mood to the nurse (or to anyone who listens). One may say that the patient's feelings are contagious. In this situation the nurse's depression tells us more about the patient than about the nurse.

The student is overwhelmed

19. I wasn't looking forward to this experience at all. Walking into this hospital and seeing the group of patients that just haven't made it floored me.

It seems that this student came to the psychiatric experience with more negative feelings than most beginners: she did not look forward "at all." Feeling overwhelmed by seeing patients who "just haven't made it" indicates that the student may be bringing a painful personal experience to the situation; perhaps she has not resolved her feelings about people diagnosed as mentally ill.

The student is "strained"

20. My patient just sits there and I feel like I have to pull the information from her. It's such a strain and I feel like I am talking to a wall.

The experience of having to "pull the information" is common in certain patient groups such as those suffering from depression. The experience of the "strain" is most probably related to the clinical situation and not to the specific characteristics of the student.

The student is interviewed by the patient

21. My patient completely reversed the situation and asked me all about myself. She was very good at questioning me and I had to stop and realize what was going on.

The experience of being interviewed by the patient is related more to the style of the patient than to the specific characteristics of the student. The patient who attempts to interview the helper wants to be in control of the situation and is having a difficult time being a patient. The student took the proper first step by stopping to realize what was going on.

The student is angered by the patient

22. I was surprised at my reaction of anger when I talked to a group of patients. It seemed they were overindulging themselves in their depression. It was as if they were each trying to say his depression was the worst.

8

23. The first time I went to see my patient, he said, "Well, here's the zoo and here's the animals in it and now you've observed it and now you can go back and tell everyone about it." I told him it wasn't a zoo and he was a human being.

The patient feels like he is an animal in a zoo. He then projects his feelings to the student whom he accuses of seeing him as an animal in a zoo. The patient, feeling uncomfortable, tries to make the student uncomfortable. The student handled the situation superbly by respectfully pointing out the reality of the situation to him. The student does not share his view of himself as an animal but perceives of him as a human being.

The student's concern about her own mental health

A common concern of student nurses and others beginning their training in psychiatry is the fear that they will discover mental illness in themselves. In addition, there is also the concern that they will "catch" the illness from the patient or that the patient will drive them crazy.

24. I was riding the subway the other day and looking around. I saw lots of people that should have been in this hospital. There's such a thin line.
25. I'm afraid I'll be left here.
26. We've all been aware of certain phrases like "it's driving me crazy or whacky or nuts."
27. I wonder how stable everyone is. At what point do people lose their ability to cope.
28. My patient said she was afraid of driving in New York City and I cut her short and changed the subject because that is a problem I have and it bothered me to hear her say it. I have all the problems my patient has and I think I should stay here.

The student is absolutely correct in observing similarities between the patient and herself. This observation, however, is not so much because of the sickness of the student but because of the health of the patient. Hospitalized psychiatric patients are healthy in many ways. Their area of illness often encompasses only a small aspect of the total personality.

Students may also be concerned about their own phobias, minor mood swings, and idiosyncracies. They should bear in mind that these symptoms and aspects of their own personalities are commonly found in normal populations. Illness is measured less by what one thinks and feels than by how one functions.

The concern that the patient will demand too much

29. I was told before seeing the patient that the last nurse had helped him so much that he developed a mother complex or oedipus complex toward her. Now I don't know if I want to be mother to him and I don't know how to avoid this.
30. First thing my patient did was to ask me to bring her a candy bar which I

did. The second meeting she immediately asked if I brought the candy bar—didn't even say good morning or anything. I think this was a test to see if I would bring it, but it is to the point where she'll ask other things of me like when she gets privileges she wants me to go down town shopping with her. I don't know how I'll react to the situation.

In statement 29 the student was concerned that the patient would expect her to be a mother or a lover. In statement 30 the patient was already expecting that the student would be more than a nurse.

Patients often have expectations of the students (and other therapeutic personnel) above and beyond their designated professional roles. Students need to understand that these needs and wishes are the patient's problem. They must set the proper limits on the relationship without offending the patient. The student will often need supervisory assistance with many patients who present requests such as described above.

The fear of hurting the patient

Hurting the patient is a common fear of students in any phase of medicine.

31. If the patient isn't there the second day, I have the fear that I drove him away.
32. I felt it was my fault when the patient walked away from me. I didn't know what to do.
33. I was afraid I'd make my patient feel on display; like making her feel she was different and that was why I was there to see her.
34. My patient started crying and talking about suicide right away. I didn't know what to do. I felt if she went home and committed suicide it would be my fault because I didn't know what to say to her.
35. Most of us are afraid of saying something wrong. We don't want to harm the patient. I think these patients are more sensitive to what we say. I was afraid to ask the patient about her illness, afraid it would upset her. I couldn't see what good I'd do . . . as a nursing student.

Patients are stronger than we often give them credit for. Furthermore, they are quite forgiving even when we do make a clumsy statement.

The patient in statement 34 who started crying and talking of suicide was merely responding with what was on her mind to an interested student. The student did not cause the patient to feel suicidal. Of course, the student should report this information to someone on the staff. If the student listens with respect and is appropriately supportive in asking questions, the patient will not be hurt.

The fear of being hurt by the patient

The students often bring to the patient contact some fears of being physically or psychologically hurt by the patient.

36. I had a fear of being clobbered. I knew it wouldn't really happen but somehow the feeling was there. While talking with this one patient I knew he

felt closed in and at times banged his fist against the wall. I had the thought, what if he banged his fist on my head.

37. After the first day I was real anxious to hear how everyone else's day went and I'd ask classmates how their day went and they would ask me back. I wanted to know if my day was like theirs. I had fears because of the stories I had heard like getting physically hurt; the stories of broken jaws and murders. But I wasn't thinking too much about it 'till I was late for class and I went to open the door to go out and it was locked. Suddenly it came to me that I was on a psychiatric ward with the door locked and no one around to let me out. I knew a moment of pure panic.

38. I was afraid the patient would yell at me if I said the wrong thing.

Although it is common for the student to fear being hurt by the patient, it is quite improbable that such an event will ever occur.

Being honest

39. I told my patient who I was and this was part of my nursing training and I wanted to talk with her and would she mind. She asked if she had to talk with me and I said no so she said she'd talk and she sure did. I didn't expect that.

This statement illustrates how a simple direct statement together with an attitude of respect can be effective in beginning a therapeutic encounter.

Differences between psychiatric and medical–surgical nursing

The nursing students discussed several aspects in which they felt psychiatric nursing differs from medical–surgical nursing.

40. We just came from medical–surgical nursing where we seemed to be able to do things for the patients. Now as I sit with my patient, I wonder what good I can be to her. By my patient's telling me of her experiences, I don't feel I am accomplishing anything.

41. In a medical problem you can always do something to make the patients feel better. You can rub their backs for instance. You are touching them and making them feel better. You cannot do that in psychiatric nursing.

These sentiments express the subjective sense of uselessness and lack of accomplishment in psychiatric nursing in contrast to the feeling of being able to do something in medical–surgical nursing. It is true that one does more for a patient in a physical way in medical–surgical nursing. These efforts prove to students that they are working and accomplishing something. In psychiatric nursing one has to be psychologically active but physically passive much of the time. It takes some time to realize that listening to that which aches in the heart of the patient may touch him more profoundly than a back rub.

42. Each experience is so new each time. After the first day I went to my text but I couldn't find my patient anywhere in the book; she wasn't written up.

43. We are so used to reading in books about patients and disease. There are certain signs and symptoms. When you come to this experience, it is so much your own judgment as to what you are going to say. It is not written in any book, per se, how you are going to treat this patient. I think there is a great deal of fear and apprehension in this. We have been taught to read before going in about the illness and treatment so we will know about the operation or what the patient will experience. In psychiatry it is the mind and the mind is so broad you can't separate direct areas you are going to work on before you meet the patient and each patient is an individual.

The above statements are both correct and incorrect. Psychiatry is a relatively new discipline as compared to medicine and surgery. Furthermore, skills and techniques in psychiatry that require the use of one's personality are difficult to transmit through textbooks. There is, however, a considerable body of knowledge that describes various psychiatric syndromes and therapeutic techniques.

44. We have been so used to having something to do to busy ourselves around the room. But in psychiatry there is just you and the patient. If the patient rejects you in med–surg, you have some place to hide. In psychiatric nursing you don't have an excuse to be in the room like to change a dressing or something.

The psychiatric nurse need not sit and stare at the patient in exquisite discomfort if the patient seems to reject her. The nurse may walk with the patient, eat with the patient, or even sit quietly on the ward with a patient in order to express caring in a comfortable and therapeutic way. Psychiatric nursing as well as medical and surgical nursing provides reason to be with and help patients.

Concerns over ending the interview

Ending the interview and leaving the patient can be a difficult task.

45. I had a fear of not being able to leave my patient. The patient was talking and I had to catch the bus. I didn't want to leave her alone. It made me feel bad and I wanted to call her when I got home to tell her I felt badly at leaving her in the middle of the story.

Leavings have special significance to certain patients in certain situations. Staff personnel may be similarly affected by leavings. The student must recognize that these feelings both in the patient and in herself may be both intense and painful.

Regardless of these feelings, the parting between student and patient described above could be made easier if at the beginning of the interview the student tells the patient how much time they will be together. Then 5–10 minutes before the interview ends the student can say, "We will have to stop in a few minutes." This will give the patient a chance to psychologically prepare herself for the end of the interview.

ROLE
APPROPRIATE
VERSUS
SUBJECTIVE
FEELINGS AND
REACTIONS

Role appropriate feelings and reactions are those that are understandable, normal, and natural for a given situation. It is appropriate for a boxer to strike his opponent in the boxing arena, for an actor to embrace a strange actress in a screen play, for an auto mechanic to lie on his back dirtying his hands in a garage, for a surgeon to open someone's abdomen in the operating room, for a physician or nurse to examine a nude body in the hospital. Yet these specific behaviors, appropriate in the contexts described above, are obviously inapppropriate to almost all other situations.

It is often an unsettling experience when one moves into a role in which new and strange feelings and behaviors become appropriate—the medical student making the first incision into a cadaver, the soldier firing his weapon during battle, the nursing student listening to a patient's most intimate personal details during a nursing interview.

Under the circumstances of assuming a new role, the student's reactions described in the preceding pages are for the most part appropriate. The students feel anxious because they do not know what will happen; they fear the worst—that they will hurt or be hurt by the patients, that they will "catch" the patients' illnesses, that they will reject or be rejected by the patients, that the patients will demand too much of them, that the patients will recognize them as beginners. The students are unsure of how to say "hello" and "goodbye," they do not know if they should be honest with the patients or if they should learn the patients' histories ahead of time.

After the initial experiences the students often feel strained, angered, embarrassed, or depressed; it seems that all their fears have been confirmed. As they become more experienced and less overwhelmed by the unpleasant worries of the beginner, the therapeutic feelings of caring, concern, compassion, sensitivity, and understanding become stronger.

Whereas role appropriate feelings and reactions are natural and understandable for given situations, subjective feelings and reactions have more to do with the special characteristics of the student. In other words, each student may react to a patient in a slightly different way because of her special personality and past experiences.

For example, the student who has had a relative suffering from alcoholism might put forth special therapeutic energies in treating an alcoholic patient. The student may also react to a patient on the basis of a physical resemblance to a friend or relative. Again, depending on the relationship, the student may react to the patient in an authoritarian, competitive, seductive, helpless, punitive, or protective manner—as if the patient were the friend or relative.

The students' reactions to patients, whether appropriate to the situation or based on their subjective reactions may either facilitate or stall the therapeutic process.

The following are examples of therapeutic responses:

1. The student or nurse in the role of a helping, caring person communicates this attitude to the patient who then feels supported and reassured.

2. The student who has had a positive relationship with her grandparents may react subjectively in an unusually supportive and respectful manner to older patients.

The following are examples of reactions that stall the therapeutic process:

1. The student in her normal concern over being a beginner makes several clumsy remarks that makes the patient more anxious.
2. The student in treating a patient who resembles her own formidable mother feels intimidated in her therapeutic attempts with older women.

**AUTO-
DIAGNOSIS**

Autodiagnosis is the process whereby clinicians understand the clinical situation by reading their own feelings and reactions.

The crucial part is knowing that these feelings exist. Diagnosing one's own feelings allows the individual to be aware of the feelings and not to be frightened by them. It prevents the nurse from overinvolvement, overreaction, and overcompensation. For example, when the nurse's attempt to rescue the patient leads to a therapeutic stall, the message received is,"Ah, I know what that feeling is. Whenever I see a patient with a drug abuse problem, I get this rescue feeling. I want to help him because I understand the problem because of my personal experiences with other friends." This insight allows the nurse not to have to act on the feelings.

The more your feelings are known to yourself, the better you will be able to control them. For example, if you are annoyed at your patient, that is all right as long as you do not act on these feelings and as long as these feelings do not interfere with your nursing care of the patient.

How does the student diagnose feelings? She first learns to pay attention to her feelings just as she pays attention to the feelings and behavior of the patient. The process is enhanced by discussing her reactions with other students, supervisors, and staff members. This process was demonstrated in this chapter.

The nurse is able to learn a great deal about patients by reading her own reactions. She learns that certain patients interest her, others elicit anger, still others arouse feelings of helplessness. Thus, when meeting a new patient, the nurse may say to herself, "I feel helpless; this patient might be suffering from a depression," or, "I feel like rescuing him; he must remind me of someone."

There are two clinical circumstances that should alert the nurse to autodiagnose feelings and reactions: (1) when nothing seems to be happening between the nurse and the patient; when she feels in a stall in the therapy with the patient; (2) when she or the patient seems to be overreacting to a situation.

When either of these situations occurs, there are two possible causes: (1) The reality of the clinical situation accounts for the problem so that the student's reaction is role appropriate. For example, a mute and withdrawn patient will make almost all clinicians feel frustrated, restless, and helpless. (2) The student's subjective reactions are responsible for the clinical stall. For instance, the patient's progress stalls because the nurse is behaving like a protective mother toward him. The nurse is fostering dependence although the patient could progress independently. Once the nurse understands her own reactions, she can begin to make therapeutic demands of the patient and therapeutic progress will continue.

By the autodiagnosis of role appropriate and subjective feelings, we are acknowledging to ourselves only what exists. We are bringing into awareness feelings that give the nurse better perspective and more control of the situation. We are making known what was unknown and conscious what was unconscious. The nurse is then freer as a human being to be therapeutic to patients.

SUMMARY There is a wide range of unpleasant but normal feelings, worries, and concerns that the nursing student experiences at the beginning of her psychiatric nursing work. A series of verbatim statements taken from a group discussion of students beginning the psychiatric nursing experience were presented to exemplify what neophytes in this clinical specialty area typically experience.

Almost all these feelings and reactions are role appropriate because they are normal or typical for the situation. If students are aware that these feelings are appropriate, they can be more comfortable with themselves and more therapeutic with patients.

In addition to role appropriate feelings, there are subjective reactions to the patient that are based more on the student's past experience than on the student's objectivity with the situation. Subjective feelings and reactions, like role appropriate feelings, may be either psychotherapeutic or may stall the therapeutic relationship.

In order to understand the feelings and reactions to clinical situations that stall the therapeutic process, students must develop the art of autodiagnosis — the ability to understand the patient by identifying and describing their own thoughts and feelings. By doing so, students gain perspective and control of the situation. Making the unknown known reduces the mystique, the fear, and the insecurity that the feeling evokes. The nurse is then free to be therapeutic.

THROUGH THE EYES
OF THE PATIENT

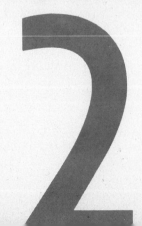

Just as students experience a wide range of intense emotional reactions as they begin to work with psychiatric patients, the person designated "patient" also undergoes considerable emotional upheaval. Being unable to cope with the emotional problems of his daily life is painful enough. Now he carries the added burden of being considered (or considering himself) a psychiatric patient. He worries about his current feelings about himself and other peoples' reactions to him. As if that were not enough, he now has to contemplate what it will be like to be a patient in a psychiatric hospital.

The nurse must have some sense of the inner experience of the patient in order to be therapeutic. If he is frightened, the nurse can be therapeutic only if she knows he is experiencing fear or anxiety, even if he gives the appearance of being brave. If the patient is sad, the nurse must respond to the sadness, even though he may amuse the staff.

To help the student understand the worries, fears, and wishes of the psychiatric patient, the authors met with two groups of patients on a psychiatric ward in a general hospital. The patients were asked how they felt about coming to the hospital, how they felt nurses were helpful, and how they felt nurses could be more helpful.

After commenting on the various patient responses, we will discuss the distinction between role appropriate and subjective feelings and reactions of the patient. Role appropriate feelings are a direct result of patienthood and are shared by many other patients. Subjective feelings, as we will describe, are determined by very special personal experiences from the patient's past.

PATIENT RESPONSES

The patient is "scared"

Reactions to becoming a patient

1. Felt very scared when my brother left and I was all alone in the hospital.
2. I was scared stiff coming in but staff reassured me and I took their word. I'm in a strange town and this is a strange hospital. I've never experienced something like this.

17

3. My fear is frustration and fright and pain — that is how I feel in this hospital.
4. I asked to be put here to get help. I'm nervous and get excited over small things. I'd never been in a place like this.
5. I was scared to death when I came in here.
6. I felt parachuted into the middle of nowhere.

The above illustrate the fear, nervousness, and scared feelings that characterize almost all patients who enter a psychiatric hospital. Statements 2, 4 and 6 vividly illustrate the profound sense of being in a strange place — something never before experienced — "parachuted into the middle of nowhere." Somewhat related to the strangeness is the sense of aloneness (see statement 1). Statement 4 illustrates the point that the patient is already troubled and nervous. As if that were not enough, she is then put "in a place like this."

These reactions to hospitalization are observed in all clinical settings: small and large wards, clean and disorganized hospitals, private and state hospitals. It is important to recognize the universality of these reactions because the nurse might attribute the patient's discomfort to the setting of a large, unpleasant ward and therefore feel there is no way that she can help.

Statement 2 indicates what the nurse can do. The supportive relationship of the nurse can be and often is everything to the new patient.

The patient is relieved

7. Home was such hell; this place is like heaven; it's no hassle.
8. I felt exhausted when I came in; physically and mentally. I was shot.
9. I came here to unwind.

Some patients are so overwhelmed by their life situations that the psychiatric ward is experienced more as a relief than a source of anxiety. These patients often elicit the reaction in staff that they are malingering, lazy, or indifferent. The nurse must keep in mind that the outside situation must have been desperate to warrant psychiatric hospitalization.

These patients may appear relatively comfortable throughout the hospitalization until the discharge approaches. As they face the return to the situation that overwhelmed them, all the anxiety that initially led to the hospitalization is reawakened. For these reasons, it is crucial to deal with the outside situation before discharge.

The patient's reaction is often colored by his experience during a previous hospitalization.

Feelings about a previous hospitalization

10. I was here before. I didn't have much choice over coming. It was here or the other hospital and that place is awful. I didn't want to be put back here and I don't want to stay.
11. I spent 6 months in a violent ward. I remember another patient slugging me. It was scary and I thought this place might be the same way.
12. I feel like a failure when I have to come here. To reenter the hospital every few years is something I can't cope with. When I come back, I know I haven't made it.

The patient may behave as if something terrible will happen to him because something terrible may have happened to him in the past. Once the nurse learns about these past experiences, they can be discussed and put into perspective.

Statement 12 illustrates the patient's feeling of failure on having to return. This feeling is certainly understandable. Often the staff also feels a sense of disappointment and failure on seeing a former patient return. This staff reaction must be guarded against so that the patient's sense of failure is not intensified. The nurse must understand that some psychiatric illnesses are chronic as are certain kinds of medical illness. That some patients need *only* to be hospitalized intermittently, not continuously, is a tribute to current methods of treatment.

Patients' advice to nurses

The patient is an acute observer of the clinical situation. We have all been a patient at some time, either in a hospital or in a doctor's office or clinic. In this situation many of us feel that if someone would only listen, we could improve clinical care.

Don't avoid human contact

13. Please talk to me rather than go to that staff meeting or into the nurse's office. When you reach out to a person at a certain moment, to another human being for help, you reach out in that moment and it becomes so important to reach out. Then to have some mundane type of staff meeting become more important than a human being . . . .

14. Don't you get sick of having to do all the clerical work of writing notes and reports?

Although the nurse must write reports and attend conferences, it is important to understand that these activities may be perceived by the patients as devices to avoid contact. In fact, nurses will acknowledge that they do use the nurse's office and the clerical work to avoid patients when they feel psychologically exhausted.

Don't depersonalize the patient

15. Please avoid labels; all labels in all forms, The white uniform, the secretary at the desk. No labels. That helped me break through a lot of inhibitions. I don't think I would have made it had I been put into a hospital bed somewhere, with the white sheets, white pillowcase, very antiseptic with a tray and the bed rolled up and the white sheet closing around it; everything white. I might have been rested but not helped with my problems. I merely would have been brought back to a state where I'd previously been treated for exhaustion and nothing more.

The patient is asking for the staff to treat him personally, to interact with him, to provide more than a sterile rest.

16. Nurses come in and immediately I am scared of a needle. Sometimes they don't use psychology; they just stick that needle in your arm like it was a piece of meat. Nothing about it; that's just it; no technique. Maybe if they came in with a green needle or a joke, it would help. I had blood taken and she hardly said hello.

The patient is asking, among other things, to be treated not like a piece of meat but like a human being.

Don't be snide

17. I'll tell you what turns me off—like cracking a joke that you can take either way. Not a ha ha joke but a snide joke like, "Why don't you get out of bed? You spend all your time in bed. Only time you get up is to take your pills." Nurses should come on with a positive remark instead of trying to be smart or funny about it.

Don't be bubbly

18. You don't have to come on as Susy Goodshoes and laugh and be bubbly all the time.

19. I hate to be told someone will talk to me later and then never does. I won't go up and mention that they promised to come and talk. Patients hate to keep after the nurses for things.

20. I get upset when I tell a nurse something and nothing seems to be done about it and I hate to repeat myself a second time. I figure if they didn't take care of it the first time, I am making a nuisance of myself to repeat it.

Clarify the communication

21. How do things get communicated about what is told. Like I know the nurse and social worker talked with my boss and I'd like to know what was said before I go in to work. I might make a damn fool out of myself if I don't know what is going on.

22. I'd like to know who tells who what. I tell the nurse I must have a certain pain or feeling and then when I ask the doctor, he said he hadn't heard about it. How do you know what is important?

The patient makes an excellent point. It is the responsibility of the staff to clarify the communication among each other.

"Don't put me down"

23. The nurses showed no compassion. Like it never occurred to them that I was scared of the place. They thought, "Why, he's just trying to be difficult," and they were thoroughly rotten about the whole thing. I wanted someone to be concerned as to why I was scared. I was in severe pain and at the time pretty well unhinged and they kept saying, "Oh, come on, at your age, scared of hospitals. Ha! Ha! Ha!" They must have thought I was an overgrown baby, but I was scared.

24. When you say "Hi" to someone and they give you a cold shoulder, it makes you feel bad. I don't like cold people and I think it is harmful.

25. Sometimes after I talk with a nurse I get this feeling and I won't talk with them again. I feel they just talk with me so that they can go out and make a joke.

26. Last Friday night I was upset and frightened and wanted to go in the quiet room. One of the staff came in and said, "There's a $20 extra charge for this room." She should have asked me what was the matter. I felt put down and won't ever talk to her again. There was a reason for my being there; I felt bad. She should have asked to talk about my fright. She wasn't the least bit sympathetic; she thought I was being capricious.

27. Too many medications are given out. Patients are "zonked out."

Don't over-medicate the patient

The "zonked out" or drugged appearance of the patient is an important clinical observation. Although this drugged appearance may be an unfortunate side effect of a therapeutic dosage of medication, it may in some clinical instances be a sign that the dosage should be lowered. The nurse should communicate this information to the physician.

The patients' advice described in statements 13–27 is reasonable and profound: Don't avoid me; *talk to me*. Don't depersonalize me; *treat me as a human being*. Don't be smart or funny; *take me seriously*. Don't be bubbly; *be yourself*. Don't break promises; *do what you say you will do*. Don't put me down; *show compassion, be friendly, trust me, have understanding*.

There are times when, because of the patient's hypersensitivity or distortion of reality, his critical remarks are not to be taken seriously. We believe that these times are few and that in general critical remarks of patients should be carefully considered.

How can we account for the facts that a bright and sensitive group of nurses can be perceived in the negative terms described above? We believe that nurses will give these impressions to patients when they do not understand the patient and when they are hindered by their own discomfort (exhaustion, for example) in the clinical situation. When these two conditions are reversed by training and experience, the nurse can be freed to give what is in her to give.

Concerns about confidentiality

28. I'm afraid people will talk about me. Do nurses have to take an oath like the doctors do? I'm afraid I might get blackmailed after I get out of here.

Although paranoid patients may have an extraordinary distrust of staff and other patients, almost all patients have an understandable concern about confidentiality. This concern is intensified in community mental health centers in which neighbors are admitted to the same ward. In another sense, when a patient is talking about confidentiality, she may be asking whether she can trust. When trust develops in the therapeutic relationship, concerns about confidentiality usually disappear.

How nurses help

29. The nurses are the shrinks around here. The doctors zip in and out. They come in for a minute to ask how you are and then you don't see them for a week. The nurses have to let the doctors know how we are doing.

30. I've had more contact with nurses this past year than I have ever had in my entire life (77 years old). I've learned you can say anything to a nurse no matter what—it is safe.

31. I can only rap with certain nurses about what really bugs me. You have to find one person to rap with or you can't stay here. You need one person to bleed on. It's a personality thing as to who you can get along with.

32. They listen. They don't interrupt you. They hear you out no matter how hard it is.

33. They try to help.

34. They give you medication.

35. They will talk to you.

36. They are there when you need them.

Statements 29 and 36 indicate the importance of the *consistency and availability* of the nurse. Statements 30, 31, and 32 illustrate the importance of the nurse's *listening*, no matter what the content. Statement 33 and others point to the importance of the attitude of *wanting to help*.

Patients' discussion about student nurses

Patient T: I think they should go through the experience of being a patient; to be on the other side of the white uniform. I'd grab them out of class one day and throw them in a state hospital and tell them they were committed.

Patient C: I don't think they would go into psychiatric nursing if you did that.

Patient T: They would understand their own little hang-ups and those of others. They'd have to look inward and be able to tell what was an idiosyncrasy and what was a major hang-up.

Patient A: If the students love people, they will go into psychiatric nursing.

ROLE APPROPRIATE VERSUS SUBJECTIVE FEELINGS AND REACTIONS

The role appropriate feelings of the psychiatric patient have been described in the previous pages. They include feeling scared, alone, frustrated, nervous, suspicious, violated, out of control, empty, and relieved. These feelings are so common that the nurse should assume that they are probably being experienced by each new patient. With this index of suspicion, the nurse is ready to respond in a supportive fashion to an otherwise difficult patient. For instance, if a patient refuses to speak and appears to be frightened, the nurse might say, "You seem terribly frightened." If the nurse was correct about the patient's feelings, these four words would be extraordinarily supportive, for now the patient would know that in this lonely and frightening place someone understands.

Subjective feelings and reactions of the patient, analogous to those feelings of the nurse, are responses to the current situation based on personal experiences of the patient in the past. In practice, the patient may respond to the nurse with a variety of subjective feelings of different intensity. He may be very angry at the nurse or be very fond of her. He may want to control her or be controlled by her. He may want to inappropriately care for her or be cared for by her. These reactions may appear at any time during the course of treatment and they may change from day to day.

It is important for the nurse to identify these subjective reactions of the patient so that she will not be overwhelmed by them. She must remind herself that these feelings are not real in that they are directed by the patient not toward her but toward someone else in the patient's life. Fortified with this knowledge, the nurse need not reject the patient because of her own anxiety. She can continue to communicate her concern for his emotional well-being.

SUMMARY

The patient's reaction to hospitalization covers a wide gamut of human emotions. Some patients feel scared, alone, frustrated, and nervous and others feel relieved to be in a psychiatric setting. These feelings are similar to those of the student beginning her psychiatric rotation and are not necessarily a part of the psychiatric illness.

The patient's reactions may be based on his feelings about previous hospitalizations, fear of physical harm from other patients, and a fear of failure on having to reenter the hospital.

Patients had suggestions for beginning nurses that were offered in the service of improving psychiatric care. They gave the following advice to the students: do not avoid them by staying in the nurse's station to write reports and by attending meetings; do not depersonalize them by labeling them; do not be snide in their comments; do not be bubbly; do not break promises; do not "put them down"; clarify communication lines between staff; do not give too much medication.

The patients stated the ways that the nurses help them: talking with them, giving them their time, listening, giving medication, being available when needed; hearing about their pain.

Role appropriate and subjective feelings of the patient were distinguished. Role appropriate feelings are usual, normal, and appropriate for someone with an emotional disorder who has recently been admitted to a psychiatric hospital. In contrast, subjective feelings are those feelings not appropriate to the situation, having their origins in the patient's past. Understanding both kinds of feelings frees the student to be therapeutic.

THEORETICAL FRAMEWORK

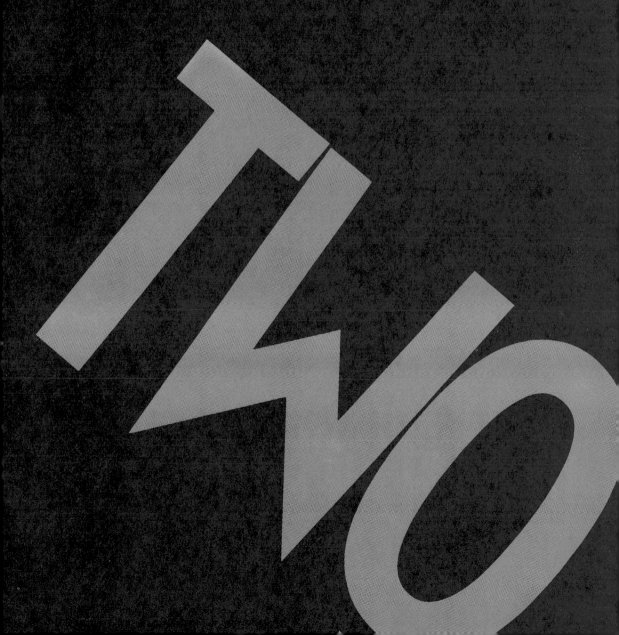

A theoretical framework is presented in order to add to the knowledge base that nurses bring with them to psychiatric—mental health nursing. A conceptual approach to patient care introduces the nurse to the four major models of patient care. Current advances in ego psychology and contemporary formulations of psychodynamic concepts present the didactic base. In addition, the authors present illustrations of a four-year course of treatment of an adolescent male patient to show the application of the concepts to nursing practice.

Chapter 3   Conceptual Models in Patient Care

Four models that are currently being used in the understanding and treatment of mental illness are described as the biologic, psychologic, social, and behavioral models of care.

Chapter 4   Psychodynamic Concepts and Ego Psychology

The theoretical formulations of the psychodynamic approach—the development and interaction of conscious and unconscious mental factors—provides a basic foundation for studying and understanding human behavior.

Chapter 5   Personality Development

The developmental tasks and phases of the life-cycle, as identified by Erik Erikson, are presented for a total view of the psychological dimensions of one's personality.

Chapter 6   Psychodynamic Concepts: A Case Illustration

Application of theory to clinical practice is made through the description and analysis of a treatment case.

CONCEPTUAL MODELS IN PATIENT CARE

3

M any people find it difficult to understand how a psychiatric nurse selects relevant clinical data, formulates a case, and decides on a treatment program. In the psychiatrically ill person, is it the symptom complex, the "unconscious conflict," the pathology in family interactions, or particular undesirable behaviors that contain the key to clinical decision making? Why does one clinician emphasize tricyclic antidepressants; another, individual therapy; a third, family therapy; and a fourth, behavior modification for apparently similar patients? Why is it apparently easier to formulate and implement a treatment plan for a patient suffering from a medical illness such as congestive heart failure?

One major reason for the difficulty in understanding psychiatric thinking is that several different conceptual models are implicitly used in the clinical formulation, but they are rarely identified as such. The four most common models are the biologic (medical), the psychological, the behavioral, and the social. When a patient is being treated, the kind of history obtained, the meaning assigned to certain historical facts, and the treatment modalities most often chosen depend on which model or combination of models is employed. These points are illustrated by 4 case histories of *one* patient, each formulated in terms of one of the four models.

BIOLOGIC MODEL

Case history

Mrs. J. is a 53-year-old widow who gives the history of a depressive syndrome. During the past few months she has lost 20 pounds, has early morning awakening, and has a diurnal variation in mood manifested by feeling better as the day goes on. She describes herself as feeling hopeless, helpless, and worthless. There is some retardation of speech. She denies suicidal intent and presents no evidence of delusions or paranoid ideation. There are obsessional trends. Twenty-three years ago there was a similar episode of depression which remitted spontaneously. The patient has a sister who was hospitalized for a depressive illness which responded positively to electroconvulsive treatments.

The modern origins of the biologic model can be traced to Emil D.

Kraepelin, born the same year (1856) as Sigmund Freud. Kraepelin's contribution was his application of the medical approach, or the *nosological conception*. By carefully observing groups of patients who exhibited similar symptom clusters through time, he was able to provide the classification of psychiatric illness which, with some modification, is still in use.

The biologic model views psychiatric illness as diseases like any others. For each disease, it is supposed that there eventually will be found a specific etiology related to the functional anatomy of the brain. The clinician using the biologic model is primarily concerned with etiology, pathogenesis, signs and symptoms, differential diagnosis, treatment and prognosis. Knowing the syndrome or disease determines the treatment. While addressing patients with proper medical respect, the clinician keeps a distance in order to maintain objectivity. This contrasts with the psychotherapeutic model in which the therapeutic relationship itself is both diagnostic and therapeutic.

The biologic model, after giving psychiatry its classification of mental illness in the late nineteenth century, has provided the conceptual foundations for (1) the development and use of the antipsychotic and antidepressant medications; (2) the development of mathematical techniques such as factor analysis which facilitates the validation of clinical syndromes and predicts the response to drugs; (3) studies of the genetic transmission of mental illness; and (4) metabolic studies of psychiatric illness, especially the depressions. The most significant events in the above four areas have occurred since 1950.

When the nurse applies the biologic model to the case history, she elicits the history of the symptom picture and observes a group of symptoms and historical data consistent with the cluster of a unipolar depression. The patient's relationship with her family, her ambivalence toward her husband, her motivation to understand her illness are interesting, and perhaps even relevant, but not central to the recognition of the illness. Antidepressant medications or electroconvulsive treatments would be the treatments of choice. The patient will be told that she is suffering from a depression, a psychiatric illness not uncommon in her age group. The illness is time limited and, with proper treatment, has a favorable prognosis.

PSYCHO-LOGICAL MODEL

Case history

Mrs. J. is a 53-year-old widow who became depressed a few months ago after the death of her husband. Although the marriage seemed happy at times, it is known that there were many stormy periods in their relationship. There have been no visible signs of grief since his death. Since the funeral, the patient has been depressed and has lost interest in her surroundings. For no apparent reason she now blames herself for apparently minor events of the past. Sometimes she criticizes herself for traits which characterized her husband more than herself. She had a similar reaction after the death of her mother 23 years ago. At that time, the patient and mother lived together. From the family history, it could be inferred that the relationship was characterized by hostile dependency. Six months after her mother's death the patient married. The patient seems intelligent, motivated for treatment, and has considered psychotherapy in the past in order to gain a better understanding of herself.

Although there are many theories of personality and many psychotherapies, the psychologic model in American psychiatry began with the work of Freud and was modified by the subsequent work of Sullivan, Fromm-Reichmann, Erikson, the existentialists, and many others. Freud's revolution depended on the "conviction that psychological events, however obscure, were understandable."[1] Through the newly developed method of free association, he was able to reconstruct childhood experience which he believed determined the adult neurosis.

In the current use of the psychological model, the developmental impasse, the early deprivation, the distortions in early relationships, and the confused communications between parent and child lead to the adult neuroses and vulnerabilities to certain stresses. As a result of these psychological determinants, we see patients who distort reality, who are prone to depression, who avoid heterosexuality, and who fear success. The social setting may be changed, psychotropic drugs may be given, but the pathology remains because the personality is pathological.

Therapy consists of clarifying the psychological meaning of events, feelings, and behaviors. The patient is taught how to experience appropriate affects and how to tolerate intolerable affects.[2] Forgotten events may be remembered, reexperienced, and then put into perspective so that the patient can be freed to see current situations as they really are. As a result, growth and maturity are enhanced.

Most important to the therapeutic situation is the nurse–patient relationship. It is the therapeutic alliance between the two that will enable the patient to remember what she has not wanted to remember and to abandon familiar but pathological ways of dealing with anxiety. It is through the vehicle of the therapeutic relationship—by experiencing these feelings toward the therapist—that the patient will relive pathological ties to important people and have the opportunity for a "corrective emotional experience."[3]

The psychological model has exerted a great influence, not only on American psychiatry, but also on everyday thinking. Its derivative, psychotherapy, has become a commonly accepted treatment of choice, especially for the neuroses and personality disorders. Advocates of the psychological model, especially since World War II, have been able to translate the clinical insights derived from classical psychoanalysis and more recent developments of ego psychology into concepts that residents in nearly all training centers in the United States can utilize in the understanding of most psychiatric patients.

Returning to the case history, the nurse, using the psychological model,

[1] L.L. Havens, "Emil Kraepelin," *Journal of Nervous and Mental Disorders,* **141** (1965), 16–28.

[2] E. V. Semrad, *Teaching Psychotherapy of Psychotic Patients—Supervision of Beginning Residents in the "Clinical Approach"* (New York: Grune and Stratton, 1969).

[3] F. Alexander and T. M. French, *Psychoanalytic Therapy* (New York: Ronald Press Company, 1946).

first takes note of the problems in the marital relationship. One pays special attention to the absence of grief [4] which has psychological meaning and is related to her ambivalent feelings toward her husband. A similar reaction after her mother's death suggests the possibility of a psychological connection between her feelings toward both her husband and mother. This is reinforced by the history that she married only 6 months after the death of her mother. The patient's criticism of herself in terms that she had used to criticize her husband suggests Freud's concept of introjection of the lost object.[5] Since the primary modality of treatment is psychotherapy, it is a favorable sign that she is motivated to gain a better understanding of herself.

BEHAVIORAL MODEL

Case history

Mrs. J. is a 53-year-old widow who gives the history of depressive behaviors of anorexia, insomnia, feelings of hopelessness, helplessness, and worthlessness. These behaviors began shortly after the death of her husband who had been the major figure in her life. Throughout the marriage he had been a continuous source of reinforcement to the patient. This quality of the husband's interaction with his wife had been evident since the marriage, at which time the patient was still depressed after her mother's death. The family stated that the husband had always ignored the patient's demands and pleas of helplessness while responding actively to the more positive aspects of her personality. After his death the patient began to complain to her children about her loss of appetite and her sense of helplessness and worthlessness. They responded to these complaints with frequent visits and phone calls, but the depressive behavior only worsened.

The behavioral model rests on the conceptualizations of Pavlov, Watson, and Guthrie (conditioned learning theory). To the behavior therapist, both neurosis and psychosis are examples of abnormal behavior which have been learned as a result of aversive events and are maintained because they either lead to positive results or because they avoid deleterious ones. The overt symptoms (the learned behavior), not the secondary manifestations of disease or unconscious conflict, are to be treated since they themselves are the problem. The typical therapeutic course includes: (1) determining the behavior to be modified; (2) establishing the conditions under which the behavior occurs; (3) determining the factors responsible for the persistence of behavior; (4) selecting a set of treatment conditions; and (5) arranging a schedule of retraining. The conditions that precede the behavior may be modified by such techniques as desensitization, reciprocal inhibition, and conditioned avoidance. The conditions resulting from the behavior may be modified by positive reinforcement, negative reinforcement, aversive conditioning, and extinction.[6]

[4] H. Deutsch, "Absence of Grief," *Psychoanalytic Quarterly,* **6** (1937), 12–22.

[5] S. Freud, "Mourning and Melancholia" (1917), *Collected Papers,* Vol. IV (New York: Basic Books, Inc., 1959), pp. 152–70.

[6] H. Urban and D. H. Ford, "Behavior Therapy," in *Comprehensive Textbook of Psychiatry,* eds., A. M. Freedman and H.I. Kaplan (Baltimore: The Williams Wilkins Co., 1967), pp. 1217–25.

The behavioral model, resting on theoretical foundations from the early twentieth century, began its rapid growth in the late 1950s. Its derivative, behavior therapy, has enjoyed considerable interest in the clinical field during the relatively brief period of its existence. Behavior therapy offers several possible advantages to other forms of treatment, including shorter duration of treatment and applicability to a broad range of patients.

Considering the case history according to the behavioral model, the nurse first identifies the behavior—anorexia, insomnia, feelings of hopelessness, helplessness, and worthlessness—which are regarded as pathological. Then the empirical relationship between the depressive behaviors and the antecedent and consequent environmental events which precipitate and maintain the depression is determined.[7] The death of the husband is interpreted as a sudden withholding of positive reinforcement of adaptive behavior. The attention received from family members inadvertently reinforces the depressive behavior.

Treatment consists of reinforcing adaptive behaviors incompatible with depression and extinguishing depressive behaviors. These therapeutic goals may be accomplished by teaching the family to respond positively to the adaptive behavior instead of to the depressive behavior[8] by purposefully encouraging the patient to express feelings incompatible with depression[9] or by establishing a period of sensory deprivation which makes the depressed patient more susceptible to positive reinforcement.[10]

SOCIAL MODEL

Case history

Mrs. J. is a 53-year-old widow who has been depressed during the past few months after the death of her husband. He had been the major figure in her life, and his loss has left her feeling lonely and isolated. After his death she moved to a small apartment some distance from her old neighborhood. Although she is satisfied with her new quarters, she finds the community strange. Furthermore, she does not have access to public transportation which would enable her to visit her old friends, children, and grandchildren. Since her husband's death, old strains between the patient and her children have been aggravated.

A social model of treatment was practiced in psychiatric hospitals in the United States from the latter part of the eighteenth century to approximately 1860. It was introduced under the name of "moral therapy" by the work of Tuke in England. During that time, social and environmental causes of mental illness were given serious consideration as moral treatment attempted to relieve the patient by "friendly association, discussion of his

[7] R. P. Liberman and D. E. Raskin, "Depression: A Behavioral Formulation," *Archives of General Psychiatry,* **24** (1971), 515–23.

[8] R. P. Liberman, "A Behavioral Approach to Family and Couple Therapy," *American Journal of Orthopsychiatry,* **40** (1970), 106–18.

[9] A. A. Lazarus, "Learning Theory and the Treatment of Depression," *Behavior Research and Therapy,* **6** (1968), 83–89.

[10] G. B. Kish, "Studies of Sensory Reinforcement," in *Operant Behavior,* ed., W. K. Honig (New York: Appleton-Century-Crofts, 1966), pp. 109–59.

difficulties, and the daily pursuit of purposeful activity."[11] Treatment results compared favorably with those for patients hospitalized today. The social model received further impetus from Adolph Meyer and Harry Stack Sullivan in the first half of this century.

The social view of psychiatric illness focuses on the way the individual functions in the social system. Symptoms are traced not to conflicts within the mind, not to manifestations of psychiatric disease, but to the "relationship of the individual to his manner of functioning in social situations, i.e., in the type and quality of his 'connectedness' to the groups which make up his life space."[12] Symptoms may thereafter be regarded as an index of social disorder.[13] Accordingly, when a socially disruptive event occurs, for example, a daughter's leaving home, a wife's dying, a geographic displacement by urban renewal, a war, or an economic depression, the resultant symptoms are seen as stemming from the social disorder.

The social model, like the medical, psychological, and behavioral models, was reawakened in the 1950s. Since then the psychiatric ward has been viewed as a social system,[14] the relationship between social class and mental illness has been established,[15] federal legislation to provide psychiatric care for catchment areas in the community has been enacted[16] and epidemiological studies have been carried out.[17] During these years, group and family therapy, day hospitals and walk-in clinics provided new ways of treating the mentally ill patient without separating him from his social milieu.

Treatment consists of either reorganizing the patient's relationship to the social system or reorganizing the social system, since the personality is neither "diseased" nor in need of fundamental restructuring. Using the social model, the therapist may help the patient better understand how she relates to the social system and how better to satisfy her needs. If others do not seem to care, how can she get them to care? If her job is not stimulating, how can she find the right one? If the patient's behavior is irrational, how can she learn to stop acting irrationally or how can her family better tolerate the behavior? If the therapist wants to restructure the "nuclear" social system, the patient may be seen with her family. The therapist who wants to

[11]T. P. Rees, "Back to Moral Treatment and Community Care," *Journal of Mental Science,* **103** (1957), 303–13.

[12]C. S. Thomas and B. J. Bergen, "Social Psychiatric View of Psychological Misfunction and Role of Psychiatry in Social Change," *Archives of General Psychiatry,* **12** (1965), 539–44.

[13]J. V. Coleman, "Social Factors Influencing the Development and Containment of Psychiatric Symptoms," in *Mental Illness and Social Processes,* ed., T. J. Scheff (New York: Harper and Row, Publishers, Inc., 1967), pp. 158–68.

[14]A. H. Stanton and M. S. Schwartz, *The Mental Hospital* (New York: Basic Books, 1954).

[15]A. B. Hollingshead and F. C. Redlich, *Social Class and Mental Illness* (New York: John Wiley and Sons, Inc., 1958).

[16]G. Caplan and R. B. Caplan, "Development of Community Psychiatry Concepts," in *Comprehensive Textbook of Psychiatry,* eds., A. M. Freedman and H. I. Kaplan (Baltimore: The Williams & Wilkins Co., 1967), pp. 1499–1516.

[17]D. C. Leighton and A. H. Leighton, "Mental Health and Social Factors," in *Comprehensive Textbook of Psychiatry* (Baltimore: The Williams & Wilkins Co., 1967), pp. 1520–33.

effect the broader social system may attempt to influence major social issues such as housing or education.

The nurse, using the social model to study the case, notices that the patient's social matrix has been altered in two ways. First, the patient has permanently lost the one person to whom she has been closest. She now feels empty and isolated. Second, by moving, she has placed herself in a situation in which she has lost access to those with whom she had previously related. In individual or group therapy one could temporarily substitute a transitional social system. Simultaneously, the therapist would attempt to reestablish a social field in which the patient could be comfortable after discharge. To do this, she might be encouraged to move to a home where she could have better access to family and old friends. Work with the family might repair any estrangement. The patient might return to work, either paid or volunteer. Continued individual or group therapy might help her acquire social skills that she may never have needed to develop in the marital situation.

DETERMINA-TION OF THE CONCEPTUAL MODEL

The nurse implicitly uses one or a combination of conceptual models to assess and plan patient care by the process referred to as clinical judgment. The selection may be made according to the results of outcome studies. It may be made on practical grounds: "This is the only available plan; let's make the best of it." Sometimes the decision rests on clinical bias. In this section we will attempt to describe some of the variables that determine the choice of conceptual models in patient care.

Clinical bias

There are physicians, nurses, psychologists, and social workers who because of training, temperament, or clinical bias see patients predominantly from one conceptual point of view. They may acknowledge the validity of other points of view, but they themselves prefer to use one model.

Sometimes there is a relationship between clinical bias and the geographic location of the psychiatric center. An association with a prominent psychiatric center leads one to identify with that point of view. This identification is also true in medicine. For example, in the insulin treatment of diabetes mellitus there are various viewpoints on how much the blood-sugar level should be controlled in the patient.

Diagnosis

Any functional psychiatric syndrome may be viewed predominantly from any one of the four major models. Certain syndromes, however, are more likely to be viewed by the biologic model than others. These are the schizophrenias, the involutional depressions, and the manic-depressive depressions. Consequently, it is from these clinical syndromes that more is known about genetics, epidemiology, symptom picture, course of illness, somatic treatment, and prognosis.

The neuroses, however, are more inclined to be viewed by the psychological model. It follows then that more is written about the psychodynamics of these syndromes than of the schizophrenias and the depressions.

Treatment

When there is an effective somatic treatment for a psychiatric illness, the biologic model is more likely to be used. Of all the syndromes, those most amenable to somatic treatment are some of the depressions and the schizophrenias. The depressions often respond to antidepressant medication and to electroconvulsive therapy. Lithium carbonate has shown great promise in the treatment of the manic phase of manic-depressive syndromes. The phenothiazines, electroconvulsive treatments, and insulin coma treatments have been used with varying degrees of success in the treatment of schizophrenia.

Social class and other attributes of the patient

A number of studies have demonstrated the importance of the patient's social class in the application of the psychotherapeutic model.[18] Patients from the middle and upper social classes are more likely to be accepted for, and to continue in, psychotherapy. In contrast, patients from the lower class and the lower middle class have a poorer chance of being accepted for therapy, and they drop out of treatment at higher rates.[19] Other patient characteristics that determine the use of the psychotherapeutic model include responsibility, verbal intelligence, psychological mindedness, the capacity to form a close personal relationship, young adult age, history of effective adaptation prior to the current difficulty, likeability, and attractiveness.[20]

Available services

The available treatment resources are an important determinant of the choice of model. Psychotherapy clinics, especially when they are not overcrowded, attempt to apply the psychotherapeutic model in understanding patients. Walk-in emergency clinics, in responding to large numbers of patients, approach the patient with social and biologic perspectives which usually require less time from staff but are effective for many clinical conditions.

There are many small, private psychiatric hospitals that specialize in electroconvulsive treatment. Many patients who have unipolar depressions receive quick, safe, and effective treatment. Some of these hospitals, however, in their persistent use of the biologic model, determined in part by the

[18]L. Schaeffer and J. K. Myers, "Psychotherapy and Social Stratification," *Psychiatry,* **17** (1954), 83–93.

[19]B. Overall and H. Aronson, "Expectations of Psychotherapy in Patients," *American Journal of Orthopsychiatry,* **33** (1963), 421–30.

[20]R. W. Heine and H. Trosman, "Initial Expectations of Doctor-patient Interaction as a Factor in Continuance in Psychotherapy," *Psychiatry,* **23** (1960), 275–78.

service that is available to them, may overlook other treatment modalities based on intrapsychic and social models.

There are some psychiatric hospitals that specialize in social techniques (family therapies, therapeutic communities) or intrapsychic techniques (intensive long-term therapy). These institutions will usually use electroconvulsive therapy infrequently or not at all.

Clinics, staffed with physicians, nurses, and social workers, that treat large numbers of patients may have little opportunity for the long-term psychotherapy that is so often necessary for personality change. Therefore, they make use of the medical and social models that require less staff but are, nevertheless, effective in many clinical situations.

The immediacy of the social situation

When the social cause is obvious, pressing, and immediate, the first consideration is rightly given to the social model. For example,

> A 30-year old married mother of three was referred for psychiatric care following an eight-month depression. Although the depression did not fit the endogenous picture, she was given electroconvulsive treatments without success (the medical model failed). It was then learned that her husband had become severely depressed just prior to the onset of the patient's depression. He arose at 4:00 A.M. each day appearing very morose. He had estranged himself from his mother and sister and spoke little with his wife. The children in their fear of him would cling to their mother. The patient complained of feeling unsupported and overwhelmed, and she developed a fear of being alone.

In this case the social model was used. The major task was to attempt to restore the relationship between the patient and husband. The social management would consist of helping the patient with a substitute social matrix (speaking to her priest, friends, family, or therapist), engaging the couple together, and helping the husband obtain psychiatric treatment. Intensive long-term psychiatric therapy for the wife at this time could have the negative effect of pulling her emotionally away from her husband and toward the therapist.

In general, a social situation in crisis can make intensive psychotherapy a near impossibility. A successful resolution of the social crisis, however, can produce such a dramatic clinical change that the patient often does not want psychotherapy. Indications for somatic treatment may likewise disappear.

It has been noted in a number of outpatient psychiatric clinics that many patients who are called to begin intensive psychotherapy after waiting several months for their turns decline to come. One of the reasons for this phenomenon may be that they had applied for treatment because of social crises, but during the waiting period the social crises were resolved and the patients no longer felt the need for help.

Failure of a model

The failure of a model to lead to the successful treatment of a psychiatric syndrome often leads to the decision to change models. For example, a patient who has not responded to electroconvulsive therapy may well respond to individual therapy, and in reverse, a patient suffering a depression who has not responded to the treatment with the group experience may well respond to antidepressants.

Mixed models

The therapist frequently uses two models simultaneously. An adolescent patient may be treated within a hospital setting by the nurse who maintains a supportive, sustaining relationship (social model) and by the psychiatrist who uses the intrapsychic model of individual psychotherapy. Without the social model provided by the nursing staff, the patient may become suicidal, need longer hospitalization, and manifest behavioral disturbances.

Social and biologic models

A chronic schizophrenic patient (biologic model) is unmistakably identified as such in the psychiatrist's office. Yet he has lived with his family, served a useful social function, and has never been identified as a patient (social model). Because of a change in his environment (his brother left for the army), he has developed an increase in his delusional thinking. He begins to feel that people are against him and therefore starts to break windows. This behavior is intolerable to his family who then brings him to the psychiatrist's office. Now he becomes a patient both socially and medically. He is given medication, becomes less delusional, and stops breaking windows. Given the original assessment of his social function, he is cured. Medically, his symptoms have been ameliorated, but he is still considered to be suffering from schizophrenia.

How the use of one model may diminish the use of another model

Clinicians who rigidly hold that one model is useful in understanding psychiatric phenomena will obviously find little use in alternative models. Even when a clinician may be equally skilled in all four approaches, the election to use one model may diminish the use of another.

For example, a psychiatric unit relies only on the principles of a therapeutic community (social model). The patient is encouraged to discuss painful issues in a group setting. Symptoms are treated with social controls and medications. Families are actively involved in the treatment program. In this situation it becomes difficult to use individual psychotherapy because the therapist–patient relationship might interfere with the group process. The discussion of painful feelings in individual therapy might communicate to the patient that the group and community are less important. Similarly, a ward that encourages individual psychotherapy implicitly discourages maximal use of a therapeutic community.

Almost all psychiatric units, especially those connected with teaching hospitals, tend to claim that they utilize individual therapy as well as the social techniques of the therapeutic community. In practice, however, teaching, research, clinical, economic, and other reasons determine which model predominates. This decision automatically determines that the other will not predominate.

The phenomenon of the decision to use one model, thereby diminishing the use of another, may also apply in outpatient settings. An example may be the question of whether to treat a patient individually, together with his wife, or to combine the two. Seeing the patient as a couple may diminish the use of the psychologic model by altering the therapeutic relationship.

Special clinical situations

There are special clinical situations in which a therapist who is knowledgeable and facile in all four conceptual models will favor a particular model.

1. In order to further the Army's goal of maintaining a fighting force in a combat situation, the therapist will find the social model extremely useful. Whenever possible, he will treat the soldier near the combat area, he will avoid defining him as sick or even as a patient, and he will return him to his military unit as soon as possible. Either defining the patient as medically ill or entering into an intensive therapeutic relationship is likely to keep him from returning to combat.
2. In treating children, whether or not the therapist directly treats this child, the parents are almost certain to receive some attention. It is clear that the patient's social milieu, the family, is having and will continue to have a major effect on the patient's problems.
3. A therapist knowledgeable in all four conceptual models is likely to use the social model if it is his job to treat a community. Economic and manpower reasons alone will justify this decision. He will become closely involved with the social agencies of the community; he will become acquainted with the problems of the school; he will do a large volume of consultation and teaching; he will see a few patients on an individual basis.

The eclectic approach

According to the eclectic approach, clinical psychiatric nursing uses information derived from all models of care. There are, however, two potential stall situations in eclecticism. First, many clinical teams may use data and methods derived from all models without knowing the models well enough to choose what is best for the patient.

Second, there is reason to believe that psychiatric nurses either become adherents to one particular model or they use bits of data from each model in an unsystematic way. At this stage of development eclectic psychiatry and psychiatric nursing can best be learned and used by making the available models already in use explicit rather than implicit. This will prevent a stall situation and will help clinicians to consciously search for data relevant to successful treatment. It will allow clinical judgments to be better understood by mental health practitioners instead of appearing as mystical conclusions.

Identifying the therapeutic leverage

In order to make a meaningful referral, it is important to know the therapist's area of expertise. The question to ask in evaluating the patient and his need is, "What model of care will give the greatest therapeutic leverage?" This leverage is essential in producing positive results. For example,

> A 64-year-old alcoholic woman was referred to a psychiatrist by an internist. Her history stated, "She always drank too much." But her drinking had become extraordinarily excessive over the past 4 years, even though she had been a heavy drinker prior to this. She was frequently intoxicated, would defecate in her underwear, lose consciousness, be socially maladaptive, and she had a liver dysfunction.

To view this problem from the biologic model, that is, having the disease of alcoholism, there would be no treatment except to stop drinking, order vitamins, or administer antabuse therapy. To view this problem as a psychologic process would prove extremely difficult. It would be difficult to treat a 64-year-old woman from a cultured, Yankee background with a treatment that concentrates on the expression of feelings because she denies feelings and insists that everything is all right.

The problem could be defined socially. Four years previously, the patient's last daughter married and left her hometown. She then was alone with her husband who also missed the daughter. In the past, the children provided the emotional support for both parents.

The therapy was designed to meet with the husband and wife as a couple in order to try to help them give to each other what in reality they were not giving. Since there was so much embarrassment in the patient's having an alcoholic problem, it was more bearable for the patient to have the problem defined as a couple problem rather than as an individual problem. The therapist, being very interested and committed to the patient, partially took the place of her daughter. This was a social maneuver because it was there that the therapeutic leverage was. The process involved introducing a new person in her life and changing her social milieu. Since personality structure of the patient could not be altered and the alcoholism could not be treated, the social model was the effective model.

Identifying the nursing approach

The nurse is an important link in the implementation of the social model of care. In this model the nurse becomes a transitional milieu for the patient in a special way which allows the patient to heal.

It is the nurse's role in the biologic model to administer medications, observe the symptom picture through time, and watch for resolution of the treatment in the medical fashion. This model is familiar to nurses because this is often the historical model under which they first learned the practice of nursing.

From an intrapsychic or psychological point of view, the nurse listens carefully to the patient for the dynamic issue even when she is not the primary therapist to the patient. The nurse's understanding and interpretation of the patient's thoughts, feelings, and actions yield valuable data for the total team planning of care. If the nurse is in a primary therapist role, this model of care takes on specific dimensions.

For the nurse's understanding of colleagues in one mental health field, these four major models of care should be familiar ones. They will enable the nurse to know which questions to ask the patient. Questions may be asked from a biologic, social, psychological, and behavioral assessment standpoint.

In summary, if nurses see themselves as eclectic in their conceptual frame of reference in psychiatric nursing, they then know what to listen for and how to interpret most effectively in the best interests of the patient.

SUMMARY This chapter focused on how the decision to use a certain model or models of care[21] is made in the psychiatric–mental health field. The health teams' variability in thinking was discussed. The decision-making process of clinical judgment was presented; this included the various conditions of clinical bias, diagnosis, treatment, demographic data, available services, the immediacy of the social situation, failure of a model, mixed models, social and medical models, how the use of one model may diminish the use of another model, and special clinical situations.

The implications for the nurse's role described the therapeutic leverage assessment and the eclectic approach. The nursing approach to the four major models was described.

[21]Adapted with permission from Aaron Lazare, "Hidden Conceptual Models in Clinical Psychiatry," *New England Journal of Medicine,* **288** (1973), 345–51.

PSYCHODYNAMIC CONCEPTS AND EGO PSYCHOLOGY

4

Chapter 3 presented the four basic approaches to psychopathology. Its major aim, in addition to presenting an overview, was to demonstrate how clinicians implicitly use various approaches in order to make sense out of clinical data. The reader can learn more about the social model by reading Part Five, The Community, and can develop a greater appreciation for the biologic approach by reading Part Four, The Clinical Syndromes. This chapter and the two that follow will describe in greater detail the psychodynamic approach.

Classical psychoanalytic theory as described by Freud and his followers is the cornerstone of the psychodynamic approach. Alternate and supplementary points of view have been presented by Adler, Jung, Horney, and Sullivan who have deemphasized the importance of instincts and (except for Jung) have emphasized social and cultural determinants of behavior. The psychodynamic approach(es) is not without its limitations. At best, it presents an incomplete understanding of human behavior. Nevertheless, many of the concepts of the psychodynamic approach have proven invaluable in understanding normal and abnormal human behavior.

BASIC DRIVES The psychodynamic approach deals with the individual's instincts or drives which seek their expression and the ways in which these instincts are dealt with by other aspects of the mind and by society. The instinct says: "I want gratification now." The other agencies of the mind, as well as society, decide whether, when, how, and in what form these drives will be gratified. Such negotiations or compromises form the basis for conflict which may ultimately result in psychopathology. An understanding of the basic drives or instincts is, therefore, important to the understanding of the psychodynamic approach.

The basic drives or instincts are psychological representations of biological processes. In other words, our basic wishes derive from biological needs in the way that the wish to eat stems from the biological state of hunger. These instincts are characterized by a *source*, an *aim*, and an *object*. The source of the instinct refers to the biophysiological state that leads to the feeling of excitation; that is, the source is biological. States of tension will result if the instinct is not discharged in some way. The aim of the instinct is satisfaction or reduction of tension. The object of the instinct is the person, situation, or condition that will satisfy the instinct. The object of sexual instincts may be a partner of the opposite sex, sublimated activity, or, in pathological states, various sexual perversions.

The classification of drives has changed throughout the history of the psychoanalytic movement. Two drives, however, that currently are believed to be essential in understanding psychological conflict are the sexual and aggressive.

The psychodynamic concept of sexual instincts includes more than those physiological states and behaviors which lead to sexual intercourse. Particularly in childhood it can be seen how excitation and pleasurable feelings are associated with various anatomical zones of the body including the oral cavity, the anal region, and the sexual organs. These infantile phenomena are regarded as sexual (1) because their fusion leads to adult sexuality; (2) because adults whose sexual expressions are blocked may revert to these childhood forms; and (3) because the child has similar emotional experiences to adults in the area of sexuality.

The aggressive instinct, like the sexual instinct, is part of a human's biological nature. This instinct can be seen in babies as they bite, push, scratch, and hurt. It has its origins in the musculoskeletal system of the body. This aggression has the potential not only for personal and social harm, but also for highly constructive and creative behavior. Like the sexual drive, aggression needs its appropriate expression.

THE TOPOGRAPHIC APPROACH TO THE MIND

The topographic approach to the mind is an early theoretical formulation of Freud which has provided important contributions relating to the dynamics of unconscious thinking, the distinction between primary and secondary process, and the dynamics of regression.

The topographic theory attempts to divide the mind into three parts: the *unconscious,* the *preconscious,* and the *conscious.* The unconscious consists of repressed ideas and repressed feelings which become partially apparent in dreams, slips of the tongue, and forgetting. The unconscious is not logical, it contains contradictory ideas and feelings, and it has no conception of time. For example, it may simultaneously love and hate, believe in irrational concepts, and feel that an event which occurred 20 years ago happened only yesterday. The unconscious is closely related to drives and instincts previously described. The sexual instincts in particular have their derivatives imbedded in unconscious process. The preconscious, which includes ideas and feelings easily made conscious, censors wishes and represses unpleasant ideas and feelings. In contrast to the unconscious, the preconscious supports the reality principle and respects logic. The conscious refers to all that is in awareness.

The above ideas, collectively referred to as the *topographic approach,* were inferred from the observation that neurotic symptoms seemed to result from the repression of unacceptable wishes which were not in the conscious mind of the patient. When these unconscious wishes were made conscious again, the neurotic symptoms would often disappear.

Freud and others realized that the topographic theory had several deficiencies in understanding psychological functioning. First, Freud discovered that there were forces (defense mechanisms) which kept the unacceptable wishes unconscious. Second, unconscious guilt—not accounted for in the topographic theory—was also a common problem in the treatment of the neuroses. Third, in psychotic conditions the idea that unconscious conflicts are at the root of the problem did not seem clinically valid. In fact, bringing to consciousness the unconscious conflict often seemed to make the condition worse. As a result of these limitations, a new theoretical framework was necessary to explain clinical phenomena—the structural approach.

THE STRUCTURAL APPROACH TO THE MIND

Contemporary psychodynamic theory divides mental functioning into three major systems or agencies, each of which has different functions. These are the *id,* the *ego,* and the *superego.* Behavior may be understood as a result of the interaction among these three systems. It must be remembered, however, that the id, ego, and superego are theoretical constructs or ways of organizing our ideas about mental functioning. Therefore, it is meaningless to ask whether or not these agencies exist. It is meaningful to ask to what degree are these concepts useful in making sense of the behaviors that we observe in health and illness.

The id

The id represents the primitive instinctual drives that seek gratification. It is the major source of psychic energy and provides the power for the functions of the superego and ego. This instinctual energy, with which the infant is endowed at birth, knows no time or logic and is unconscious. It wants its wishful and irrational impulses to be immediately and totally discharged according to the pleasure principle.

The ego

As the instinctual demands of the growing infant become incapable of reducing tension, the ego emerges. Wanting something is not enough. The ego then brings the reality principle to bear. It mediates the demands of the environment and the demands for instinctual satisfaction. It sees to it that the discharge of tension is appropriate. It decides how to act and when to act. Whereas the id originally comes into conflict with external reality, eventually conflict occurs within the mind—between ego and id. In this situation, the ego may prevent the id's instinctual discharge.

The superego

The superego is the last of the three systems to develop. In contrast to the id which strives for pleasure, the superego strives for perfection and morality.

It is little wonder that these two systems are often in conflict. The standards of right and wrong adopted by the superego result from rewards and punishments, approving and disapproving behaviors by the parents and other important people in a person's early years. An important part of superego development arises from an attempt to please parents and not lose their affection. "I will do the right thing and they will love me." With superego formation, it might be said that the child has internalized the parent's beliefs as to what is right so that now there is an automatic signal inside. The ego must now deal with the superego, a force which is sometimes as irrational and unreasonable in its standard of right and wrong as the id is in its demands for pleasure. When these standards are not met, a person may experience terrible guilt, a fear of punishment, diminished self-esteem, and remorse. The superego may oppose both the id and the ego.

The dimensions of the superego described above resemble the conscience. There is a less well-described subsystem of the superego, the *ego-ideal,* which is an incorporation of that which a person has been approved of and rewarded for. A person does what is right not only out of fear of punishment but out of a desire to please and be rewarded.

EGO PSYCHOLOGY

During the past two decades, the attention of psychoanalytic theorists turned from studies of instincts and their vicissitudes to a careful and comprehensive study of the ego. The structural approach which set the ego apart as a distinct agency set the stage for these later formulations. The major contributors to writings on ego psychology include A. Freud, Kris, Hartmann, Erikson, and many other contemporary theorists. Studies of the ego have taken two major directions, each of which has considerable clinical importance. The first is the study of the mechanisms of defense. The second is the study of various ego functions which are primary conflict free and result from maturational aspects of intellectual functioning.

EGO FUNCTIONS

In common usage, the concept of the ego is grossly oversimplified, its meaning global and vague. The related concepts of ego strength and ego weakness suffer similar limitations in clinical practice.

By the efforts of Freud and the ego psychologists who followed him, it is now possible to begin to define the ego by a finite number of functions which necessarily overlap and have a dynamic relationship with one another. Understanding these discrete functions, at least from a descriptive and, hopefully, from a dynamic point of view, has the potential for increasing our abilities to treat patients.

Attempts to categorize ego functions is still in a pioneering stage. We will present the twelve functions described by Bellak et al. in their recent comprehensive study. We believe that the nurse will benefit by becoming at least familiar with the following concepts which will assume greater importance in the future.

Reality testing

Reality testing refers to one's ability to distinguish what is happening in one's thoughts and feelings from events in the outside world. People who are hallucinating, are delusional, or disoriented are suffering from the severest degree of impaired reality testing. They define the world as consisting of their mistaken beliefs and perceptions. For many psychotic patients, this distortion of reality serves a defensive function in protecting the ego from a feared disintegration of personality. Impaired reality testing can also occur in normal people. For example, in the phenomenon of prejudice, a person may attribute behaviors and attitudes to another person regardless of whether these behaviors or attitudes are actually present. One of the most acute abilities to test reality is seen in psychological mindedness, the ability to observe one's own psychological operations. In clinical conditions characterized by disturbances in reality testing, the nurse functions as an auxiliary ego. Specific therapeutic tasks may include teaching the patient to recognize internal reality (the perception of feelings within himself), pointing out distortions at clinically appropriate times, providing educative information which may rectify distorted ideas, arranging group therapy situations for social feedback, and administering psychotropic agents to help reverse the psychotic process.

Judgment

Judgment, as an ego function, includes (1) the ability to anticipate the consequence of one's behavior and not to repeat maladaptive behaviors, (2) the ability to behave appropriately in terms of external reality, and (3) the ability to discriminate. Having good judgment assumes good reality testing, but it goes beyond it. Judgment may be impaired in the presence of organic states, functional psychoses, mental deficiency, or powerful drives. It is possible for people who have adequate reality testing to suffer from impairment of judgment. We see this phenomenon in impulse prone people and in politicians whose serious mistakes in judgment may ruin otherwise promising careers. Fatigue, superego pressure, and powerful impulses also lead to impairment of judgment. Treatment of impairment of judgment depends on the factors that cause it. Postponement of action may be helpful. During the time now available, the patient can more carefully review his conflicting goals while the powerful impulses originally leading to the desire for action have a chance to subside. During long-term work, the patient can be taught to recognize various circumstances which lead to poor judgment.

Sense of reality of the world and of the self

Sense of reality, as reviewed by Bellak, refers to the subjective experience of external events as real, the sense of one's body and parts of it as belonging to or emanating from oneself, the sense of individuality and uniqueness, and the sense of separation of one's self representations from one's object representations. Disturbances in the sense of reality include feelings of alienation, hypnagogic phenomena, depersonalization, derealization, dreamlike states, trances, fugues, world destruction fantasies, and identity diffusion. Sense of reality is a separate ego function from reality testing. In reality testing, the patient can come to the proper conclusion as to what is internal reality and external reality regardless of his subjective experience. Sense of reality, however, has to do with the person's subjective experience. A person with the subjective feeling that the world is about to be destroyed has an impaired sense of reality. If he knows that this experience is subjective and not a part of the external world, then reality testing is still intact. Treatment of faulty sense of reality depends on an understanding of the underlying condition.

Regulation and control of drives, affects, and impulses

This regulatory function of the ego relates to a person's ability to postpone gratification rather than to act impulsively to achieve it and to the ability to tolerate painful affects such as anxiety and depression rather than to act them out or regress. Psychopathic characters, inadequate personalities, alcoholics, and drug addicts are among the patients who have defective regulatory mechanisms for the control of drives, affects, and impulses. Impairment of regulation and control of drives is the most common cause for hospitalization of psychotic patients. Treatments of impaired regulatory and control mechanisms include the use of psychotropic agents, strengthening of the superego, interpretation, limit setting, education, changes in environment, and the development of better signal functions of the ego so that a dangerous buildup of excessive drive becomes apparent.

Object relations

Object relations is a complex and important dimension of ego functioning which refers to the quality of an individual's relatedness to others. The many concepts used to describe object relations include narcissistic vs. anaclitic, object constancy, symbiosis-separation-individuation, degree of separation or fusion of good and bad object representations, primitivity-maturity of object relations. Under optimal conditions, a person is able to sustain meaningful relationships with a minimum of inappropriate hostility. With seriously impaired object relations, relationships are few, detached, unstable, and characterized by self-centeredness, unreasonable dependency and entitlement, and inappropriate hostility.

Thought processes

The ego function referred to as *thought processes* refers to those processes that sustain and facilitate the processes of attention, memory, concentration, anticipation, and concept formation. It also refers to the use of language for primary vs. secondary process thinking. In the ego-psychological framework, these impairments are seen as attempts to respond adaptively to stresses in a person's internal and external reality. Patients with impairment of thought processes are characterized by concreteness, impairment of memory, magical and autistic thinking, and primary process thinking. Various organic states as well as functional psychoses can produce these disordered ego states. Any measures that diminish anxiety will improve thought processes. Such measures include psychotherapeutic intervention as well as medication.

Adaptive Regression in the Service of the Ego (ARISE)

Regression in the service of the ego refers to a lowering of some of the ego's functions to better accomplish some of its tasks. These regressions may put one in better touch with his unconscious or with his earlier experiences, therefore enabling him to see things differently, perhaps more creatively. A considerable amount of stability of ego functioning is necessary to let down the guard. These controlled regressions, however, permit one to better enjoy and participate in artistic endeavors, creative insights, sex, humor, and imagination. The ability of the ego to regress adaptively is probably unrelated to intelligence. With disturbances in adaptive regression, one sees a rigid character structure in which ego regression leads to considerable anxiety. There is stereotyped thinking, an inability to tolerate ambiguity, difficulty enjoying fantasy and play.

Defensive functioning

Defensive functioning refers to the ways in which mechanisms of defense, character defenses, and other defensive operations of the ego (1) affect ideation and behavior and (2) succeed or fail in responding to anxiety, depression, or other painful feelings. With inadequate defensive functioning, the patient experiences extreme anxiety which may lead to an impaired ability to concentrate and function. In other words, unsuccessful defensive functioning can lead to impairment of other ego functions.

Stimulus barrier

Stimulus barrier refers to a person's ability to organize and integrate responses to various degrees of sensory stimulation. People on one end of the stimulus barrier continuum may be oversensitive to excesses of light, sound, temperature, or pain with subsequent withdrawal, physical symptoms, or irritability. People on the other end of the continuum may be oblivious to minimal but adequate stimuli resulting in a general underresponsiveness. Deficiencies in the stimulus barrier may be congenital in origin or they may result from early development. It is postulated that the healthy ego is able to adapt by increasing the stimulus barrier when bombarded (for instance, falling asleep) and by decreasing the stimulus barrier when sensory input is minimal.

Autonomous functioning

Autonomous ego functioning includes attention, concentration, memory, learning, perception, motor function, intention, various habit patterns, learned complex skills, work routines, hobbies, and interests. Although these functions may be impaired in mental illness, it is not uncommon for many of them to be intact in the midst of a florid psychosis. These functions, when intact, facilitate the recovery of other ego functions.

Synthetic-integrative functioning

Synthetic-integrative functioning of the ego refers to the ability to integrate potentially contradictory attitudes, values, affects, and behaviors. When this function is impaired, there is an absence of consistent life goals, poor planning, and difficulty in relating different experiences.

Mastery-competence

The ego function of *mastery-competence* refers to (1) the person's ability to perform in relationship to his capacity so that he can actively master and affect his environment, (2) the subjective sense of competence reflecting how the person feels about what he can master and accomplish, and (3) the discrepancy between (1) and (2). In significant disorders of this ego function, the person feels powerless or helpless to act. He feels impotent and behaves passively, feeling at the mercy of powerful forces.

Regression

DEFENSE MECHANISMS OF THE EGO

Regression refers to the ego's attempt to retreat in the face of conflict and anxiety to ways of feeling, thinking, and behaving from an earlier level of development. The path of regression is usually determined by the various places in which the person had been fixated as a child. Some examples of regression to points of fixation include the regression of a person confronted with a sexual situation to drinking (an oral mode) or to cleaning (an anal mode). An adaptive form of regression, described previously, is regression in the service of the ego.

Repression

Repression refers to the forgetting of unconscious wishes, feelings, or impulses. Most important of the repressed material are sexual in nature, usually derivatives of the phallic or genital levels of development. This defense mechanism is particularly important in the development of hysterical phenomena. Repression may be illustrated in everyday life (1) by forgetting material that the person ought to know and (2) by forgetting dreams that may expose unconscious material that produces anxiety. Patients who have had traumatic medical experiences, especially in their early years, may repress much of the feelings and thoughts associated with these experiences.

Reaction formation

In *reaction formation* the person expresses unacceptable feelings and impulses by expressing the very opposite. Feelings of hate may be dealt with by expressions of affection. The desire to be cared for may be dealt with by expressions of autonomy and independence. Although reaction formation is seen in all neuroses, it is especially characteristic of the obsessional states.

Isolation

Isolation is characterized by the separation or isolation of an idea from the emotions connected to it. Most commonly, the idea is remembered and the affect is repressed. Obsessional patients commonly use this defense to the detriment of therapy. The nurse can see the defense in operation when the patient reports important content in a boring or shallow manner.

Undoing

In *undoing,* a defense mechanism closely related to reaction formation, a person undoes or cancels an act by behavior which is the opposite of what was done before. In reaction formation, the attitude changes. In undoing, the behavior changes. This mechanism, like isolation and reaction formation, is characteristic of many obsessional patients.

Projection

Projection refers to attributing one's feelings, impulses, thoughts, or wishes to the external world instead of to oneself. If a person feels bad, aggressive, or sexually excited in ways which overwhelm the ego with anxiety, these feelings may be projected. The person may then be able to say that others are sexually interested in him, hostile toward him, or wanting him to do bad things. With projection, not only can the person rid himself of undesirable feelings, he also can discharge emotions against the outside. Projection is used in a wide variety of normal conditions. For instance, a beginning nurse who feels insecure and inadequate may project these painful feelings to a patient or supervisor. It is then the patient or the supervisor who regards the nurse as insecure or inadequate. The nurse may then become indignant over this alleged treatment instead of bearing the pain of her own feelings. Projection is most pronounced in paranoid conditions in which there is an actual break with reality.

Introjection

Introjection refers to the taking in, the internalization, or the "swallowing up" of the object (the other person) in order to avoid the distinction and separateness between the object and the self. The two become one. This mechanism, first developed during the oral phase of development, may be called into operation in certain pathological states in order to avoid the trauma of loss or separation.

Sublimation

Sublimation refers not to one particular mechanism of defense but to various defenses which lead to the successful outcome of translating sexual energies to alternative socially valuable outcomes. The activity, its aim, or its object may be changed, but, ultimately, the energy is discharged without blocking. The other defense mechanisms do block instincts with the result that the ego is continuously working at warding off unacceptable impulses. Various forms of work and play may represent sublimations of unacceptable impulses.

Denial

Denial refers to the ego's total failure to acknowledge the reality of an affect, an experience, an idea, or a memory. The young child whose ego is under-developed can fulfill his wish that unpleasant realities do not exist by denying them. In later childhood and even in adulthood, when a more developed ego is functioning, denial is likely to be carried out in fantasy, day-dreaming, or games. Here, there is a temporary pushing aside of reality with the full knowledge that the fantasy is not real. It is in the psychoses that serious denials continue to exist in adults.

Displacement

In *displacement,* an alternative object for a person's instinctual desires is found which permits a release of emotions or drives. The substitute object never yields complete satisfaction. However, these various displacements do yield the creative and productive activities of society.

Identification

In *identification,* the person reduces anxiety by taking over someone else's traits and behaviors and making them his own. He may identify with loved ones, with hated aggressors in order to avoid the feelings of helplessness, with persons who are gone in order to avoid the pain of the loss, and with therapists. One's personality consists ultimately of multiple identifications that have been tested for their ability to reduce anxiety.

Rationalization

Rationalization is the mind's way of justifying one's behavior by stating motives other than the genuine ones. This is often used to avoid bearing the full honesty of the situation. Generally, there is an element of truth in the rationalization. The person takes one small aspect of the truth and enlarges it. For example, a student fails a course and says that the teacher was ineffective. Or a person cancels a doctor's appointment because the car has a flat tire. Or a student is late passing in an assignment because she says a snowstorm kept her from going to the library.

In clinical practice, the following terms and concepts have considerable utility. The nurse will hear these terms and should be able to translate them into observable clinical behaviors.

Fixation and regression

From infancy on, a person proceeds through a regular progression of psychological stages, each of which represents an attempt to master particular developmental tasks. No stage or phase of development is entirely mastered. Many people have a tendency to cling to a particular phase because of their failure to resolve the phase specific issues at the appropriate period in their lives. This tendency is referred to as *fixation*. In periods of stress, the individual manifests behaviors and takes on defenses associated with that particular level of development. This process is called *regression*. In general nursing, as well as in psychiatric nursing, we see patients whose regressive behaviors are a result of psychological or physical traumas which have upset their equilibriums. The style of regressive behaviors can be understood in terms of childhood fixations. These behaviors may take the form of nontrusting, sullen withdrawal, annoying demands, withholding, or a bragging denial of distress.

Narcissism

The concept of *narcissism* is attracting considerable interest in contemporary psychoanalysis as an important tool in understanding psychopathology. The word "narcissism," however, means many things to many people and is a source of serious confusion. Clinicians should make sure that they agree on definitions when discussing the subject.

Primary narcissism refers to the state of an infant in which he is unable to distinguish between himself and the outside world. He is psychologically incapable of relating to an object (another person). When the infant is able to recognize the mother as a separate person, he can invest energy or libido in that person (object libido). A duality between *narcissistic libido* (investment in the self) and *object libido* (investment in others) can be observed throughout life. In psychological or physical trauma, a person may withdraw libido from others and reinvest it in himself, a state referred to as *secondary narcissism*. People suffering from *narcissistic personality disorder* assume grandiose conceptions of themselves. They have serious difficulty in relating empathically with others since they perceive others as existing only to serve them. A *narcissistic conflict* or *trauma* refers to an event which threatens one's self-esteem. *Normal or healthy narcissism* refers to a basic sense of acceptance of oneself despite knowledge of one's realistic limitations.

Nurses deal every day with patients suffering narcissistic trauma, regressed to states of secondary narcissism, or manifesting narcissistic personality traits. It is hoped that the nurse has enough healthy narcissism to withstand the psychological assaults of these and other patients.

Primary gain and secondary gain

Secondary gain refers to the social and psychological uses the patient makes of his symptoms. He may gain sympathy, psychological support, or even financial gain. The labels of mentally ill, physically ill, or patienthood itself are associated with particular roles which communicate expectations to others. *Primary gain* refers to the unconscious significance of the symptoms themselves. A functional paralysis, for instance, may have the primary gain of symbolically castrating the patient for unconscious misdeeds.

SUMMARY   Psychodynamic concepts were discussed in terms of basic drives, the topographic approach to the mind, the structural approach to the mind, and ego psychology. Bellak's twelve ego functions and the defense mechanisms of the ego were identified.

REFERENCES   Bellak, Leopold, Marvin Hurvick, and Helen K. Gediman (1973). *Ego Functions in Schizophrenics, Neurotics, and Normals.* New York: John Wiley & Sons, Inc.

Fenichel, Otto (1945). *The Psychoanalytic Theory of Neurosis.* New York: W. W. Norton & Company, Inc.

Mack, John E., and Elvin V. Semrad (1967). "Classical Psychoanalysis" in *Comprehensive Textbook of Psychiatry,* eds. Alfred M. Freedman and Harold Kaplan. Baltimore, Md.: The Williams & Wilkins Co.

PERSONALITY DEVELOPMENT

5

Developmental phases and the crises that are associated with each form an important cornerstone of personality theory. Mastery or failure at each phase influences the adaptive behavior of the person and ultimately one's personality style. Two key clinical contributions to this theory include Sigmund Freud's psychosexual scheme which links early drive characteristics and object relationships and Erik Erikson's further expansion of these concepts to include the total life cycle of humans. We will discuss personality development both in terms of the individual and the stages of the life cycle and the interaction of the individual to his environment, specifically to parental interaction.

Infanthood: "I am what I am given"

DEVELOP-MENTAL PHASES AND CRISES

The infant is truly a dependent individual in that his total existence depends on resources outside himself. Since the basic zone of contact is the mouth, the psychosexual term of *oral phase* of development is commonly used. As Schwartz and Schwartz state:

> The baby needs to take in nourishment in order to survive. He expresses pain or physical discomfort by crying, and derives pleasure and comfort from sucking. The mouth area is richly supplied with sensory nerve endings and becomes the main focus for the relief of tension and the achievement of gratification through early infancy.[1]

The infant's behavior gradually becomes more discrete in terms of finding the food, discriminating what goes into the mouth, learning to delay immediate gratification and putting other objects into the mouth. In effect, the pattern of parenting determines the ways the infant learns to give, to get, and to demand.

As infants gain in motor development (at the oral, biting phase), they

[1]Lawrence H. Schwartz and Jane L. Schwartz, *The Psychodynamics of Patient Care* (Englewood Cliffs, N. J.: Prentice-Hall, Inc., 1972), p. 59.

55

progress to oral, visual, and manual grasping and to letting go and holding on to objects. One sees the beginning signs of self-stability and continuity through attention, focus, concentration, and discrimination of objects in depth and dimension.[2]

The positive reinforcement of the parent encourages the infant in his development. He develops self-trust by trusting in what he sees and hears. The beginning feelings of confidence and faith develop from the learning that he will receive or get done what is needed. Mastery of the task implies that as he achieves, he is weaned; he loses as he gains.[3] Erikson views this developmental crisis as the origin of optimism or pessimism. Erikson clearly states, "The firm establishment of enduring patterns for the solution of the nuclear conflict of basic trust versus basic mistrust in mere existence is the first task of the ego and thus first of all a task for maternal care."

Failure to master this first ego task leads to varying forms of psychopathology. Behavior disorders in adults termed *oral behaviors* include: clinging and demanding behavior, impulsive greed; deep feelings of internal division; distrust (giving up) and reactive rage; needs to bite, fight, and take rather than receive.

The absence of basic trust can be seen in infantile schizophrenia, and lifelong underlying weakness of such trust is seen in adult personalities in whom withdrawal into schizoid and depressive states is frequent. Erikson comments on this psychopathology:

> The re-establishment of a state of trust has been found to be the basic requirement for therapy in such cases. For no matter what conditions may have caused a psychotic break, the bizarreness and withdrawal in the behavior of many very sick individuals hides an attempt to recover social mutuality by a testing of the borderlines between senses and physical reality, between words and social meanings.[4]

Toddlerhood: "I am what I will"

The infant progresses from the earliest months of passive intake and dependent receptiveness through the end of the first year to active and aggressive oral behavior. In this second phase of the life cycle, Erikson describes muscular maturation as setting the scene for two simultaneous sets of social modalities: holding on and letting go. The resolution of these two conflicts may be hostile or benign. That is, to hold can become a destructive and cruel retaining or restraining, and it can be a pattern of care. To let go may also be destructive or it may be a relaxed "to let pass."[5]

Continued verbal and motor development result in beginning communication by the child and upright walking. As children experiment with

[2]Fredrick C. Redlich and Daniel X. Freedman, *The Theory and Practice of Psychiatry* (New York: Basic Books, Inc., 1966), pp. 141–42.

[3]Ibid., p. 152.

[4]Erikson, *Childhood and Society,* 2nd ed. (New York: W. W. Norton and Company, 1963), p. 248.

[5]Ibid., p. 251.

autonomy, they try to assess control through negativism, self-will, compliance, and dawdling. The basic zone for retention-elimination is termed the *anal phase* of development since the socializing task for this period is toilet training. The developmental crisis of the 2–3 year-old is shame and doubt about control and loss of autonomy.

Erikson further discusses this phase:

> What enduring qualities are rooted in this muscular and anal stage? From the sense of inner goodness emanates autonomy and pride; from the sense of badness, shame and doubt. To develop autonomy a firmly developed and convincingly continued state of early trust is necessary. . . . Firmness must protect him against the potential anarchy of his yet untrained judgment, his inability to hold on and to let go with discrimination. His environment must back him up in his wish to "stand on his own two feet" lest he be overcome by that sense of having exposed himself prematurely and foolishly, which we call shame, or that secondary mistrust, that looking back which we call doubt . . . .[6]

The second nuclear conflict to be resolved is autonomy versus shame and doubt. Phase-related adult characteristics of this task are putting things into their place, being organized, meticulous, compliant, or rebellious. If feelings of shame and doubt are strong, adults may be characterized by stubbornness and overcompensatory control, jealous reform or compulsive cleanliness. Failure to resolve this basic conflict may result in adult traits of cleanliness or dirtiness, orderliness or sloppiness, punctuality or disregard for time, rebellion or defeat and avoidance.

Oedipal: "I am what I can imagine I will be"

The child now has a growing cognitive ability with the capacity to conceptualize and internalize relationships. Children can express feelings, and they can anticipate, worry, grieve, and brood. Their ability to imagine and wish is increased. They frequently project all blame onto others, for example, mother or a sibling. There is a heightened awareness and curiosity of the self. This interest and love for the self is called *narcissism* and is at its height between the ages of 3 and 6.

In locating themselves in respect to their family, they focus specifically on the parents and thus the development of the family triangle relationship. The major source of conflict in children from age 3 to 6 evolves from what Freud describes as the *Oedipus complex*. Erikson comments on this phase:

> . . . the increased locomotor mastery and the pride of being big now and almost as good as father and mother, receives its severest setback in the clear fact that in the genital sphere, one is vastly inferior; and furthermore that not even in the distant future is one ever going to be the father in sexual relationship to the mother or the mother in sexual relationship to the father. The very deep consequences of this insight make up what Freud has called the oedipus complex.[7]

It is from this phase of development that the psychoanalytic theory of sexuality has its origin. The previous two psychosexual phases of infantile

[6]Ibid., p. 84–85.
[7]Ibid., p. 86–87.

sexuality (oral and anal) each contribute in the infantile sexual development from the respective zones of development. Now in the oedipal phase, which Freud labeled the *phallic urethral stage,* the sexual orientation more fully develops. Infantile genitality, as Erikson says, is destined to remain rudimentary, a mere promise of things to come.

The issue of sexuality overtly develops. Girls tend to seek out a new element in the relationship with the father and boys with the mother. The oedipal child becomes interested not only in his body, but also in the bodies of those around him. The main focus of pleasurable feelings shifts to the genitals. The genital differences of people are particularly heightened and children enjoy seeing the nude bodies of other children, and, in addition, they are excited about showing off their own bodies.

Psychoanalysts write of the fears that the male child develops in his dread of losing his genital organ or being "castrated." The concept of castration anxiety comes from this developmental phase. Erikson states:

> Infantile sexuality and incest taboo, castration complex and superego all unite here to bring about that specifically human crisis during which the child must turn from an exclusive, pre-genital attachment to his parents to the slow process of becoming a parent, a carrier of tradition.[8]

The phase-specific crisis is between initiative and guilt. Mastery of the crisis implies identification with the parent of the same sex and subsequently internalization of values and sanctions in the form of conscience, superego, and ego ideal. The resolution of the Oedipus complex occurs at about age six or seven, at which time the child gradually renounces many of the rivalrous sexual wishes toward the parent. Sexual fulfillment becomes postponed until after physical maturation occurs.

As Schwartz and Schwartz cite:

> Before the Oedipus stage passes, the child tends to behave obediently or to misbehave mainly on the basis of whether he will be punished or will receive love and approval from his parents. As the Oedipus complex passes, the child's psychic development permits him to "internalize" approval and disapproval. From that time on, he begins to be able to "know" within himself the difference between right and wrong and to lay down standards of behavior and rules of conscience that will thereafter guide much of his behavior.[9]

Failure of task performance at this stage of development may produce serious consequences in adult life. Erikson states that the resolution of the basic conflict is a split between "potential human glory and potential human destruction." The child becomes divided within himself. When the superego becomes cruel and uncompromising, deep rooted resentments and regressions may develop toward the parent who did not live up to the new conscience the child set up for himself. As Erikson points out, one of the "deepest conflicts in life is hate for a parent who served as a model . . . but who was found trying to get away with the very transgressions which the child can no

---

[8]Ibid., p. 256

[9]Schwartz and Schwartz, *The Psychodynamics of Patient Care,* p. 140.

longer tolerate in himself." Other important results of task failure in this period of development result in hysterical behavior, intense anxiety or guilt, and antisocial personalities.

Latency: "I am what I learn"

With the resolution of the Oedipus phase, the stages of infantile psychosexual development are completed and the child now enters into the first major social system outside the family; this period of development is called *latency*. This phase usually lasts from age six through eleven. The expression of infantile sexual energies into nonsexual energies is termed *sublimation*. This mechanism remains active throughout life as the ego rechannels drive energies into socially acceptable means of discharge. It is during latency that the resolution of the three previous phases of development results in increased ego control over instinctual drives.

One can see this process by observing in grammar school children how personality traits and patterns reflect reactions against earlier infantile sexual and aggressive drives. For example, aggression and cruelty are replaced by sympathy and concern for others; messiness gradually eases into cleanliness; exhibitionistic tendencies give way to modesty; and selfishness and greediness are replaced by cooperation and willingness to share.[10]

Tasks in this developmental period are the acquisition of special skills, incorporating social values and patterns, and competition and interaction with peers and authority figures. The child looks beyond the family and begins to interact with another social system.

School presents a new challenge to children in that it puts to the test the preparation they have for learning. It has been found that neurotic, deprived, or abused children do not listen or use the kind of communication that teachers depend on for their work with children. The child may be poorly prepared to learn or may lack pleasure in learning. This may be complicated by attitudes of passivity and defiance which may lead to underachievement. This, in turn, leads to inferiority and low self-esteem.[11] As Erikson describes the task of this phase:

> The child's danger, at this stage, lies in a sense of inadequacy and inferiority. If he despairs of his tools and skills or of his status among his tool partners, he may become discouraged from identification with them and with a section of the tool world. To lose the hope of such "industrial" association may pull him back to the more isolated, less tool-conscious familial rivalry of the oedipal time . . . . Many a child's development is disrupted when family life has failed to prepare him for school life, or when school life fails to sustain the promises of earlier stages.[12]

Failures in mastery of the task of industry will result in problems of latency-aged children that can be grouped under three headings. The most frequently heard term for problems of this age is *immaturity*. Anderson and

---

[10]Ibid., p. 175.
[11]Redlich and Freedman, *Theory and Practice of Psychiatry,* p. 146.
[12]Erikson, *Childhood and Society,* p. 260.

Carter cite the three kinds of problems most frequently referred to a child guidance clinic or school special service as follows:[13]

1. *Poor school performance.* The achievement of mastery of cultural technology does not measure up to the standards of school and/or parents. The child's school behavior disrupts his learning or the learning of others.

2. *Persistence of certain symptoms.* Symptoms persist that are not unusual in younger children but are not expected at this age period. These are such symptoms as fears, short attention span, daydreaming, hyperactivity, enuresis, and not assuming expected responsibilities.

3. *Social inferiority.* A symptom is found in the isolated child or the child who constantly associates with younger children. A sense of social inferiority might be manifested by overcompensatory behavior, for example, bullying or bragging excessively. In the event that societal expectations are too demanding or opportunities for development of competence are too limited, a kind of cultural inferiority may result.

Adolescence

Adolescence may be described as an action-oriented phase of life in which feelings and thoughts are primarily expressed through behavior. This phase is a very significant developmental period in the life of an individual. As a result of rapid physical, psychological, and physiological growth, the adolescent is compelled to face new and stunning emotions. In the search for equilibrium, the adolescent must struggle against many of the crises of earlier years. Ernest Jones says that the way an individual passes through the stages of development in adolescence is to a very great extent determined by the form of his infantile development.[14]

Edith Jacobson[15] comments on the reactivation of the family triangle issue during adolescence. This phase is thought to be a natural consequence of the revival of the oedipal instinctual strivings. The reawakened oedipal wishes are intensified not only by the impact of puberty, but also by fears of the outside world. This resolution differs from the Oedipus complex in that in adolescence the identification with the patient of the same sex is abandoned in the service of separation from home and cathexis of new relationships.[16]

The adolescent has the task of giving up old incestual ties with the parents. He has the pain of losing his original love objects, of dealing with this mourning process, and of resolving old patterns of restriction and prohibition.[17] The final solution to oedipal issues and the final establishment of the

---

[13]Ralph E. Anderson and Irl E. Carter, *Human Behavior in the Social Environment* (Chicago: Aldine Publishing Company, 1974), p. 143.

[14]Ernest Jones, "Some Problems of Adolescence," *British Journal of Psychology,* **13** (1922), 44–45.

[15]Edith Jacobson, "Adolescent Moods and the Remodeling of Psychic Structure in Adolescence," in *Psychoanalytic Study of the Child,* Vol. 16 (New York: International Press, Inc., 1961), pp. 164–83.

[16]Irene Josselyn, "The Ego in Adolescence," *American Journal of Orthopsychiatry,* **24** (1954), 233–37.

[17]Jeanne Lampl-DeGroot, "On Adolescence," *The Psychoanalytic Study of the Child,* Vol. 15 (New York: International Universities Press, Inc., 1960), p. 100.

necessary independence of ego and superego is undertaken in adolescence. It is a farewell to childhood in which the adolescent now has to redelineate himself and thus expand his identity.[18]

The intensity of the adolescent phase of development and the vehemence of its external expression have made understanding of the individual difficult. Anna Freud[19] describes and explains the swinging pendulum that characterizes adolescence as:

> The elusive mood swings of the adolescent — the height of elation or the depth of despair, the quickly rising enthusiasms, the burning (or at other times sterile) intellectual and philosophical preoccupations, the yearning for freedom, the sense of loneliness and the avid desire for companionship, the rebellion against authority yet the pledge to some leader or idol of his choosing, the marked selfishness and materialistic craving co-existent with high idealism, the inconsiderate behavior toward others and the extreme sensitivity toward himself — are all explained by the war between the id, the ego and superego.

The major task in adolescenthood, as described by Erikson, is the development of a sense of identity. The phase-specific tasks for the adolescent may be identified as gaining independence from the family, integrating new-found sexual maturity, establishing meaningful and working relationships with peers of both sexes, and making decisions about life work and goals.

Clinicians generally prefer to divide adolescenthood into at least two subcategories. Early adolescence is the period from age 11 to 14 and includes puberty and the ensuing physical and psychosocial development. So many physiological and anatomical changes occur during this period that the young person becomes understandably preoccupied with changing body image. For example, primary and secondary sex characteristics appear along with changes in height, weight, muscular development, and body proportions. Changes also occur in coordination and strength. The time period for these changes is individual with some rapidly occurring within two years and with other young people within five to six years.

Later adolescence is the period from age 15 to 19; the issues of this period are related to career, marriage, and parenthood. This is the period when there is a consolidation of the personality and a beginning sense of identity as a mature person.

Schwartz and Schwartz describe this phase:

> During later adolescence, the young person begins to assume more adult responsibilities and manifests increased control of his impulses. Prepubertal anxieties, with their sexual and aggressive conflicts, begin to yield to a growing biological (and especially hormonal) stability and to new-found ego capacities, which in turn increasingly control the sexual and aggressive impulses.... Conflicts ... are derived from ... physical changes ... and the upsurge of sexual feelings that accompanies the onset of menses in girls and the genital changes

---

[18]E. Jacobson, "Adolescent Moods," p. 165.

[19]Anna Freud, "Adolescence," *The Psychoanalytic Study of the Child,* Vol. 15 (New York: International Universities Press, Inc., 1958), pp. 255–78.

in boys and arouses in them echoes of conflicts about sexuality which existed during the oedipal stage.[20]

Erikson defines this fifth stage of personality development as identity vs. role confusion. He points out that the form of ego identity is more than the sum of the childhood identifications, that it is the accrued experience of the "ego's ability to integrate all identifications with the vicissitudes of the libido, with the aptitudes developed out of endowment and with the opportunities offered in social roles." The danger of this stage is in role confusion.

Many problems in adolescence can be understood in terms of the reawakened oedipal conflict which, in turn, often has its roots in a failure to resolve the original triangular situation. George Gardner describes the four major task areas in which problems frequently arise during adolescenthood.[21]

1. The problem of the drive for relative independence and autonomy.
2. The problem of inner control of sexual impulses and the establishment of a moral code.
3. The problem of identification with the same sex.
4. The problem of educational and vocation choices.

Erikson states that when role identity is based on strong previous doubt as to one's sexual identity, delinquent and outright psychotic episodes may present themselves. He advises that if these incidents are diagnosed and treated correctly, they do not have the same pessimistic significance that they have at other ages.[22]

Anderson and Carter further identify the characteristic troubles of the adolescent identity crisis which mental health professionals need to understand.[23]

1. *Psychosis,* usually in the form of schizophrenia. This is a condition of identity confusion in the extreme and the traits may be considered as exaggerations of "normal" traits:
   a. Feelings of dislocation and estrangement.
   b. Total docility or exaggerated rebelliousness.
   c. Emotional lability, rapid mood swings.
   d. Feelings of everyone being against one.
   e. Idealism that seems to be a denial of reality.
   f. Confused body image and sexual identification.
2. *Neurosis,* usually described as identity confusion as a conflict between the ideal self and other selves. The alternating excitability and lethargy of adolescents may well be examples of this tendency.
3. *Delinquency,* as a socially defined deviant adaptation to inner demands and outer expectations. It may be the result of particular internal conflicts or it may be an individual or group rejection of cultural values of a larger system.

[20] Schwartz and Schwartz, *The Psychodynamics of Patient Care,* p. 198.

[21] George Gardner, "Psychiatric Problems of Adolescence," in *American Handbook of Psychiatry,* ed. Silvano Arieti (New York: Basic Books, Inc., 1959), pp. 870–92.

[22] Erikson, *Childhood and Society,* p. 262.

[23] Anderson and Carter, *Human Behavior,* p. 148.

Adulthood

The personality development phase of adulthood is generally divided into two subcategories: young adulthood and middle adulthood. For each of these stages, Erikson has identified tasks to be mastered. The critical task for the young adult is to enter in an involved, reciprocal way with others sexually, occupationally, and socially.[24] The mastery of this phase results in intimacy and solidarity; the failure results in isolation. Essentially, the person completes the transition from the family of origin to the family of procreation. It is in this period that the young adult strives to achieve the first phase of sexual (genital) maturity and he seeks a sense of intimacy with a partner of his choosing. Erikson further defines this stage:

> Body and ego must now be masters of the organ modes and of the nuclear conflicts, in order to be able to face the fear of ego loss. . . .[25]

To date, the psychoanalytic writings place a heavy emphasis on adult genitality as the utopia of the concept of organismic sexuality. Erikson does qualify this concept by adding, "It is integral to a culture's style of sexual selection, cooperation, and competition."[26]

The second stage of adulthood is achieved during the middle years of adulthood, the years 30 to 60. It is during this period that a sense of generativity leads to productive and creative work. In past decades, this has meant child-rearing for women. In contemporary times, both women and men are increasingly sharing parenting functions so that both may pursue meaningful careers outside the family structure.

This stage of adulthood is important in terms of the physical and physiological body changes. The main theme of the age period 45 to 60 for both men and women is that of hormonal change. There are certain issues which many people in this age period face and which have implication for continued mental health. They are identified by Hamburg, Coelho, and Adams.[27]

1. The vulnerability and likelihood of a serious illness is greater at this time than it has been previously. People often identify with a family member or friend who is ill and of the same age range.
2. There is a high probability of parents becoming chronically ill and dying at this age period.
3. Individuals become concerned over the aging process and find this personally threatening.
4. Children become increasingly independent and leave home. This is especially difficult for parents who have placed their main role value in life as being a mother or father.

[24]Ibid., p. 149.

[25]Erikson, *Childhood and Society,* p. 263.

[26]Ibid., p. 266.

[27]D. A. Hamburg, G. V. Coelho, and J. E. Adams, eds., "Coping and Adaptation: Steps toward a Synthesis of Biological and Social Perspectives," in *Coping and Adaptation* (New York: Basic Books, Inc., 1974), pp. 403–41.

5. There is a need to reorganize one's time and interests and energies due to the changing family structure.
6. Careers may be undergoing transition either up or down as people take time to reevaluate where they have been and what they have accomplished in terms of future years left to achieve previously planned goals.

Anderson and Carter comment on other approaches in describing personality development in the mature years. They define four major social expectations or tasks for the adult.

1. *Sexuality.* Adult sexuality is an important aspect of intimacy and the sharing of identity. Genitality, in the sense of the capacity for full and mutual consummation of sexual potential, is only characteristic of adulthood. Sexual mutuality forms the foundation of the family system.
2. *Generativity and child-rearing.* The assumption of responsibility for transfer of the culture and nurturance of the young fulfils the destiny of the adult of a species. This requirement is particularly stressful for those without a firm sexual identity and the capacity to merge self-interest with the interest of others. This is not confined to being a biological child-rearing parent. It includes a participatory generative role that is gratifying to self and others, such as child care, teaching, or a role that benefits future generations.
3. *Participation in social processes.* This function furthers the purposes of society and culture. This requires a measure of subordination of personal needs to the needs of others. This is particularly stressful to those who isolate and retain a primarily self-indulgent orientation.
4. *Work.* A work function is required that is gratifying to self and to society. In our culture, work has become a major organizing theme and we construct our life styles around it. The usual response of an adult to "who are you" results in an occupational role function.[28]

Failure to master or achieve these developmental tasks usually shows up as external or situational crises of adulthood in terms of marital, social, or occupational conflict and failure. Disordered personality styles express themselves in the person's inability to function in adult tasks.

Older adulthood

The crisis of aging confronts the person with the finite boundary of the personal life cycle which is death. The predominant theme in this stage of development is ego integrity vs. despair. As Erikson states:

Only in him who in some way has taken care of things and people and has adapted himself to the triumphs and disappointments adherent to being, the originator of others or the generator of products and ideas—only in him may gradually ripen the fruit of these seven stages. . . . It is the acceptance of one's one and only life cycle as something that had to be . . . and that for him all human integrity stands or falls with the one style of integrity of which he partakes.[29]

Failure to achieve ego integrity is identified by Erikson as despair. The

[28]Anderson and Carter, *Human Behavior,* p. 150.
[29]Erikson, *Childhood and Society,* p. 268.

theme of this age period is loss, and thus without adequate emotional support to sustain and bear the losses, it is understandable why the older adult is vulnerable to despair. The losses of this period may be identified as follows.[30]

1. Loss of work role and occupational identification.
2. Loss of intimate ties as friends, acquaintances and spouse die.
3. Loss of sexual interest as defined in recent research that sexual activity gradually declines in frequency.
4. Loss of physical abilities, particularly sensory and motor.
5. Loss of intellectual processes.
6. Intellectually, the person may become more of a closed system.
7. Despair and disgust include the feeling that time is running out and there are no alternatives possible at this late date.

In defining the full cycle of human life, Erikson cites the parallel of trust as the first of the ego values, with adult integrity as the last of the ego values, by saying, "Healthy children will not fear life if their elders have integrity enough not to fear death."[31]

PERSONALITY DEVELOPMENT: ENVIRONMENTAL EFFECTS Discussion of the personality development of an individual includes mastery or failure of the developmental tasks of the life cycle *and* interaction of the individual and the environment, specifically the parents' adaptive behavior to the developing child. This chapter would not be complete without brief mention of the situations that can influence the child. Developmental problems of children will be discussed in a separate chapter, but here we identify parental behavior patterns and family disorganization that can affect the child. It is becoming increasingly clear that certain patterns of child-rearing have a definite negative effect on the developing personality. These patterns are identified as follows.

PARENTAL DEPRIVATION. This parental behavior includes not only gross neglect of the child but parental overcontrol, masking of feelings, and attitudes of indifference to the child. Early rejections, the psychological loss and separation of parent and child, may show their effects later in severe behavior disorders.

PARENTAL OVERPROTECTION. This behavior interferes with the ability of the child to learn to master anxieties, tends to keep the person tied to the parents, and fosters a poor self-identity.

INCONSISTENCIES. Inconsistent behavior in child-rearing is especially noticeable in such parental tasks as reward and punishment and the setting of behavioral limits.

SEXUAL CHILD ABUSE. Reports are increasingly indicating that the sexual abuse of children by adults who may also be family members is a traumatizing crisis for the child.

CRUEL AND ABUSIVE PUNISHMENT. The punished child not only fears and fights the punitive parents, but he also identifies with them. Studies have traced overt personality traits of aggression, defiance, and passivity, as well as the

[30]Anderson and Carter, *Human Behavior*, pp. 154–55.
[31]Erikson, *Childhood and Society,* p. 269.

stern, self-punitive attitudes derived from unconscious identification with a harsh, unloving parent.

Family disorganization

So that the nurse may gain a better understanding of why noxious conditions exist in a family structure, three of the potential areas in the marital relationship are described below.[32]

Inability of parents to form a coalition

In the successful parental role each parent supports the other. The child then sees marriage as a relationship in which one partner works for the other's satisfaction as well as for his own.

Marriages in which spouses criticize and devalue each other place a heavy burden on the child. For example, if the boy is identifying with his father and father is constantly devalued by the mother, whose love the boy also wants, the child naturally becomes confused. For example, the mother might say to the father, "All you do is sit around the house, watch television, and drink beer. Can't you do anything besides be a nothing?"

If the mother puts the father in a helpless position in the family, she can interfere with a healthy identification process. Or the father can do the same thing to the mother. Children react when the family environment is heavy with arguing and fighting. If the children are unaware of the reason for the argument, they may interpret that it has to do with them which, in turn, may make them feel responsible and guilty. Children who participate in this kind of family atmosphere will also learn this behavior and will be considerably more prone to enforcing this same kind of marital interaction in their own marriages.

Inability to maintain the essential boundaries between parents and child

When one parent is upset or angered by the other parent, the child may be used to meet the angered parent's needs. For example, after a family fight, the wife may gather the children around her and ignore the husband. She may allow such behavior as the children's sleeping with her at night.

Or a parent may feel that he is competing for the other parent's love and affection. The father who shows preference to his teen-age daughter may place his wife in a competitive position with the daughter. This, in turn, has implications for the manner in which the parents and child relate.

SUMMARY

This chapter discussed personality development in terms of the developmental phases and crisis identified by Erikson and the psychosexual theory. A description of the individual, as well as the phase-specific task, was identified for the following phases of the life cycle: infanthood, toddlerhood, oedipal phase, latency, adolescenthood, adulthood, and older adulthood. Failures in task achievement were discussed in relation to the phase. The negative aspects of parenting were included in order to complete the picture of personality development of the individual through the environment of adults.

[32]Julius Segal, ed., *The Mental Health of the Child,* Public Health Service Publication No. 2168 (Rockville, Md.: National Institute of Mental Health, 1971), pp. 270–73.

PSYCHODYNAMIC CONCEPTS
a case illustration

The two previous chapters presented the basic concepts of psycho-dynamic theory. This chapter will illustrate many of these concepts by presenting a case report of an 18-year-old male who received 27 months of intensive psychotherapeutic treatment. The principal therapist was author A. W. B.; the administrator during the final year of treatment was author A. L.

Current history

CASE HISTORY An 18-year-old male was referred to a psychiatric hospital for evaluation and treatment following his third serious suicidal attempt in a one-year period. His chief complaint on admission was: "I'm not able to concentrate on my work at school. My mind goes blank. My thoughts keep swimming. I can't use my potential."

The symptoms began to develop 3 years prior to admission when he first experienced difficulty in concentrating. He began drinking and developed an inverted sleep pattern manifested by sleeping during the day and remaining awake most of the night. His school grades plummeted in his sophomore year from honors standing to failure. He experienced uncontrollable rages which resulted in destruction of property, usually his personal possessions. He stopped dating girls and gradually lost all interest in former activities. During the 3-year period, there was a progressive withdrawal from others. There were no delusions, hallucinations, or ideas of reference.

The suicide attempts took place in the early hours of the morning when the patient was socially isolated. Although there was no obvious precipitating event, the first attempt followed increasing discouragement over school grades. He experienced irritability and anorexia with a 30-pound weight loss, felt that nothing mattered, and that there was little reason for him

A. Burgess and A. Lazare, "Dual Therapy by Nurse and Psychiatrist," *American Journal of Nursing,* **70** (6), 1292–98. Copyright June 1970 by The American Journal of Nursing Company. Sections quoted with permission from the *American Journal of Nursing.*

to live. He attempted to kill himself with carbon monoxide but was found unconscious in the garage by his mother who accepted the explanation that this was an accident. Three months later the patient ran his car off a dangerous curve. This too he explained as an accident. Shortly thereafter, the patient took a 3-month car trip across the country with the hope of getting away from all who knew him. He said this was the first time he felt at peace with himself. The police found him out of gas and money and sent him home. The third suicide attempt, occurring one year after the first, followed an argument with his mother over his not attending school. According to the patient, he saw himself as a failure, uncomfortable at home and with others. Death, he said, was his only solution. The patient again used carbon monoxide and was unconscious for 3 hours; his legs were partially frozen because of the 30-degree below zero temperature.

After a short stay in a general hospital, the patient was transferred to a psychiatric hospital for evaluation. His referral for definitive psychiatric care was accompanied by the following psychological report:

> Test results suggest there is good reason to be concerned over suicidal intent. There is a significant withdrawal from a commitment to life, a real retreat to solitude, and a refusal to get involved in any interaction with the world, people, or even himself. . . . There is a complete negation of all feelings; the patient believes that people ruin everything. This position is not a form of adolescent rebellion against authority but goes much further in that death is seen as the only possible resolution. . . . There is considerable thought disorder. Our diagnostic impression is of a schizophrenic process[1] with paranoid and depressive features.

Past history

The father, a college graduate in his early fifties, met the mother while in the military service. He was being treated for psychosomatic problems in an army hospital where she worked. Following a brief courtship, they were married after the father received a medical discharge for uncontrollable vomiting. The patient was born at the end of the first year of marriage. For the first year of the patient's life, he lived with his mother and maternal grandparents while the father lived with his own parents, presumably seeking employment. The family was reunited when the father began work. Early childhood recollections include the patient's playing by himself or helping mother with housework or baking. Father seemed to be either with his friends or at work. The patient slept in his parents' room until age 4. After he moved into his own bedroom, he often awoke at night, would go to the bathroom, and, fearing to return to his own room, would go to his parents' room and sleep between them. At the age of 6 the patient vividly remembers a family argument during which his mother cried and screamed while the patient hid his head under the pillows to stifle his own crying. When the

---

[1]Although psychological testing demonstrated pathology seen in schizophrenic patients, it was the authors' working formulation that these findings are better understood as manifestations of a regressed adolescent ego. See Discussion on page 79.

patient was 11 years of age, the father fell and injured his back. He subsequently retired from his job on complete disability. Since then, the father is said to have spent his time at home criticizing his wife for the way she did her housework and for not making her sons behave. There is a report of an attempt by the father to hang himself in the basement. The mother is described by the social worker as a controlled woman who has had difficulty in expressing any feelings. She works hard in the home but gets few satisfactions from it. Since her husband's retirement, the mother has returned to work.

The patient characterizes the interaction of his parents as one constant argument. He becomes angry at his father for antagonizing his mother and then feels sorry for his mother. Once one party has initiated the argument, the other always continues. The mother has said many times that she would have been better off if she had never married. The patient agrees. In the midst of the marital strife, the patient feels that neither parent is seriously interested in him. He is especially critical of his father for his lack of ambition and for his failure as a disciplinarian.

The patient was an only child until age 6 when a brother was born. Two years later a second brother was born. With the birth of the first sibling, the patient began stuttering and stealing. The stealing continued until the current hospitalization. The stuttering continued until his mid-teens when the preoccupation with suicide began. Because of his inability to speak clearly, he described himself as a "blundering idiot." He generally avoided the presence of others and focused his attention on solitary activities, such as fishing, walking in the woods, and driving alone at night.

HOSPITAL COURSE Although this chapter will review 27 months of hospitalization and psychotherapy, the emphasis will be placed on the final 12 months, during which the primary therapeutic figures were the nurse-therapist and the psychiatrist administrator. The first 15 months of the hospitalization will be reviewed more briefly; special attention will be paid to the role of the nurse who was to become the central and most constant therapeutic figure throughout the treatment.

The first 15 months of hospitalization

The first 15 months of treatment were tumultuous. Many variations in the treatment approach involving several staff members characterized this period. This pattern was seen not only as staff reaction to the obvious depth of the patient's despair and to his failure to respond to treatment but also as a manifestation of his ability to manipulate others and to engage them in conflict.

During the first 2 months of hospitalization, the patient was seen 3 times weekly for 45-minute interviews by a resident psychiatrist who assumed total therapeutic and administrative responsibilities. This endeavor to engage the patient was unsuccessful, for he saw any attempt by the staff to relate to him as an invasion of his privacy. "This is all much ado about nothing. I just want to die." Because of his unabated wish to kill himself, a course of 21 electroconvulsive treatments were given. The treatments were started during the seventh week of hospitalization and were administered 3 times each week for 7 consecutive weeks. Although there were no dramatic changes in the patient's behavior or affective responses, his obsession with death lessened slightly.

Beginning with the third month of hospitalization, co-therapy was instituted. The second therapist was a psychiatric nurse. She was in frequent contact with the first therapist as well as with the nursing staff, and she met with the patient 5 times each week for 45-minute interviews. (During the first several weeks of therapy, interviews were as brief as 10 minutes.) The psychiatrist and the nurse shared the therapeutic responsibilities and the psychiatrist alone handled administrative matters. It was anticipated that the two therapists would have a better chance of reaching the patient than one. It was conjectured that if the patient became overwhelmed in his relationship with one therapist, he might turn to the other in order to work out the impasse.

During the first 6 months of the co-therapy arrangement, the patient showed little desire to become involved. For many weeks he said he could remember neither the name of the nurse-therapist nor the hour for the appointments. He later acknowledged that during the long silences in the therapy hour, he was planning just what he wanted the therapist to hear. The patient was controlled both in speech and in motor action. He walked with robotlike body movements. For the first 3 months of this period, he was well behaved and passively compliant in his ward behavior. For the next 3 months he actively avoided contact by being late or absent for appointments or by leaving the hospital without permission. Throughout this 6-month period he continually talked and wrote about death as his only solution. He wrote:

> *Alone on the hill, by the sea,*
> *A grave stands, populated joyfully by me.*
> *Here I lay, under the ground*
> *Never again to see the sun*
> *Forgotten by man, a long time ago*
> *Which is the way it should be.*

In the seventh month of co-therapy (the ninth month of hospitalization), the patient verbalized for the first time his positive feelings toward the nurse-therapist:

> Last night I was just overwhelmed. This will sound silly. I just felt like putting my head in your lap and bawling. I don't have anything to cry about. I'm not sorry for myself.

As the patient showed further evidence in subsequent weeks that he trusted, cared about, and depended on his nurse-therapist, he also became increasingly anxious about the relationship:

I was feeling too close. I was almost happy about things . . . . If I could get everyone to despise me, then I could go ahead and kill myself.

In an apparent reaction to the anxiety generated by the intensity of his feelings toward the nurse-therapist, the patient demanded that she stop seeing him, expressed homicidal feelings toward her, and then requested transfer to another hospital. When the transfer was refused he poured glue on the ward typewriter keys, smeared furniture with paint, and set fires in the hospital. It was at this point in therapy that the relationship between the two therapists became strained. He would be rebellious and hostile with one therapist and tractable and compliant with the other; and in this manner he was able to pit one against the other.

Who was the "real therapist"? How was co-therapy affecting the patient? These questions were difficult to ask and even more difficult to answer. Meanwhile, by his behavior, the patient was effectively setting therapist against therapist, doctor against nurse, and chief-of-service against resident psychiatrist. He had succeeded in creating utter confusion on the ward. Treatment plans were reorganized; the chief-of-service assumed the administrative role; and the resident psychiatrist and the nurse therapist continued as co-therapists. The antisocial behavior of the patient and the intrastaff conflict continued.

At the end of 15 months of hospitalization, the patient was still playing the nurse and psychiatrist off against each other. He had been unable to come to terms with a male in a position of authority and was still struggling with his feelings toward the maternal female. Suicide remained a possibility for him. Nevertheless, the patient did acknowledge his dependence on and positive feelings for the nurse-therapist. It was on the strength of this relationship, together with the patient's being liked by those working with him (this was one of his greatest strengths), that the hospital now committed itself to an additional 12 months of treatment, despite the fact that the male therapist and the chief-of-service were terminating their relationships with the patient upon completion of their hospital training.

At this time psychological tests were administered:

The test results indicate a schizophrenic process that appears to be both stabilized and of some standing. The patient is able to put up a fairly orderly front in situations that are structured and nonstimulating; he apparently has an awareness of what responses one should make in social situations and is able to act as if he had the appropriate reactions. Yet, underlying a rather brittle facade are indications of severe pathology revealed in significant thought disorder, impaired reality testing, a grandiose paranoid orientation, and considerable emotional withdrawal.

. . . Establishing an identity as a male is almost impossible for the patient. He sees masculinity as terrifying since it involves being brutal and violent—the male is a sexual beast without a mind and without any control over his impulses. Women, on the other hand, are extremely devalued; they are "crude," "barbaric," "helpless," and objects of contempt . . . . He perceives of himself as rotten, ugly, loathsome, and ultimately as castrated.

. . . In contrasting the present results with those on admission, the patient has further developed the ability for firmer ego boundaries in formally defined situations. He is better able to keep pathological elements from intruding on his cognitive functioning. He has a better appreciation of social expectations and can perform more adequately in a conventional way, although these responses are not genuine but "as if" reactions. Underlying the more acceptable clinical facade, peculiar and autistic thinking and emotional withdrawal remain.

The sixteenth to the twenty-seventh month of hospitalization

During this 12-month period, the nurse became the sole therapist and continued to meet with the patient 5 times each week. She was active and supportive; the focus of therapy was on the clarification of day-to-day feelings and events and their relation to former modes of adaptation. Interpretation of unconscious material was minimized. The new chief-of-service assumed the role of administrator. He met with the patient 15 minutes twice each week to discuss and deal with rules, schedules, school progress, medical problems, medications, and visits home. The nurse-therapist, psychiatrist-administrator, ward head nurse, and social worker met together for 30 minutes each week to review the case and especially to note how the patient might be manipulating one member of the treatment team against another. Throughout this period the only medication used was 100 mg of thorazine which the patient took 3 to 4 times weekly for sleep.

During the first few months of this new treatment arrangement, the patient's behavior seemed to be aimed at disrupting the relationship between the therapist and administrator. In addition, he deviously attempted to destroy the limit-setting authority of this new male with whom he had to contend. After one month of the new therapeutic arrangement, the patient informed the nurse-therapist that he had recently held up a gasoline station. She discussed this with the administrator who in turn confronted the patient with the story. He responded, "You really believed that? Women sure are gullible. I'm surprised at Mrs. B. for believing a story like that." The administrator made clear to the patient that this was an important matter and would be taken seriously. The police were telephoned and it was learned that there had been no crime. The patient then expressed his anger at the therapist for "squealing" and demanded to know what in their relationship was confidential. He added, "The fact that you believed the story showed your lack of trust." The patient later confessed that the purpose of the whole maneuver was to confuse the administrator. "I knew you would tell Dr. L. When he finds out there was no hold up, he won't know what to believe." Despite his protestations, the patient seemed relieved that the therapist and administrator handled the situation in a coordinated and consistent manner. In therapy there followed a discussion of past antisocial behavior:

> If I were caught for all the things I've done in my life, I'd have quite a police record. No one would want to have anything to do with me. That's the part of me that comes to the surface when I'm all alone. No one knows about it; except you are beginning to. How can I do so many things that are wrong? I used to like it for the trouble it made for other people; doing things I shouldn't

and getting away with it . . . . Sometimes I lay awake at night just thinking of things to do. I can see why Oswald did what he did; kind of could be like me. Going out for a walk with a gun and just shooting someone . . . . I could do it because I never get caught for anything.

In subsequent interviews the patient began to discuss his delinquent behavior which had occurred during the earlier part of the hospitalization. The patient repeatedly brought up this issue in therapy by saying, "Don't tell Dr. L., but . . . ." This communication was seen as an attempt on the part of the patient to have both the therapist and administrator know about and control his delinquent behavior. At the administrator's insistence the patient returned or replaced all stolen items and repaired damaged property.

After 3 months of the therapist-administrator work, the patient made plans to begin his senior year of high school in the community. During the first year of hospitalization, he attended the hospital school. As he was about to resume his studies, he verbalized (for the first time) his feelings about the weekly meetings between therapist and administrator.

. . . sometimes it's jealousy, sometimes it's frustration. I guess it's mostly feeling sad. Whatever the feelings, I end up feeling sad, even if I'm angry.

The patient reacted to these stresses with destructive fantasies and dreams. He saw himself murdering, raping, and mutilating various people, especially the therapist. His dreams were filled with headless people, with blood flowing from all directions. He began minor self-destructive acts which included fasting, drinking mouth wash and cough syrup, and eating nutmeg. School, he said, was impossible.

It isn't going to work. Got a headache as soon as I got to school. Then went to chemistry and just couldn't understand or concentrate on what the teacher was saying and the headache got worse. By the next class I was having trouble walking, trouble hearing what people were saying. I cut out before lunch; couldn't even stay the day . . . . Felt like before. Could hear the teacher's voice droning in the background and it didn't mean anything to me and I couldn't concentrate. I'm not going back there and torture myself. I know my limitations. I just want to stay in the hospital; put me on ward restrictions; anything. I knew it would be hard getting back in this world but I never remember it being so hard. And I don't want anything to do with it.

He refused to attend classes and, within a few days, turned in his books to the high school. At this time he became involved with a married female patient who physically resembled the therapist. He utilized this situation to play therapist against administrator.

If I tell you what I'm doing, and my feelings, you'll tell Dr. L. and he'll restrict me. You said to try and do more things with people and I do and want to talk about them, but I get restricted.

The patient's bizarre fantasies, his inability to attend school, his inappropriate sexual behavior, and his general hostility were seen as reactions to (1) a new task demanded of him—school, (2) partial separation from the warmth and protection of the hospital and therapist, (3) concern about the relationship between the therapist and administrator, especially with his being away at school. These issues were not interpreted to the patient. Instead, the therapist clearly verbalized her feelings of concern by saying, "The point is that you should be attending school every day and not be spending your time thinking of not going. . . . School is serious business and your getting better is most serious." Simultaneously, the administrator offered to coach the patient in chemistry. The offer was readily accepted. With these joint therapeutic efforts, the patient's school difficulties came to an abrupt end. He began attending school regularly and told the female patient to stop bothering him since he would not be able to finish high school unless he stopped seeing her.

During the sixth month of the therapist-administrator work, the dream material changed from destructive, gruesome rapes, murders, and beheadings to dreams of wolves and lions pursuing him. In one specific dream a wolf was chasing him while he carried his father's gun. When he attempted to shoot the wolf, the gun would not fire. At the same time he began to talk openly and frequently about his hostility toward the administrator. The weekly meetings between the therapist and administrator especially infuriated the patient. He would stand in front of the office during the meetings and peer through a scratch in the frosted surface of the window. In discussing his feelings about these meetings during the therapy hour, the patient spoke with a freedom of expression not previously noted:

> You probably can't wait till Wednesdays. You save every tidbit I tell you and hand it over to Dr. L. like a bucket of shit. . . . You can bet I'm not going to tell you anything else. I've told you enough and it just gets me in trouble. If no one else knows what's going on, it's like it never happened. I can forget about it. It is hard to forget if everyone knows something so I'm not going to give you anything any more. Dr. L. is concerned with my actions and what is the sense of him getting it second hand. I can tell him my actions myself.

At the end of this interview, the patient began to smoke a cigar. This was the first overt sign of identification with the administrator who frequently smoked cigars. In later interviews it became clearer what the weekly meetings meant in terms of his own parents' interaction.

> My parents are the only other people who have talked about me, but they'd always argue. My parents were never united toward me. In fact, I used to play my parents one against the other. I'd ask my mother for something and she'd say to ask my father. If one said no, I'd go to the other and get him to say yes. But my parents didn't work together. All they do is fight. Even if they thought the same thing, one would change their mind just to make an argument. You and Dr. L. are different. He is always asking me how you and I are doing and won't let me do anything unless he talks with you first.

With the patient's acknowledging the solidity of the relationship between the therapist and administrator, his anger toward the administrator heightened. He was filled with hate and rage, but there was no evidence of bizarre thoughts or dreams. The therapy interviews at this time were dominated by his thoughts and feelings toward the administrator:

I can't stand him; I can't deal with him. Seems I'm always having to go to him for something and I've never had to do that . . . . He's a man and I haven't found a man yet that I've liked. I can't even talk to him. I don't think it's right he has so much authority over me and I won't go along with it. . . . I'll rebel, do things to show he can't control me, like lying and acting different than I am. I'm not used to people controlling me. My parents never did. Dr. L. is the only one who can regulate me — or tries to. He even tries to get in on what's going on between us.

(Therapist: He's the boss and that is something new to you.)

At home my mother was the boss and I got around her by being stubborn and she gave up. They weren't very effective in controlling me. They didn't know how to deal with me. I never went to them for anything . . . . That Dr. L. really gets to me, and I don't want to deal with him. He won't stay rejected and that makes me mad. I'm just his responsibility. He got assigned to me. Things didn't work out with Dr. R. so I got Dr. G., and Dr. L. inherited me as a legacy. Had to take me and I'm trying to get rid of him. He's like my father; just doesn't come into the picture. If it weren't for him I could talk to you about anything. I can't stand his breaking in; he has no business with you. Your business is with me, not him. I don't like your having to deal with him and I don't want to spend my interview time talking about him. It just gives me a headache.

The rebellion was a relatively feeble one, taking the form of leaving the ward without informing the staff of his whereabouts. The administrator responded by insisting on a schedule of his daily activities. The patient left a note for the administrator accompanied by a schedule. The note further elucidated the dynamics of the evolving relationship between patient and administrator:

I am very angry to have to admit your existence and I would not except Mrs. B. seems to think you are around and have to be dealt with. You are wrong when you say I think you are a tyrant. That is not the case. You are just an annoyance like a sore pimple on the buttock. You try to saddle me with red tape which I do not care to bother with. You try to make trouble for me and you are trying to come between Mrs. B. and myself. I respect you as a doctor and a person but you are like a third leg to me. A leg which makes things difficult for the other two, one being myself and the other Mrs. B. You are not important in my treatment but you have succeeded in making yourself known. All right, I recognize you if that will make you happy. But I don't need you. Things are going well for me and things are well at school and this is all independent of you. You could screw things up I grant you, but why don't you try to make things easier for me instead of trying to prove your existence by binding my arms. I guess you are saddled with me just as I am saddled with you so maybe we can get along somehow.

Although it was apparent that the patient was finally coming to terms with the two therapeutic objects, one further crisis was to occur in the ninth month of the therapist-administrator work which would resolve with relative completeness the triangular conflict. The patient missed two appointments with the administrator, and after 3 months of perfect attendance, he skipped 2 days at school. Simultaneously, the administrator had been informed of serious family illness and was hurriedly completing his duties before leaving town. Preoccupied himself, he found the patient and abruptly informed him that he was on ward restrictions until he could meet his responsibilities. The administrator was rather arbitrary and set the restriction with inappropriate anger without discussing it with the patient. In the therapy hour that followed, the patient talked of his rage and murderous feelings over what he rightfully interpreted as the administrator's "taking out his anger" on him. He felt rejected, helpless, and impotent. He wanted to stick a knife in Dr. L.'s back or lock him in his office and tell him a bomb would go off in 5 minutes. This incident occurred on Friday and the administrator was away for the weekend. By Sunday evening the patient was extremely depressed as well as explosively angry. Upon his return that evening, the administrator discussed the situation with the therapist and then went to the hospital. In the discussion that ensued, the patient said that he was angriest over the inconsistency of the administrator's not talking to him before placing him on restrictions. The administrator apologized for the way in which he handled the situation, told him what had happened in his personal life, and acknowledged that the patient was justified in being angry. Commenting on the situation in the next therapy hours, the patient said:

> Friday all my nerves were telling me to do something: strike back, kill, destroy, burn up the place, maim, wreck. I didn't know what to do. When I get angry, it's a symptom of my illness; with other people, they are just human. Dr. L. can be a big prick and tell every one what he's thinking and it's OK. I try to be a big prick and I'm told I'm upset or manic or high . . . . After Dr. L. came in and explained what happened, I felt differently. For some reason things don't seem so bad now. Now I can go ahead with my plans . . . .

Several weeks after this incident the patient had his hair cut for the first time in 3 months. At the same time he discussed his fantasies about having wanted to be a girl. He also dropped and shattered his glasses and the following week began wearing frames similar to those of the administrator. During the subsequent months, there was a sharp increase in the patient's activities and interests. For the first time in the 25 months of hospitalization he began to use the hospital facilities. He did some oil paintings which were later entered in the hospital art exhibit. He began using the hospital swimming pool in an attempt to "get back into the physical shape I was in before I got sick." On the ward he assumed a supervisory role with other patients. After learning of a planned panty raid, he admonished the male adolescents in words that might have been used by the administrator:

> This is a mental hospital, not a college. Some of those female patients might get pretty upset if a lot of boys came dashing into their dorm in the middle of the night. And besides the staff, especially Dr. L. would take this very seriously and probably transfer you out. So you had better think about it twice.

The school year was coming to a successful conclusion. After school he began to socialize with the boys in his class; and his interest in girls was reactivated when he met a nursing student during one of his visits home. He spent several hours talking with her, found he enjoyed her company, and was pleased that she accepted his invitation for a date. Turning his attention to vocational plans, the patient found a job where he could work part time after high school and then full time during the summer. He considered entering college in the fall. On his twentieth birthday he commented, "I feel like Rip Van Winkle waking up after 20 years."

A subsequent visit home proved highly successful, especially in the interaction between patient and father. For the first time in the patient's memory they sat together and talked. Father brought out his college books and shared some of his college experiences. In the next therapy session the patient discussed for the first time his positive feelings toward his father:

> You know, my father isn't as unimaginative as I always thought. He seems more interested in things and really has some good ideas. Maybe he feels I'm worth talking to now. My father had many things for me to do when I went home and he stayed around and supervised. And he seems interested in my going to school and what I'm doing now . . . . The only problem is my mother. She still thinks I'd be happiest at home. I told her I wasn't the same person I used to be. She said when I straightened out I would be. She still doesn't know I never was in very good condition; that I was such a mess inside and all tied up in knots.

Psychological testing was repeated in the twenty-seventh month of hospitalization, 12 months after the previous testing. The clinical changes noted during the 12 months of the therapist-administrator work were corroborated by the testing which is summarized below:

> The patient has made impressive gains in ego strength during the past year. There was a marked improvement in the ego's ability to deal with libidinal material, better reality testing, notable evidence of a stronger observing ego, better impulse control and more effective use of intellectual defenses . . . . At the expense of this ego improvement, certain problems still remain. There is still a moving away from people. The patient clings to a position of moral superiority which keeps him estranged from others . . . . The patient has made strides in establishing an appropriate sexual identification. He shows a definite healthy phallic striving, though there are still strong feelings of weakness and inadequacy . . . . The test indicates that definite changes have occurred in the psychic structure. The "as if" type facade formerly seen has been integrated into his personality.

Eighteen-month follow-up

After the 27 months of hospitalization reported above, the administrator, upon completion of his training, terminated with the patient. This separation led to an upsurge of libidinal material in therapy which lasted for several weeks. Three months later the patient was discharged from the hospital. As an outpatient, he continued to see the nurse-therapist. Eighteen months after the completion of the therapist-administrator work (15 months after discharge from the hospital and 12 months after termination with the therapist) the patient was sharing an apartment with a roommate, had several healthy male friends, and was dating frequently. He visited his parents and found these trips rewarding. After he was discharged from the hospital, the patient abruptly decided not to attend college but continued with the job he had begun while still a patient — working as an orderly at a general hospital one block away from the psychiatric hospital. During the 18 months after the completion of the therapist-administrator work, the patient took no psychiatric medication, and there was no recurrence of depressive, psychotic, or antisocial symptoms.

DISCUSSION During the first 15 months of therapy, several trends became evident. The patient was more able to trust and be dependent on people; he was less insistent that all humans be excluded from his life; he could better cope with his feelings of desperation and hopelessness. It could be said that oral issues were negotiated. It was not until 6 months of therapy had elapsed before any of these changes became evident. At this time, when the patient acknowledged his positive feelings toward the nurse-therapist, he began to act excited, frightened, and angry. This reaction was seen both as a result of anxiety over his hostility to one so close with the subsequent threat of dissolution of ego boundaries[2] and also as a response to the sexual excitement he was experiencing toward an incestual object. The oedipal drama was to begin. The patient now sought out the male therapist to challenge his authority on one hand and to seek control and support from him on the other. During this phase of treatment (the seventh through the fifteenth month), the patient, an expert at promoting family discord, paralyzed the staff's attempts to manage his behavior by rendering the male figure impotent in the limit-setting tasks. This behavior was an acting out of the oedipal situation in which the patient was permitted to have mother through father's ineffectualness. In the interview material he demonstrated how he played a significant role in provoking parental fights in which father would invariably lose.

The final 12 months of therapy began with a new administrative arrangement in which there was a nurse as therapist and a psychiatrist as administrator. At first the patient tried to set these two therapeutic figures against each other. When this failed, he encouraged their working together in the service of controlling his behavior by leaking information to them about his delinquent behavior. As he became aware of the joint involvement of the therapist and administrator in his treatment, he became "jealous," "frustrated," "angry," and "sad." He reacted to these feelings by fasting, drinking mouth wash, refusing to attend school, and experiencing bizarre fantasies and dreams. Because of the school difficulties, the administrator began to tutor the patient in his school work. This sharing of interest preceded concrete signs of identification with the administrator, a dynamic shift that enabled the patient to tolerate his instinctual frustrations. Soon thereafter, a change in the quality of the patient's psychopathology was noted. He no longer experienced bizarre and gruesome fantasies, and he simultaneously reported typical oedipal dreams of animals chasing him.

It can be inferred from the patient's behavior that he was creating a series of crises in an attempt to recapitulate to the original oedipal situation. The clinical changes emerged from the resolution of these crises which demonstrated that:

> 1. He could not disrupt the relationship between therapist and administrator. (Mother and father cannot be separated; they talk together rather than fight.)

[2]F. Fromm-Reichman, "Basic Problems in the Psychotherapy of Schizophrenia," *Psychiatry,* **21** (1958), 1–6.

2. The administrator would hold firm, take him seriously, and help him with controls. (Father cannot be ignored or rendered passive and impotent; father will protect him from his feelings toward mother.)

3. The administrator could like him and want to give him something. (He can be acceptable to father and father to him.)

Changes in the patient's manifest behavior and fantasy life were consistent with the resolution of oedipal issues. In addition to phobic animal dreams, the patient began to dream of crime and punishment themes, and he simultaneously resolved never to lie or steal again. There were castration fantasies of the administrator holding the patient's hands behind his back. Fortification of the superego was occurring. Meanwhile, the administrator became a "third leg" as well as a "big prick" with the power to do anything. There were progressive signs of the patient's identifying with the male authority— wearing similar glasses, smoking cigars, becoming interested in chemistry, advising other patients against panty raids, and working in a hospital. While these changes progressed, minor crises and testing continued until the administrator unwittingly erred in his handling of the patient. After this episode the patient asked, "Now I can go ahead with my plans?" Only with a father who was approachable could identification and final resolution be a possibility. The crises ceased. The patient became dedicated to his school work; he obtained employment; he enjoyed female companionship, and he developed an appreciation for his father. Having renegotiated oedipal issues, the patient could make use of more mature defenses and employ them to cope with conflicts appropriate to his age.

The reactivation of oedipal issues is a natural consequence of the sexual maturation process in adolescence and is expressed in the relationship with the parent of the opposite sex. Its importance both in the normal development and in the pathology of adolescence is well established.[3] This reactivation of earlier conflicts has led Eisler[4] to comment that "Adolescence appears to afford the individual a second chance; it is a kind of lease permitting revision of the solutions found during latency which had been formed in direct reaction to the oedipal conflict."

These general considerations help explain the relative facility with which the therapeutic changes in the patient were effected. By dealing with particular issues during this stage of the patient's development, when the final oedipal resolution was still negotiable, the therapeutic impact was greatly enhanced.

It remains to be explained how changes in the patient's bizarre preoccupations and fantasies and faulty reality testing were effected, since this pathology (at least in adults) is not usually related to the oedipal conflict.

[3] I. M. Josselyn, "The Ego in Adolescence," *American Journal of Orthopsychiatry,* **24** (1954), 223–37; E. Jacobson, "Adolescent Moods and the Remodeling of Psychic Structure in Adolescence," *The Psychoanalytic Study of the Child,* **16** (1961), 164–84; and A. Freud, "Adolescence," *The Psychoanalytic Study of the Child,* **13** (1958), 255–78.

[4] K. R. Eissler, "Notes on Problems of Technique in the Psychoanalytic Treatment of Adolescents; With Some Remarks on Perversions," *Psychoanal,* **13** (1958), 223–54.

This phenomenon must again be understood in terms of the ego in adolescence. In reaction to any upset producing great anxiety, according to Anna Freud "impulses from all pregenital phases rise to the surface and defense mechanisms from all levels of crudity or complexity come into use. . . . Consequently, the pathological results—although identical in structure—are more varied and less stabilized than at other times of life."[5] Following Anna Freud's reasoning, we see that the adolescent upset will have the appearance of a psychosis when the increased powers of the id threaten the existence or integrity of the ego. This process appears to be the case in the patient described in this report. The therapeutic resolution fostered repression and strengthened the ego.

The course of treatment illustrated the way in which the joint work of the nurse-therapist and the psychiatrist-administrator facilitated the reawakening and resolution of oedipal issues. The separate functions of each of these therapeutic figures will be briefly considered in the context of current role models.

The therapeutic efforts of the nurse have been referred to as "nursing therapy."[6] Work in this field has consisted of intensive psychotherapy of severely regressed patients. Although nursing therapy closely resembles and has been influenced by psychoanalytically oriented psychotherapy, it also claims an independent line of evolution—the nursing care process. Nurse-therapists, as a result of the nursing tradition, can supply the needs of the severely regressed patient with facility. They can be parental and supportive, a real object supplying real needs.

The administrator traditionally relieves the therapist of decision making burdens which interfere with the freedom of therapist and patient.[7] Whether or not the opportunities of this arrangement outweigh the pitfalls is a subject of current debate. Cohen and Grimspoon[8] added a dimension to the role of administrator in the treatment of impulsive adolescents. Through his limit-setting function the administrator serves as an important object of identification for the patient. Although the administrator in the present case served both as a decision maker and as an object of identification, neither of these roles fully describes his function.

The model which best describes the interaction between therapist and administrator in the present case is that of dual therapy or multiple therapy. (Strictly speaking, *dual* or *multiple therapy* refers to two or more therapists who are present in the interview *simultaneously*.) In dual or multiple ther-

[5]A. Freud, "Adolescence," pp. 255–78.

[6]J. Mellow, "The Evolution of Nursing Therapy and Its Implication for Education." Unpublished doctoral dissertation, Boston University School of Education, 1965; and J. Mellow, "Nursing Therapy as a Treatment and Clinically Investigative Approach to Mental Illness," *Nursing Forum,* **3** (1966), 64–73.

[7]A. H. Stanton and M. S. Schwartz, *The Mental Hospital* (New York: Basic Books, Inc., 1954).

[8]R. E. Cohen and Lester Grinspoon, "Limit Setting as a Corrective Ego Experience," *Archives of General Psychiatry,* **8** (1963), 74–79.

apy, a treatment not infrequently described since 1950,[9] multiple transferences are established and dealt with. In this case, the patient's reaction to the two therapeutic figures was enhanced by the roles they assumed. The therapist was a nurse, a caring parental figure; the administrator held the power and assumed the authoritative role. In addition, the relative amounts of time spent by the nurse and administrator with the patient are not unlike the relative amounts of time a mother and father spend with a small child. Several of the advantages which have been attributed to dual therapy are useful in understanding the therapeutic process in the present case.

1. Multiple transferences can vividly and rapidly recreate family themes. One common theme is the oedipal situation.
2. Transference feelings are developed more quickly and can have more range and ease of abreaction.
3. When the therapeutic figures are of the opposite sex, each serves as chaperone in defending against both homosexual and heterosexual panic.
4. Because the patient can split his feelings and express them to both therapeutic figures, overwhelming hostility can be diffused.[10]

A major pitfall of dual therapy, intrastaff competition, was observed in the early phases of the hospitalization.

The collaborative therapeutic efforts of nurse and psychiatrist is of special interest in the current search for role definition among mental health workers. Not only nurses, but also psychologists and social workers have begun to take increasing therapeutic responsibility. In the hospital setting the psychiatrist will continue to assume medical responsibility. We feel then that further exploration of the therapeutic possibilities of these new treatment arrangements will be of value.

SUMMARY This chapter reported the course of the 27 months of psychiatric hospitalization and psychotherapy of a severely disturbed 18-year-old male. The focus is on the final 12 months of treatment during which time the major therapeutic figures were a nurse-therapist and a psychiatrist-administrator. It was illustrated how this variation of dual therapy served as a catalyst in the reawakening and resolution of oedipal issues. Changes in manifest behavior, fantasy life, and psychological testing, reflecting shifts in identification patterns, superego fortification, and ego integration traced the effects of the therapeutic process. It was suggested that the patient's being an adolescent explained both the fluidity of the ego as well as the importance of oedipal issues in therapy. The functions of the nurse-therapist and the psychiatrist-administrator were discussed in terms of current role models.

[9]M. L. Hayward, J. J. Peters, and J. E. Taylor, "Some Values of the Use of Multiple Therapists in the Treatment of the Psychoses," *Psychiatric Quarterly,* **26** (1952), 244–49; R. K. Greenbank, "Psychotherapy Using Two Therapists," *American Journal of Psychotherapy,* **18** (1964), 488–99; and J. Warkentin, N. L. Johnson, and C. A. Whitaker, "A Comparison of Individual and Multiple Psychotherapy," *Psychiatry,* **14** (1951), 415–18.

[10]Greenbank, "Psychotherapy Using Two Therapists," pp. 488–99.

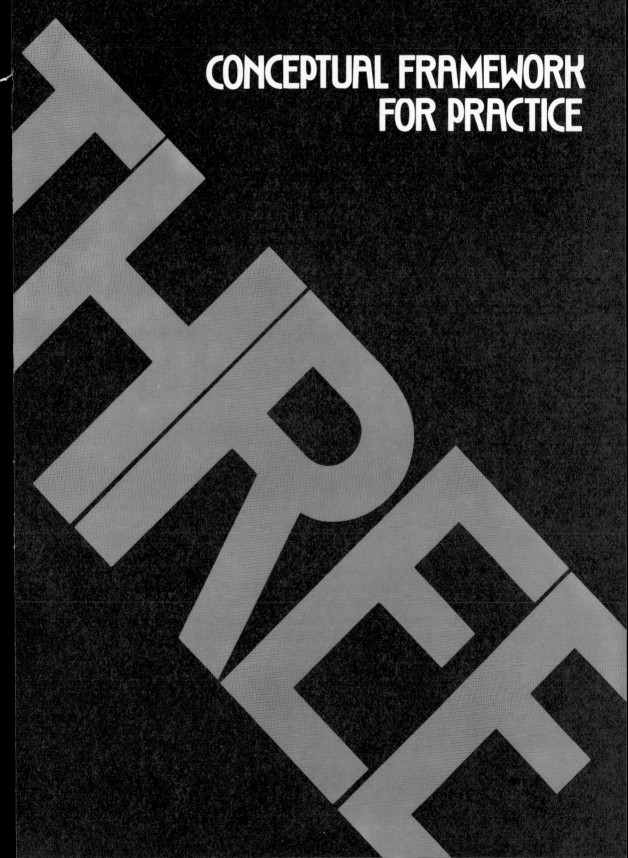

CONCEPTUAL FRAMEWORK FOR PRACTICE

THREE

An important step in nursing practice has been the development and acceptance of a framework for practice called the *nursing process*. Subsequent chapters deal with the basic approaches and concepts that are part of the nurse's inventory of resources in caring for a troubled human being. Standards of nursing practice are highlighted in the sections in which they are most applicable.

THE NURSING PROCESS

7

T he nursing process is the systematic ordering of cognitive steps that provide the basis for nursing practice. It is a method of careful perception and observation, critical thinking, and analysis which leads to a nursing plan for action with a client or patient. The steps forming the basis for the standards of psychiatric-mental health practice as described by the Congress for Nursing Practice include the assessment of the client's status, the plan of nursing actions, the implementation of the plan, and the evaluation. For optimal care, these sequential steps are used concurrently and recurrently in nursing practice. This chapter will describe the application of the nursing process as it is applied in psychiatric nursing.

ASSESSMENT The primary purpose of this step of the nursing process is to collect data on the mental health of the client in order to make a formulation of the health concerns and problems. The nurse uses such skills as observation, encouraging the patient to talk, listening, and keeping the interview focused on collecting essential data. This step is systematic and continuous.

Standard I of the *Standards of Psychiatric-Mental Health Practice* describes this step of assessment.[1]

Methods of Data Collecting

Data is collected from the patient, the family, the physician, the social network (which includes extended family, neighbors, and significant people), and from the health team who knows the patient. The format for collecting the necessary information on the person and his reason for seeking care may be made by the individual nurse or the admission team. Data may be obtained from a formal interview, informal observation, records, and talking with family and health team members.

[1]Congress for Nursing Practice, *Standards of Psychiatric-Mental Health Nursing Practice* (Kansas City, Mo.: American Nurses' Association, 1973), p. 3.

The individual nurse In many cases, the nurse is the most available staff member when a patient is admitted to an in-patient unit. At this time the assessment and plans for the initial care are made. In the community, a patient may present himself at a mental health clinic where the interview is the situation in which the nurse learns the nature of the patient's problem. Home visits by the community nurse often provide clinically rich data.

The admission team In some in-patient psychiatric settings or psychiatric out-patient settings, the initial assessment is performed by a clinical team consisting of nurse, physician, social worker, psychologist, psychiatric technicians, occupational therapists, and students. At the time the patient is admitted, a member of the admission team meets with the patient and family or whoever accompanies the patient to the clinic. In this way, the family is immediately involved in the treatment of the patient and is asked to share the responsibility for treatment.

Some of the goals of the admission team are to prepare the family to work with social service, to communicate the hospital's concern for family problems (financial, child-rearing), and to allow the patient to participate in these decisions. The team also presents precisely what the hospital can do. This action minimizes the fear to the patient, family, and staff that treatment

STANDARD I

DATA ARE COLLECTED THROUGH PERTINENT CLINICAL OBSERVATIONS BASED ON KNOWLEDGE OF THE ARTS AND SCIENCES, WITH PARTICULAR EMPHASIS UPON PSYCHOSOCIAL AND BIOPHYSICAL SCIENCES.

RATIONALE: Clinical observation is a prerequisite to realistic assessment of a client's needs and for the formulation of appropriate intervention. Observations can be facilitated through knowledge derived from a broad general education. In addition, scholarship acquired in the study of psychosocial and biophysical sciences fosters acuity of perception and alerts the nurse to psychologic, cultural, social, and other relevant clinical data.

Assessment Factors:
1. Data collecting activities involve observation, analysis, and interpretation of behavior patterns of clients which indicate a need for growth promoting relationships.
2. Data collecting activities involve identification of significant areas in which clinical data are needed.
3. Data collecting activities involve utilization of knowledge derived from appropriate sources to gain a comprehensive grasp of the client's experience.
4. Data collecting activities involve inferences drawn from observations which contribute to a formulation of therapeutic intervention.
5. Data collecting activities involve inferences and treatment observations which are shared and validated with appropriate others.

or hospitalization is forever or indefinite. Clearly stating the goals of the hospitalization and exploring rehabilitation after discharge present reality to the patient and family.

Other useful goals of the team conference are to evaluate the suicidal, destructive, or regressive potential of the patient and to determine to what extent the family can exercise control or to what extent the family is encouraging the behavior of the patient.

The patient and family usually are reassured by the hospital's being frank and open about hospitalization. If there is the nontherapeutic action of signing legal papers before the treatment begins or if the family is hustled away, the observation of important dynamics is avoided and the family, which could be used as an ally in the treatment, is alienated.

The convening of the treatment team sets the tone for the patient and staff and establishes the functional structures and roles of the unit. This places the nurse in a special relationship to the patient. It is especially useful when the patient, who may need extra support in a crisis, can turn with confidence to the nurse.

Once the admission conference is over, the nurse usually escorts the patient to the ward and introduces him to the other patients and staff members.

Basic Data

How the person comes for help How is the decision made for the person to come to the hospital or clinic? How does he finally come to the attention of a physician or nurse? People arriving for psychiatric care come by various ways. For example:

A 19-year-old boy arrived at the emergency room of a general hospital asking to be admitted to the psychiatric unit because he felt depressed and had suicidal thoughts. He had come to the hospital after asking the police for assistance. The police, believing that the young man might kill himself, drove him to the hospital. This person did not ask his parents to bring him, but he did not come alone. He felt the police would help. They did. The way in which this person came for help is the significant point: he sought out the police, an authority figure, a symbol of limit setting, perhaps even a symbol of punishment.

A 16-year-old male arrived at the psychiatric unit of a general hospital on a stretcher. Although he was visibly agitated and shaking, he kept saying, "I'm all right." His parents were with him. He needed both physical assistance and his parents to come to the hospital. The way in which this patient came for help is the significant point: he sought out a community service, the ambulance service, and his parents to bring him to the hospital. For some reason, the parents were unable to manage their son themselves in order to bring him for help.

A 21-year-old woman arrived at a state hospital accompanied by her father, her boyfriend, and her parish priest. This young woman came for help with three males: one from her family network, one from her peer group, and one from a community group. The significant point is that this young woman sought out males rather than females, males with different roles and different symbolic meanings, when she was in distress and also included members from her total social network group.

A 72-year-old woman arrived at a mental health clinic and stated, "I have to talk with someone. I am so lonesome." This woman came for help by herself and her opening remark stated her need for human contact. The significant point is that this woman had no one else for support in her social network group.

The above examples show the various ways in which people come for mental health services. Sometimes people come independently, dependently, and interdependently for help. The people who accompany the person are significant clues to whom the person is able to seek out. All the data may be of significant diagnostic value.

The person's perception of the problem

When the person is asked why he came to the hospital or clinic, his first words often tell more about him than the several paragraphs that follow. For example, when the person says, "I am here because my father said I had to come," the person is saying that he is here because his problem was uncomfortable for his father, not because it was primarily distressful to himself.

As stated in the above example, many people have been *advised* or *convinced* that they should come to a hospital. The family physician, a psychiatrist, a community agency, such as the police, school, or court, may be responsible for advising the person to seek psychiatric help. The person may be relieved to be in the hospital; he may be indifferent; or he may be angry and resentful. Many acutely ill psychotic people are brought in who do not see the need for hospitalization. They say, "I don't need to be here. I'm not sick."

Other reasons for a person's being advised to seek help are: "It was more my wife's request than anything else." "I'm here to appease my family." "I'm here because my brother beat me and took me to the cop station and found tracks on my arms and took me to a doctor and the cops took me to this hospital."

A 16-year-old male is admitted because his behavior is a problem to his foster parents. His problems revolve around his being truant from school, feeling suppressed by his foster parents because of the friends he chooses and the outside activities in which he can participate. He had a bad experience with marijuana in which he misinterpreted a water tank for a flying saucer. He resents babysitting for his foster brothers and sisters and says that they do not mind him. He says, "I feel like killing them."

Some patients seek hospitalization because of a *control issue*. In the above example, the 16-year-old was expressing a need for controls, although this was not his reason for coming to the hospital: his foster parents brought him to the hospital because they felt unable to control him and were advised by the family physician to do so. When people who have difficulty controlling their thoughts, feelings, and actions are admitted to the psychiatric unit, they may say: "I lit a fire in the school trash can." "I felt there was something wrong with me. Mostly I had the feeling of wanting to kill myself." "I took an overdose of sleeping pills and my roommate found me."

Some people seek hospitalization because they are looking for *protection and comfort* in exchange for the noxious environment in which they are currently living. On admission these people may say: "I was afraid of my husband. Because my fear was so great, I wanted to be safe for the night." "I had to get away from the family bickering and my father's beating me. I couldn't stand it any longer. I was going out of my mind." "I need a rest physically and mentally and wanted to survive without sleeping pills at night."

Some people come to the hospital requesting help because they perceive the hospital as a place to obtain help for *psychiatric symptoms*. These people realize that they have psychic distress and will say: "I was depressed; running in circles and had to stop." "I felt sick and strange." "I think people are watching me." "I feel I am mentally ill."

Some people perceive having emotional difficulties, but they state their reasons for being in the hospital in terms of a *specific problem* to be solved. These people may say: "I have a drug problem." "I need help in talking to people." "I want to cut down on my medication and to determine the cause of my stomach ailment and headaches."

In summary, people may perceive the psychiatric unit as a place they have been advised to come, a place to help them with control, a place of protection and comfort, a place to come to receive help with psychic distress, or a place for an environmental change.

The family's perception of the problem

The way the family perceives the patient's problem may be either similar to or dissimilar to the way in which the person perceives his problem. For example, the father may say, "Susan is so depressed. She lies around all day and cries." This may be exactly how the patient describes her problem.

Or the family may say, "Joe is such a problem. He argues and fights with everyone and if he is going to do that and keep us all upset, we don't want him at home." This family perceives the patient's problem as unacceptable behavior to them. They want the hospital to take their son and make him not a problem at home.

The family may say, "Mary is so bad. She runs with a wild group and takes drugs." This family views the daughter's problem in moralistic terms.

The family may be divided on how they see a problem. The mother may say, "I cannot stand to even see my daughter. She told me she was a homosexual and I could never talk with her again." The father may say, "My daughter told me her problem and that she does not intend to change. That is her decision and what can I do about it? What she does in her personal life is not going to affect my talking with her as my daughter." If the goal is to repair any estrangements in the family structure, it will be necessary to work with the mother in the situation.

When there is a conflict either between how the family and patient view the problem or a conflict between parents or how each views the child's problem, it indicates a need for negotiating goals in order not to stall the therapeutic process. The following example illustrates the patient's perception, the family's perception, and the formulated nursing care plan that resulted from a negotiation of goals.

A 17-year-old young man presents with the complaint, "my thoughts are all screwed up and I don't know what to do." The admission followed an episode in which the young man was truant from school, later dropped out of school, and then ran away to a commune in a large city. He was brought to the hospital by members of the commune after he experienced a bad drug trip.

The conflict between the father and son was noted during the admission conference. When the social worker was discussing the hospital bill, the father said, "If my son becomes so incompetent that he cannot face the realities of life and speaks of suicide, who is going to miss him?" The father felt that the son had become a "vegetable" since being hospitalized. The father felt that the cause of the son's difficulty was an "act put on because he did not want to go to school or work." The mother said that the son always had a low tolerance for extended involvement in school, sports, or general activities.

The patient felt that his difficulties came from experimenting with drugs and this complicated his situation and intensified his feelings of disinterest and noninvolvement.

The father wanted the hospital to project how long the son would be hospitalized. He felt that the hospital was too expensive and wanted the son out. The son felt that the hospital was helping and wanted to stay.

The conflict between the father and son is obvious. The hospital staff formulated a patient care plan to focus on the social model of care. They met with the parents and son during the course of hospitalization. They helped the father with his feelings of anger and disappointment in the son who did not measure up to the ideal of the strong, independent, productive college graduate son he had wished for. The staff helped the patient with his feelings of anger and disappointment over his parents not measuring up to his idea of concerned, caring, and understanding parents. A compromise to the realities of each other's unique style was the goal of family therapy.

The person's goals and requests for treatment

It is important to ask people who come for mental health services how they hope that they might feel and behave and how they hope that the facility might help with these goals. The patient may never be satisfied until the goal(s) is accomplished. For example, a person's problem may have been medically defined as schizophrenia. The person might say, "I am here because of my husband." When you ask her what she thinks the hospital can do for her, she says, "You have to tell him to stop coming home and beating me because when he does, my hallucinations start up again." All the antipsychotic medicine will not change the situation because the husband keeps coming home and beating her. The goal would have to include healthier communication between husband and wife. Somehow, the husband would have to stop beating his wife in order for the hallucinations to cease.

When people are asked, "What do you want to accomplish while you are in treatment here?" they respond in a number of ways. Some responses are specific. For example, hospitalized patients have given the following responses.

School-related: "I want to get better so I can go back to school."

Work-related: "I need to be able to go home and go to work when I leave."

Social-related: "I want to be able to speak up in groups."

Family-related: "I want to get on the right track with my husband, cooperating with him and with each other, and to stop hurting myself and him."

"My husband and I have to get some marriage counseling and try to have a better marriage. If this does not work, I will have to cope with the situation the way it is."

Self-related: "I need to be as good as I was before I started taking drugs."

"I have to stop shaking, stammering, and having headaches."

"I have to get my memory back."

"I want to live normally without this driving need to wash."

"I need to be able to control my actions.'"

"I want to overcome my depression and understand why I am depressed and to deal with my problems accordingly."

"I want to be able to know what I am thinking about."

For treatment to be successful, it is important to have the patient's complete cooperation. In order to obtain cooperation, goals and requests must be elicited, acknowledged, and responded to. Many of the failures in psychiatry may be traced to the basic fact that the patient did not feel that he was psychiatrically ill, did not want treatment, and did not want help. The person preferred to stay the way he was.

The family's goal for treatment The assessment of patient and family goals is essential. It is important to ask the following questions: Are the goals for the patient and family different? If they are different, does this mean that goals are couched in interpersonal terms rather than in intrapsychic terms? Do they really want something different? Are they aware of this? Does the family want the patient to recover? If so, recover to what?

Some of these questions may not make sense until some histories are looked at, especially histories of alcoholics who have recovered from their addiction. For example, many times the wife who had complained bitterly during the course of the husband's long drinking history will leave or divorce the husband when he is in good health. For dynamic reasons, his being an alcoholic met some of her psychological needs and when he returned to health, he presented new and intolerable difficulties and demands.

It is important to assess the family members who are important to the patient. Who comes with the patient to the hospital and who visits the patient? Who is present and who is not and why? Are the missing people important to the goals for treatment? The following example shows that the mother and daughter at the admission conference feel angry toward the missing father:

An 18-year-old young woman presents at the psychiatric clinic accompanied by her mother. She states, "My father is not here because he cares more about his teaching and his students than he does about me."

Later in the interview it became apparent that the triad relationship of mother, father, and daughter was significant in the daughter's problem.

> The daughter stated that after an injury to her neck 19 months previously, she had not been the same since. The patient dropped out of school and was then tutored. She changed tutors because the first one "told me I was dumb and he never gave me a chance."
>
> After she dropped out of school, the patient's somatic symptoms appeared concerning her neck and stomach. The symptoms pointed to appendicitis, but she was "too uptight" to have surgery.
>
> Father doubts the daughter's somatic complaints. Mother and daughter blame father for poor communication. The daughter's relationship with mother is better, but she doubts mother's ability to deal with the father.
>
> The daughter is angry with the father and his treatment of the mother. She gets irritated with mother's "crumbling to father's wishes." She gets depressed and speaks of suicide.

The daughter is in conflict because she feels disappointed that the father does not show care or concern for either her or the mother and because she feels frustrated in her own attempts to feel secure, to be able to attend school, and to be able to develop her own friends. Because conflict immobilizes her, she can see no alternative except suicide. Patient, family, and hospital goals have to be well negotiated in order for therapeutic progress to be made.

Psychological Assessment

Assessment of emotional status, life-style and methods of coping, dynamic issue, and interaction patterns are key data to collect on the psychological assessment of the patient.

In the interview, the nurse should observe the verbal style of the person. Is the person verbal, quiet, guarded? Does the person spontaneously offer information or merely answer the questions being asked? Is the emotional style of the person controlled and masked or is the person able to express feelings? One must determine whether or not this observation is part of the emotional life-style of the person or is caused by the stress being experienced by the interview or the emotional situation? What are the interaction patterns? Who does the person seek out when troubled? Who is important to the person?

The dynamic issue Part of the psychological assessment is the determination of the precipitating cause or event that led to the patient's hospitalization or request for help. By listening for the "last straw," one can assess the critical dynamic issue that is problematic to the person. The issue or reason is called dynamic because there is meaning in why it has occurred.

There is a psychodynamic issue to every situation. For example, did the "last straw" present a threat of a loss of love or of a loss of people giving to the person in an emotional way? Or is the person one who needs to feel good but now feels that he is a bad person? Or is the person one who needs to feel in control but now feels out of control? Or is the person one who needs to win and now feels that he is going to lose? Or is the person one who needs to be admired but no longer feels that anyone admires her?

The same precipitating event for two patients could have two different meanings. For example, a person dies. To one patient this means the loss of someone who cared and gave him something he needed. To another patient it means that because he had been so angry at the person he has contributed to that person's death and now the patient feels that he is a bad person. He may feel that he could have done more to prevent the death.

The dynamic issues may be viewed as follows:

To be cared about, loved, and protected. People who have strong needs for security, acceptance, and protection are prone to develop psychiatric symptoms when threats to these needs occur.

A person who has these needs predominating may become ill because of the loss of someone who provided them. The person may not return to normal health until the sources for succor are reestablished. These needs are often referred to as the *external supplies of life*. For example, it often happens that the death of one mate leads to the death of the surviving mate within a short period of time. This is more frequently the case in elderly couples. It is felt that the emotional needs met by each mate are so great that no one else could substitute for the surviving mate.

An example of this dynamic issue is a 45-year-old single teacher from the East Coast who moved to the West Coast to accept an excellent teaching position. Her move required that she leave her mother with whom she had lived all her life. This was a very difficult decision to make. Shortly after assuming her new role, she became severely depressed. She required hospitalization and electroconvulsive therapy before she was able to return to her community and her work. The loss of her mother's caring, coupled with a strange and unfamiliar environment, placed too great a strain on her emotionally. Until she was able to adjust to the new location, the new people, and the new interests, she needed support and succor from the hospital milieu and staff.

Patients suffering from schizophrenia are known to have reacted unfavorably to situations in which genuine caring and succor were lacking. When they are unable to take it upon themselves to find the replacement, someone else must provide this model of care. For example, a bright 18-year-old male student who managed to achieve well academically in his small hometown high school becomes disorganized and lost under the pressures of the large and impersonal university in which competition is high. The student was fifth in his high school class of fifty, but now he must compete in college with the best graduates from all high schools. The pressure increases his feelings of inadequacy and social failure and he becomes ill over the issue of needed security, comfort, and protection.

The resolution of this issue calls for returning the person to a situation in which he can depend on a caring person.

To be in control, to be good. People who place a high value on being good, conscientious, and in control may become symptomatic when there is a threat of the possibility of their being wrong or bad. Sometimes the "bad" is only in the form of thoughts or wishes, but even this is intolerable for them. For example:

> A 39-year-old woman became severely depressed after the birth of her fifth child. The baby was a great strain emotionally, physically, and financially. Although she said she was happy to have the baby, her inner thoughts were saying she wished she did not have the baby. She felt guilty because of these thoughts and became depressed.

Psychological assessment of this issue implies providing a model of care aimed at helping the person feel more secure in being a responsible and conscientious woman.

The therapeutic task is to help her bear the painful feeling over which she feels guilty. The exploration of her thoughts and feelings is an attempt to free the "bad" thoughts. If she is encouraged to talk, she may be able to see the reality of the ambivalent feelings that mothers have from time to time toward their children. By listening, the nurse shows that she is not afraid to hear these thoughts and feelings. The human element is stressed with this mother so that she may understand the ideal and the real. No one can be good and perfect all the time. The mother has to make peace within herself about her ambivalent feelings.

Another example of this dynamic issue is a 23-year-old single female who is admitted for attempted suicide. When she is asked, "What do you hope to accomplish while you are here?" the patient responds, "To get better and be a good person again." The issue of being good and not bad is significant in planning treatment to help her to see her suicidal behavior in realistic terms rather than just in moralistic terms. People whose dynamic issue is to be in control tend to be logical and orderly in their approach to problems. They are conscientious and punctual. When there is a threat to the loss of control over their bodies or their abilities to function effectively, they may develop psychiatric symptoms.

To be strong, secure, and to achieve. The need for achievement and to be strong and secure is the important issue. People become upset when they are in situations in which they feel weak and insecure. For example, victims of rape whose dynamic issue is to be strong become upset when they believe they were not aggressive or strong enough to avert the rape. A victim with this dynamic issue would not talk to a nurse about her concerns as to whether people were helpful to her after the rape (as with the dynamic issue of being protected and loved) nor about feeling bad in a moral sense (as the dynamic issue of to be good and in control) but instead would discuss feeling defeated and powerless.[2]

[2]A. W. Burgess and L. L. Holmstrom, *Rape: Victims of Crisis* (Bowie, Md.: Robert J. Brady Co., 1974), p. 231.

Defense mechanisms In the assessment picture, it is helpful to identify the psychological defense that a person uses in coping with the environment. People use defenses chronically (over a long period of time) and acutely (specific to the crisis).

Ego defenses are related to the assessment of the dynamic issue. People locked in psychological struggles or fights are concerned with the issue of not giving in and having autonomy. These people use the defense mechanisms with the compulsive phase of psychological development such as doing and undoing. For example, the person will say, "I can't stand Joe. He is just terrible and he steps all over people, but then he is nice to his family. Yet, on the other hand, he yells at all his friends." The person initially takes a stand, later behavior changes this stand.

Some symptoms indicate a way of dealing with difficult feelings and defending against those feelings. For example, conversion symptoms represent physical ways of dealing with feelings. A patient who says she cannot walk and falls down every time she tries may have a conversion symptom if an organic basis causing the symptom cannot be found. Walking may symbolically represent moving out of a situation, for example, a pending divorce that she had tried to deny for years.

Strengths of the person What does the patient have to ally himself with in the treatment process? If the nurse assumes that there is some kind of alliance to be made, then the therapeutic task is to be allied, as the therapeutic person, with these strengths in order to obtain the patient's full cooperation. Essentially, the nurse emphasizes the patient's strengths in order to maximize the therapeutic process. This action helps to avoid infantalizing the patient or doing for him what he can do for himself.

When it is ascertained from the patient's history that he does have a certain amount of strength, this should give confidence that, no matter what the regressions are, the prognosis can be good. By the same token, if the patient has a minimal number of strengths, the nurse cannot necessarily expect great advances.

Strengths are assessed by looking at how successful the person has been in his life. How has he done in academic situations, family situations, work situations, recreational situations? How does he relate to other people on the unit? Assertive and outgoing behavior is consistent with strength.

It is essential for the nurse to find the aspect of the person's personality that joins the nurse in the therapeutic alliance. It is this healthy aspect with which one can make important therapeutic progress.

Social Assessment

The assessment of social factors includes some knowledge of the person's cultural, religious, and socioeconomic background. These data may be learned from the direct interview with the person or family and from the patient's history of education and employment.

The assessment of the person's social network provides important information on the people with whom the person is involved: his family, his peers, his community.

It is important for the nurse to observe who comes to visit the patient and what the visiting style is. Some families visit the patient singly; other families gather the entire clan for the visit. Often cultural mores determine visiting customs. Friends, peers, or community people may visit only when the family is not there or they may prefer to come in their own group.

It is important to assess the patient's mood and his reaction to visitors before, during, and after the visit. Occasionally, it may be observed that the visits are so upsetting to the patient that visits must be limited or possibly restricted to certain people. The nurse usually can determine this and may set limits on visitors.

The nurse should observe how the visitors physically act when they are with the patient, for this can indicate the patient's position in the group. Is there physical contact, for example, shaking hands, kissing, or embracing when they meet or end the visit.

> During one admission conference, the 17-year-old daughter being admitted sat right next to the mother. The daughter cried and held the mother's hand during the entire conference.
>
> A 20-year-old college sophomore presents in an extremely agitated and confused state at a general hospital emergency ward. He keeps saying, "They will kill me if you leave." The father made arrangements to stay all night with the son. The mother, after her son's admission to the psychiatric unit, was observed sitting next to her son's bed, cradling his head in her lap, stroking his head, and saying, "Everything will be all right."

These examples show the patients' extreme dependence on parental figures. The issue of succor or needing to be cared about will undoubtedly come up in the nursing care plans. In these particular examples, healthier ways of dealing with dependent needs would be recommended and implemented.

In the general hospital, patients can put great demands on family members and often make them feel guilty. An example is an 80-year-old woman hospitalized with pneumonia. She holds her son's hand as he prepares to leave at the end of visiting hours and says, "Please don't leave me. I get so lonely at night and the nurses don't pay any attention to me at night."

The nurse's observations of these situations can be most helpful. The patient makes increasing demands on the visitor and plays upon his guilt feelings in order to make him stay. The nurse can say to both family and patient, "It is time for the visit to end. I want to prepare Mrs. Smith for the evening and it is important for you to be home with your own family." The nurse should then talk with family members to ensure that they have the opportunity to express their feelings about how they feel the hospitalization is progressing.

Another important observation point is where and how visitors sit in relation to the patient. Does the patient sit alone? Is there any ally in the group? Is there an alliance against the patient? The nurse should observe how the patient is shut out of conversations by a domineering person.

What are the communication styles within the family? Every family has its own special rules, channels, and styles of communication. Various family constellations form the family structure. In the sibling world, which brothers and sisters form an alliance? In the parent-child world, which child or children do the parents favor or differentiate between? In the grand-parents-child world, which child do the grandparents single out? In the aunt-uncle world, which niece or nephew do they single out?

Which members of the family talk to whom and when? Often, communication between patient and family is neither very distinct nor clear, and it can be easily identified as a problem during the admission process. For example:

> An 18-year-old female is brought to the clinic by her father who says, "I can't communicate with her at all. I'm not easy to get along with myself, let alone talk with her." The stepmother says, "I don't understand the girl either. Ever since she has been on drugs I know less what to talk to her about."

The father expressed his guilt about not being more involved with her, but since his remarriage his interest in his daughter's activities has markedly declined. The history shows that the parents were divorced when the patient was 9 years old and that she lived with her mother until her mother remarried. She then lived with various relatives until she became pregnant at age 16 at which time she went to live at the home for unwed mothers. After her daughter was born, she lived with the baby in an apartment and supported herself on money received from Aid to Dependent Children. She has been on drugs for the past year, receiving LSD, marijuana, speed, and mescaline from three "Hells Angels" men in the next apartment. She made three suicide attempts in the last year primarily because someone had rejected her. Her main symptom developed when she felt that the "neighbors were trying to get her." She then became frightened and called her father.

Much of this patient's difficulty centers around her feeling rejected—that no one cares. There is reality in both feelings because no one directly shows that he cares. She has no direct communication with anyone who is important to her. One of the main goals of hospitalization is to strengthen and repair ties with family and important people so that they can provide care and the succor that she vitally needs in order to stay alive.

It is very helpful to be able to observe and have the patient and family talk about the patient's illness and hospitalization. If there is an opportunity to view this, the nurse should try to assess the answers to the following questions: What is the affective response when the patient describes her illness? At the same time, what is the response of the family? Is there evidence of blame and responsibility? What does the patient expect of the family and vice versa? Who is doing what to whom? Who is trying to accomplish what? Who has disappointed whom? Is there something specific that the patient wants from the family or the family from the patient before the patient can progress?

Behavioral Assessment

The behavioral model views mental health problems or distress as unacceptable or noneffective behavior, as behavior learned in a maladaptive way. For example, overweight people who are unable to control their eating patterns would have "learned" noneffective behavior in maintaining average weight. Similarly, smoking and drinking behavior may be classified as maladaptive behavior patterns.

In assessing maladaptive behavior patterns, the nurse looks for the problem behavior and then identifies the antecedent and the reinforcing event. For example, one 45-year-old man only started on a drinking episode after a failure in his work situation or after an interpersonal rejection. While the patient was hospitalized for depression he was helped to see the relationship between the failure, his need to drink, and the resulting behavior.

If the patient is observed in the clinical setting, the nature of the patient's relationships with other patients in the hospital can be assessed. The nurse should seek answers to the following questions: Does the patient engage with people or does he withdraw? With which sex does he relate most freely? Are the relationships on a give-and-take basis? Or are they domineering or being dominated relationships? Are they taking care of or are they being cared for, hurting or being hurt, manipulating or being manipulated, destroying or being destroyed?

Medical Assessment

The psychiatric nurse must always maintain an awareness of the patient's medical needs. It is especially helpful to note any changes in the following biophysical status of the patient:

NEUROSENSORY SYSTEM: vision, hearing, speech, touch, taste, state of consciousness.

CIRCULATORY SYSTEM: skin color, palpitations.

RESPIRATORY SYSTEM: Breathing, cough, chest pain.

GASTROINTESTINAL SYSTEM: appetite, bowel habits.

GENITOURINARY SYSTEM: urinary and sexual functioning.

The above observations may be exceedingly important in a variety of situations:

1. Physical illness such as thyrotocese or brain tumor may mimic psychiatric illness.
2. Physical illness may preclude the use of certain psychiatric medications.
3. Physical illness (symptoms) may result from the withdrawal of many medications including alcohol, barbiturates, and many tranquilizers.
4. Physical symptoms may result from untoward effects of psychiatric medications.

In the above situations, the nurse's observations may be lifesaving.

Case Formulation

The final step in the assessment process is to pull together all the data collected and to make a statement on how the data fit together. This statement, or case formulation, is a bio-psycho-social-behavioral summary of patient problems. The following summary statement is one example:

> This is a 60-year-old woman with depressive symptoms with no acute physical problems who is socially isolated, whose depressive behavior seems to be rewarded by staff, and who possesses good ego strength evidenced by considerable accomplishments by pre-hospital adjustments.

Nursing diagnosis

The term *nursing diagnosis* has been in the nursing literature since 1963.[3] However, it was not until October, 1973, that the First National Conference on the Classification of Nursing Diagnoses was held. At this conference the first tentative list of nursing diagnoses was developed and the pledge was made for nurses to continue to participate in its refinement and expansion.[4]

The data we have been talking about will ultimately be used as nursing diagnoses as nursing develops its standard nomenclature. Meanwhile, however, while the diagnostic categories are being standardized, in this text the term *nursing diagnosis* refers to the statement of the patient's mental health or psychiatric problem.

Stages of Care Plans

PLANNING   Care plans may be divided into three phases: the preliminary initial care plan, the total assessment care plan, and the revised care plan.

Preliminary initial care plan   In this phase, a care plan is made to include the essential nursing interventions while the full assessment is being completed. Very often various members of the team contribute data to this plan. For example, nursing students who have a limited clinical time might contribute data from one nursing assessment area. This data would be included in either the total assessment (initial) plan or in the revised nursing plan.

Total assessment care plan   This plan includes the total assessment described in the beginning section of this chapter. Understandably, it may take several days to complete, depending on the nature of the patient's impulse control or mental status.

Two steps are generally needed to develop this care plan: The first step is to review all data from patient, family, social network, and health team. This includes the basic identifying data of patient requests and goals and the bio-social-psycho-behavioral assessment. The second step is to plan and implement the direct services that can be provided immediately to the maladaptive behavior.

[3]Nori I. Komorita, "Nursing Diagnoses," *American Journal of Nursing,* **63,** No. 12 (1963), 83–86.

[4]Kristine Gebbie and Mary Ann Levin, "Classifying Nursing Diagnoses," *American Journal of Nursing,* **74,** No. 2 (1974), 250–53.

STANDARD III

THE PROBLEM-SOLVING APPROACH IS UTILIZED IN DEVELOPING NURSING CARE PLANS.

RATIONALE: A nursing diagnosis is based on pertinent theories of human behavior. It is used to plan therapeutic intervention taking into consideration the characteristics and capacities of the individual and his environment in order to maximize the treatment program for the client.

Assessment Factors:
1. The individual's reaction to the environment is observed and assessed.
2. Themes and patterns of the behavior are observed and assessed.
3. Nursing care plans are used as a guide to nursing intervention.
4. Nursing care plans are interpreted to professional and nonprofessional persons giving care.
5. Observations and reports of others are incorporated in the nursing care plans.
6. Nursing care plans are designed, implemented and reviewed systematically by the nursing staff.[5]

The following case illustrates an initial care plan. The patient did not wish to be hospitalized which involved further negotiations. However, this care plan shows how the nurses assessed the patient and stated direct interventions.

Sean, a 25-year-old dark haired, neatly dressed young man was accompanied to the psychiatric unit by his mother and uncle. The mother was first to respond to the question asked by the admission team, "What brings you here to the hospital?" She was nervous, agitated, and on the verge of tears. She constantly asked how she could handle Sean, reassuring staff that she cared for him, but reiterating his need for financial independence from her because she could not support him any longer. She insisted on showing the staff her take-home check of $65.00. She also stated she wanted to move to a one-room apartment closer to her work.

She stated the difficulty as, "This is the son of my second marriage. He has been bothering the neighbors during the day when I am at work because he does not want to be alone. He comes in my room at night because he does not want to be alone and I can't get any sleep. The neighbors have threatened to have us evicted because of the trouble Sean makes. He refuses to eat the food I cook, but goes out and buys his own."

Sean was asked how he saw the difficulty. He said, "I have trouble sustaining myself physically, breathing and eating. Have felt this way for several months. Haven't been able to work this whole past year." The conversation after this point became confusing and difficult to follow.

The uncle then volunteered the following information:

[5]Congress for Nursing Practice, *Standards of Psychiatric-Mental Health Nursing Practice* (Kansas City, Mo.: American Nurses' Association, 1973), p. 3.

"One month ago, the half brother Ed (by the mother's first marriage) also moved in. He ridiculed Sean for not working. He also opposes this hospitalization. My sister can't deal with Ed and he came to live with us last week. Sean's father left the family 15 months ago for another woman. Both my sister and nephew say this didn't matter to them at all."

The following highlights of past history were obtained from the answers to the question of what had gone well for Sean. Sean was active in high-school sports and dated occasionally. He worked after high school until he had enough money for college. He lived in his own apartment while working. He earned a scholarship to a well-known college and went there for one year. He made dean's list that year. Sean said that he felt inferior socially and financially. He went to a clinic for this once, but he did not return for further appointments.

The observations of communication and support between the family and Sean were felt to be minimal during the admission conference. The mother said she wanted to help Sean. There was little verbal communication between mother and son.

The attitude toward hospitalization was seen with the mother hoping that the hospital would cure Sean. Sean, however, could not accept that he was at the hospital for psychiatric help. He refused to sign a voluntary paper.

The following table shows the nursing assessment and initial patient care plan formulated for immediate care:

Nursing Assessment	Initial Patient Care Plan
1. How the patient comes for help: (What brings you to the hospital?) Accompanied by mother and uncle.	1. Encourage patient to talk about his family. (What does your family say to you or talk to you about?)
2. The patient's perception of the problem: "I have trouble sustaining myself physically, breathing and eating."	2. Be supportive: "It must be uncomfortable for you to be here. I am here to help you and to talk with you about being here."
3. The family's perception of the problem: "He can't be handled; he won't sleep or eat alone."	3. Social service to see mother during patient's hospitalization to work on separation issue between herself and son; arrangements made and patient told of this service. "A social worker will be talking with your family about future plans."
4. The patient's request for treatment: Could not see the hospital helping him and would not sign voluntary paper.	4. Negotiate subgoals: what the patient wishes for himself and the importance of signing the paper so that hospitalization is goal directed. "What do you wish the hospital to do for you?"
5. The family's request for treatment: "Make him financially independent from mother."	5. Begin working on Halfway House referral when discharge becomes a reality. Nurse in contact with team members.

6. Psychological assessment:
   Dynamic issue: to be cared
   about. Defenses: denial.

6. Structure day's activities to provide
   security and consistency through
   establishment of the nurse-patient
   relationship. "I'd like to talk with you
   for 30 minutes twice a week about
   your progress in the hospital."

7. Social assessment:
   Patient is involved with the
   family.

7. Occupational therapy for one-to-one
   activity; interactions with male
   psychiatric counselors. "Lets spend
   some time in the OT room and
   decide on an activity to do."

8. Medical assessment:
   Feels weak, not eating,
   trouble breathing.

8. Physician prescribes phenothiazines.
   Nurse assesses symptom reaction to
   medication. Nurse with him at mealtime. "Be sure to tell me how the
   medicine makes you feel."

9. Behavioral assessment:
   Makes trouble; the
   neighbors complain.

9. Ignore behavior that disturbs other
   patients on the unit and reward
   behavior that is constructive. "Can
   we talk about what you feel prior to
   your behavior which makes people
   complain? Let's try some alternatives."

10. Strengths of the person:
    Interest in sports; work record;
    earned scholarship; attended
    college one year.

10. Rehabilitation for vocational testing
    and/or job placement. Include patient
    in sports activities of the ward.
    Encourage patient to talk of college
    experience and academic plans.

The Revised Care Plan   The revised care plan develops over time as new data emerge in the identification of further issues. Two steps are necessary to update the conceptualization of patients' distress. First, review the immediate care plan and evaluate how the plan is working. Second, as new issues arise, make them part of the care plan revision.

IMPLEMENTA-TION   The implementation of the nursing care plan refers to nursing intervention or nursing management, the aim of which is to restore bio-social-psycho-equilibrium.

Before the plan is implemented, however, the nurse should try to come to an agreement through negotiating with the patient on the treatment goals and on the means for achieving these goals. If an agreement cannot be reached, perhaps an open discussion will lead to the nurse's educating, and being educated by, the patient, thus leading to a stronger therapeutic alliance. This interaction is called the *clinical negotiation*. It depends upon the nurse's eliciting the request, a task requiring persistence and compassion.[6]

The implementation of the nursing plan is always very different for each patient, depending on the problem behaviors, social matrix, psychological functioning, the syndrome, and the medical situation.

[6]See Chapter 22.

Standard IX further delineates the importance of nursing interventions as psychotherapeutic steps.[7]

STANDARD IX

PSYCHOTHERAPEUTIC INTERVENTIONS ARE USED TO ASSIST CLIENTS TO ACHIEVE THEIR MAXIMUM DEVELOPMENT.

RATIONALE: People with mental health problems fashion many of their patterns of living and relating to others on a psychopathologic basis. In order to help clients achieve better adaptation and improved health, a nurse assists them to identify that which is useful and that which is not useful in their modes of living and relating. Alternatives available to them are identified.

Assessment Factors:

1. Useful patterns and themes in the client's interactions with others are re-enforced.
2. Clients are assisted to identify, test out, and evaluate more constructive alternatives to unsatisfactory patterns of living.
3. Principles of communication, problem solving, interviewing, and crisis intervention are employed in carrying through psychotherapeutic intervention.
4. Knowledge of psychopathology and its healthy adaptive counterparts are used in planning and implementing programs of care.
5. Limits are set on behavior that is destructive to self or others, with the ultimate goal of assisting clients to develop their own internal controls and more constructive ways of dealing with feelings.
6. Crises intervention is used to reduce panic of disturbed patients.
7. Long-term psychotherapeutic relationships with clients are undertaken.
8. Colleagues are utilized in evaluating the progress of the psychotherapeutic relationships and in formulating modification of intervention techniques.
9. Nursing participation in the therapeutic relationship is evaluated and modified as necessary.

The discussion of the clinical syndromes in Part Four will include detailed discussion of the nursing intervention for the various situations.

EVALUATION Once the plan for care has been formulated and implemented, there is a need for constant evaluation of the results. These results must be examined in relation to the patient's requests and goals, the family's requests and goals, and the nurse's judgment of sound clinical objectives. Failure to meet reasonable objectives should lead to a reassessment of the data, a reformulation of a care plan, and new methods of implementation.

Standard II of the *Standards of Psychiatric-Mental Health Practice* is

[7]Congress for Nursing Practice, *Standards of Psychiatric-Mental Health Nursing Practice* (Kansas City, Mo.: American Nurses' Association, 1973), p. 5.

cited as a summary for the evaluation step of the nursing process as it applies in psychiatric nursing.[8]

STANDARD II

CLIENTS ARE INVOLVED IN THE ASSESSMENT, PLANNING, IMPLEMENTATION AND EVALUATION OF THEIR NURSING CARE PROGRAM TO THE FULLEST EXTENT OF THEIR CAPABILITIES.

RATIONALE: To a very large degree, the therapeutic process is a learning process. The same principle that applies to learning also applies to therapy; that is, the learner or client must be an active participant in the process. The ability to participate in such a process will vary from person to person and, at times, even within the same person. The word "therapy" is used here in its broadest sense; that is, any behavior or planned activity that promotes growth and well-being. Thus, "nursing care program" and "nursing therapy" are interchangeably used, although it is recognized that many other forms of therapy exist.

Assessment Factors:
1. Clients' capabilities to participate at any given time are assessed, always keeping in mind the ultimate goals mutually determined by the client and nurse.
2. Plans for achieving and re-examining the goals are developed with the client, making whatever readjustments are necessary to progress toward them.
3. Problems are identified in collaboration with the client to determine needs and to set goals.
4. Progress of clients toward mutual goal achievement is assessed.

SUMMARY This chapter discussed the nursing process in terms of the individual nurse assessing the patient or the admission team assessing the patient upon admission to a psychiatric unit.

The areas for assessment were described as: how the patient comes for help; the patient's perception of the problem; the family's perception of the problem; the patient's goal for treatment; the family's goal for treatment; the psychological assessment; defense mechanisms; the social assessment; relationships with the hospital setting; the medical assessment; and the strengths of the patient. The final step in the assessment process is to make a case formulation which includes the nursing diagnosis or statement of the patient's mental health problem.

Planning patient care is discussed and applied to a specific case. Implementation, negotiation and evaluation of the care plan completes the steps of the nursing process.

This chapter includes Standards I, III, IX, and II of *Psychiatric-Mental Health Nursing Practice.*

[8]Congress for Nursing Practice, *Standards of Psychiatric-Mental Health Nursing Practice* (Kansas City, Mo.: American Nurses' Association, 1973), p. 3.

REFERENCES AND SUGGESTED READINGS

Bower, Fay Louise (1972). *The Process of Planning Nursing Care.* St. Louis: The C. V. Mosby Co.

Holmstrom, Lynda Lytle, and Ann Wolbert Burgess (1975). "Developing Diagnostic Categories," *American Journal of Nursing,* **75,** No. 8., pp. 1288–91.

Kalkman, Marion E. (1968). "Recognizing Emotional Problems," *American Journal of Nursing,* **68,** 536–39.

Keegan, Lynn G. (1970). "Changes in Action," *Nursing Outlook,* **18,** No. 12, 42–43.

Komorita, Nori I. (1963). "Nursing Diagnosis," *American Journal of Nursing,* **63,** No. 12, 83–86.

Mundinger, Mary O'Neil, and Grace Dotterer Jauron (1975). "Developing a Nursing Diagnosis," *Nursing Outlook,* **23,** No. 2, 94–98.

Peterson, Linda W. (1967). "Operant Approach to Observation and Recording," *Nursing Outlook,* **15,** No. 3, 28–32.

Roy, Sister Callista (1975). "A Diagnostic Classification System for Nursing," *Nursing Outlook,* **23,** No. 2, 90–94.

Unangst, Carol (1971). "The Clinician's Use of Nursing Rounds," *American Journal of Nursing,* **71,** No. 8, 1566–67.

Wagner, Bernice (1969). "Care Plans: Right, Reasonable and Reachable," *American Journal of Nursing,* **69,** No. 5, 986–90.

TECHNIQUES IN THE THERAPEUTIC PROCESS

8

The primary goals of nursing include health promotion, health maintenance, health restoration, and health reorganization. Some nursing curriculums are designed to teach nursing as primary nursing intervention, secondary nursing intervention, and tertiary nursing intervention, depending on the person's state of health.

It may seem easier to teach or to learn the concepts and interventions for achieving these goals in general nursing situations, for example, in medical surgical areas. Yet, for the psychiatric patient or for the medical patient under emotional stress (a common situation), the nurse asks, "What can I do? What can I say? How do I help?"

The Congress for Nursing Practice has defined psychiatric nursing as "a specialized area of nursing practice employing theories of human behavior as its scientific aspect and purposeful use of self as its art."[1] This chapter will describe some general concepts of being therapeutic: therapeutic attitudes, as well as the human qualities required of the nurse, and specific therapeutic tasks.

Self-assessment

ATTITUDES AND HUMAN QUALITIES OF THE HELPER

Examining one's attitudes and style is a very personal affair for we are talking about our very self, our personality, and our unique identity. Self-assessing is, therefore, a difficult task. It involves being aware of the interpersonal assets and talents that the nurse brings to the situation. It further involves knowing what qualities and skills must be further developed within nurses in order for them to provide a more therapeutic interchange with patients.

From the very start it is essential to understand that this self-assessment process—the constant examination of feelings, attitudes, and actions—is a basic tool of psychiatric nursing. It is as basic and fundamental as the stethoscope is to the medical nurse.

[1]Congress for Nursing Practice, *Standards of Psychiatric-Mental Health Nursing Practice,* (Kansas City, Mo.: American Nurses' Association, 1973), p. 2.

For some it may be more difficult to examine one's attitudes than to analyze the expressions of one's feelings or to view one's behavior. Attitude is the statement of one's position or stand on an issue. Ideally, each new situation should be started with a completely open mind. But how often is that the case? Take, for example, the student's original attitude toward the psychiatric nursing course. Some students still have the attitude that psychiatry is the answer to the human dilemma, and others still have the attitude that psychiatry is the reason for our dilemma.

It is essential that the student adopt the position that when examining feelings, attitudes, and actions or having them examined by an instructor or classmates, it is not to be a blaming or a breast-beating process. The nurse who is angry out of all proportion to the situation is not to be blamed. There is something to be examined and understood. If a patient will not speak to a nurse, again there is something to be understood. Unless we adopt this attitude, we would be pretending that we are always loving, kind, and understanding in order to avoid criticism. Not only would this attitude be sheer pretense, but it would also be hard to tolerate or justify.

Being natural

Personality represents our unique identity. Those distinct personal character traits that distinguish us from every other human being establish us as an individual. During the years of personal growth, a stylistic pattern of communication and relating to people emerges as part of the behavioral style.

Many people pass through life only dimly aware of their behavioral style and how it affects others. Yet people are aware of the principle that everyone is different and unique. Literature abounds in material on personality and behavioral styles, and colleges are well catalogued with courses on personality development and psychology. Understanding the human phenomenon of the uniqueness of a person is one step in the self-assessment process. The importance of understanding and developing one's natural behavioral style is to facilitate feeling secure and being therapeutic in nursing situations.

Extracting the very best of humanness within oneself is to accent natural talents and to make use of one's special qualities.

Students should trust their natural behavioral style. Twenty years of living has taught interpersonal skills that others have perceived as therapeutic in the broadest sense. Unless one has absolutely no friends and all relatives completely avoid you, one does have natural talents.

Each of us has a natural style that in itself is so unique that it separates us from all other human beings. The student should ask: what are some of the characteristic and understanding ways that I have in dealing with people and what is it that people especially like about me and respond to?

Students should start out by simply being natural and then seeing how much of their everyday interaction is therapeutic. They will find many aspects of their style that are perfectly acceptable in a social situation but may be inappropriate in a professional setting. It is these particular aspects of style that will be important to critically examine. However, unless one starts by being natural, one may lose valuable traits such as charm, softness, and warmth in the attempt to be very "professional."

The professional style that a nurse finally adopts will be a special mixture of the natural self together with some traits of several instructors and colleagues whose style and manner "feels right" to her.

Professional comfort

To be therapeutic, nurses should be comfortable in their professional role. Professional comfort comes most naturally from experience. Unfortunately, the discomfort of the inexperienced student is hard to conceal. This is illustrated by two nursing students during their first day on a ward.

> The nursing student was in a four-bed unit carefully checking her patient's name from her assignment list when one of the patients said, "Hello, nurse." The student promptly said, "Just a minute, sir, and I will get you one."

> The same day, another nursing student was taking the blood pressure of her patient when the patient, not knowing the status of the student, said, "How long have you been in nursing?" The student anxiously looked at her watch and said, "Exactly 10 minutes."

It may be helpful for you to think back to the time you first talked with a patient and remember your own degree of "professional comfort."

Students should be fully aware of the importance of professional comfort in the therapeutic process. At the same time they must be patient with themselves, for it takes time to acquire the experience.

Respect

Respect for the other person is crucial in all human interaction. It is of particular importance in the therapy of psychiatric patients. The term *respect* is used in the sense of paying attention to, observing carefully, and appreciating the worth and dignity of another person. The nurse communicates respect by taking the person seriously, by being honest, by listening well, and by regarding the patient as a person instead of an object. Failing to do the above by giving false reassurance or by infantilizing the patient is equal to saying, "I ignore your strength, I do not take you seriously, I am not interested in you, and I do not respect you."

Psychiatric patients commonly suffer from lowered self-esteem or even experience feelings of self-hate as part of their illness. Medical-surgical patients may share similar feelings because of their "lying around" and not being able to do an "honest day's work." Being able to communicate respect to the patient is therefore a powerful therapeutic tool.

Optimism (every patient can be helped)

In order to be therapeutic, the nurse must believe that each patient can be helped. This may be hard to accept when a patient is seriously regressed, when he has been sick for a long time, or when he is grossly demanding and trying. Nevertheless, many regressed patients do make dramatic recoveries; patients who have been sick for a long time have been known to respond amazingly well, and demanding patients often become delightful when they recover.

Even in the most desperate of situations we must hold to our initial assumption that every human interaction has the potential for being therapeutic. Not everyone can be cured and not everyone can be rehabilitated, but some suffering can be relieved. The patient can be helped if he has hope; he can only sustain a feeling of hope if the helper communicates that feeling to him.

There are positive aspects to all people

Patients whom students like and find interesting will usually respond to treatment more rapidly than patients whom they dislike. If this is true, students may face the seemingly impossible task of learning to like or at least finding something positive about an unpleasant, unattractive, hostile, uncooperative, or withdrawn patient. How can this be done? First, students must acknowledge to themselves how much they dislike the patient. You try to determine what it is about the patient that bothers you: his withdrawal, his hostility, or perhaps his personal grooming. Then you try to understand what it is about yourself that is bothered: possibly feelings of helplessness or anxiety about failing. If necessary you should discuss your feelings with a classmate or instructor. At this point you may more calmly take another look at the patient. You should attempt to understand the aspects of the patients' behavior that you dislike. You will find meaning. If the patient is trying to push you away, you will undoubtedly find a good reason for it if you review his past history. If he is withdrawn, you must feel this behavior is doing something for him. If the student enters into the world of the patient, his behavior will have meaning. At the same time you will find a real suffering human being, struggling in the best way he knows to survive. Using this approach, students are likely to find something about the patient to respect.

Sensitivity

Being sensitive is becoming acutely aware of the subtle changes in thought, mood, or behavior in another person. It is a feeling or a hunch that something is not right. It is listening, looking, and feeling more carefully and more intently than does the nonprofessional. In a sense, it is having one's own radar.

For example, the nurse enters the patient's room and senses that something is wrong. The atmosphere in the room feels different to the nurse. Perhaps the patient is more reserved and thoughtful. Instead of saying, "Good morning. How are you this morning?", the nurse might enter the room and just say, "Good morning." After a pause, if the patient does not respond, she might say, "I have the feeling there is something on your mind." Using the human quality of sensitivity, the nurse is able to communicate to the patient that she knows something is on his mind and that she is interested in listening to him. Almost all patients in this situation will respond favorably.

In another situation:

> A patient group was gathering for an informal meeting and one patient remarked that Mary was missing. Other patients ignored the absence and the group started talking.

> The nurse attending the meeting felt something was not right about Mary's being missing. She went to the patient's room and saw that no one was there. Knocking on the bathroom door within the room brought Mary's response of "leave me alone." The nurse heard a cracking noise and tried the door handle, telling Mary she was doing this because she was concerned about her. The door was locked. The nurse asked Mary to open the door but no further talk was exchanged. The nurse then went to get the master key to unlock the door and when she did, she found Mary cutting her wrists with a piece of broken glass.

The nurse was paying attention to her own feelings of discomfort. This situation was picked up not only by the nurse but also by another patient who had first noticed Mary's absence at the group meeting. Because the nurse acted on her hunch that something was wrong, a problem situation was discovered that could be handled and resolved in time.

Involvement

One of the characteristics that distinguishes the nurse from other mental health professionals is the degree of involvement associated with patient care. The nurse has traditionally stood by the patient on a 24-hour basis through life threatening situations and through chronic suffering. By continuing with this tradition, psychiatric nurses make their own unique contribution in the treatment of mental illness.

Involvement often takes the form of direct action. Listening and understanding may not be enough.

> A nursing student was helping patients wash and dress for the day. Two teen-age girls started fighting over a bottle of shampoo. In the struggle for the bottle, it fell and shattered. One of the girls grabbed the broken bottle and disappeared into the bathroom, closing the door behind her. The nursing student opened the door in time to see the girl ingesting the contents of the bottle as well as the broken pieces of glass. The student forced the girl's mouth open and pulled out the pieces of broken glass.

After the incident was reported and the patient was examined for any remaining glass in her mouth, the patient was X-rayed for any ingested glass. The student's action was important to the therapeutic relationship with this particular patient as well as with the other patients who witnessed the event. The student was available at a critical time to intervene and resolve an upsetting situation with the patients. The emergency nature of the situation required immediate action. The nurse acted on the basis of her caring. She would not allow the patient to destroy herself. She involved herself by direct action in a way that instantly identified herself as a caring, protecting, significant therapeutic person. Discussing the incident immediately after it happened put the situation in perspective for all patients involved.

Caring

A 17-year-old high-school girl on her admission to a psychiatric unit raised some questions about caring:

> . . . walking down the street and I said "hello" to a face I know. But no reply came. Probably in a hurry. Nobody has time anymore. Went to the beach . . . . The sun dominated the sky; it has a way of making you feel wanted. . . . As I left, I called "goodby" to the sun, but it didn't answer. I know it has other places to shine on. Now even my footsteps leave no traces. As my "hello" to a face, and a "goodby" to the sun: Will I leave a trace? Will anybody care?

The patient is describing her sense of insignificance: the feeling that she does not matter and that nobody cares. Her feelings of isolation and alienation are felt.

The quality of caring, as a genuine human concern, is important in the therapeutic alliance made with the patient. The patient must be made aware of the nurse's caring and be convinced of the sincerity in order that definite progress may be made.

Feeling responsible for a person in terms of being involved with his well-being and by helping him to reach for mutually agreed upon goals is in reality caring for the patient. As the patient works with the nurse on goals for recovery, he will use the nurse's humanness and strength to build back his own resources. In giving of oneself, through one's own uniqueness, coupled with an attitude of being genuinely interested in the patient and trying to understand and help him, the nurse will find developing, the fundamentals of relating with the patient. Initially, one should start by just listening and trying to understand the human process within the person instead of trying to concentrate on specific interviewing techniques contained in some textbooks. Interest and caring about an individual are not technical skills; they are the basic arts of psychic healing.

Nurses do not need to tell the patient they care. They show concern for the patient by listening and by trying to understand the anguish or loneliness in the patient's heart. When nurses are comfortable enough to enable them not to worry about interview technique, posture, facial expression, and speech, the natural concerns for people will begin to show. It is then that the patient will know that the nurse cares.

The patient must know that the nurse is aware of his goals, his strivings, and his wishes and that the nurse is working hard with him in order to accomplish these goals.

Patience and persistence

The importance of the patience that is required in the healing process of the mind is frequently underestimated in the psychiatric setting.

Working with severely depressed or regressed patients or those with grave character disorders requires considerable (sometimes infinite) patience. This quality, coupled with the physical presence of the nurse, often provides the first affirmative therapeutic results. There are often days and weeks when the nurse does not feel any progress is being made. The patient just sits or lies around and says, "Everything makes me depressed. I just want to be alone." An approach of value in this situation is the patience that is demonstrated through the physical presence of the nurse. This approach can and often does set the stage for therapeutic success.

The ability to wait until the patient is ready to move may yield high dividends. As one patient put it, "I thought I could wait you out but your patience won out and I decided to try it your way."

In another example involving a medical student:

> The student was assigned to a depressed patient who was mute. He said absolutely nothing. The student sat with him each day for two weeks. Technically, the student did not know the proper thing to say. He sometimes just sat with the patient. Sometimes he said things such as, "You must feel terribly low." Mostly he just persisted. On the fifteenth day, the patient turned to the bewildered student and uttered his first words: "You sure know what you are doing." Two weeks later the patient had recovered and was discharged.

It is important to remember that the therapeutic process must not be rushed and miracles shouldn't be expected; the nurse must persist with the therapeutic attempts.

Although nurses may have all the necessary therapeutic attributes, they may still fail to be therapeutic if they can neither persevere nor persist. The patient who is emotionally ill has often been neglected, deprived, or even humiliated for many years. Why should he then assume that after a day or even a week the nurse will treat him differently? Despite the nurse's therapeutic goals, she will be as suspect as someone who is intending to harm him physically. This is especially true of the patient in the midst of a psychosis who misperceives reality. He may perceive that "*all* nurses are part of a conspiracy." His nurse may then be perceived as part of the conspiracy.

Persistence and patience usually win out in the end. The disturbed patient remembers that no matter how he has provoked the nurse, rejected her, or harassed her, she will continue to be respectful, hopeful, honest, sensitive, and involved. She is both patient and persistent. How else can one better demonstrate concern, interest, and caring?

THERAPEUTIC TASKS Even though nurses may be comfortable with their attitudes, feelings, and style, they may still ask, "What do I do? How do I help?" The nurse may be comfortable within the tension and drama of the operating room, but that does not make her an effective operating room nurse. There are specific and particular tasks to be performed.

The following examples illustrate situations that occur in a general hospital in which nurses must perform specific psychological tasks in order to help:

A 14-year-old girl is admitted unconscious to the intensive care unit after taking an overdose of 64 assorted bromides, pain relievers, barbiturates, and amphetamines. Two days later she starts to respond and says, "Why didn't you let me die?"

A 30-year-old woman states after the birth of her fourth baby, "I didn't want this baby. Two were enough. My husband left me 3 months ago. I can't even stand to look at this child."

A 35-year-old married fireman with three children is admitted with the diagnosis of myocardial infarction after he collapsed at the scene of a fire. He says he has not had a heart attack, but rather the smoke overcame him. He refuses to stay in bed as part of the coronary precautions.

A 22-year-old pregnant wife sits by the nurse's station waiting for her 27-year-old husband to return from his radiation treatment for metastatic cancer of the bone.

In this section we will discuss some of the important therapeutic tasks to be performed by the nurse. Once the nurse is acquainted with these tasks, the clinical situations described above will no longer seem overwhelming.

Observation

In developing therapeutic attitudes and behaviors we set forth how you must learn to observe yourself. In a similar manner the nurse must also learn to observe the patient and understand his environment before therapeutic tasks can be performed.

One observes through the five senses. *Visual observing* means seeing the person and his environment. Judgment developed through clinical practice is needed in order to know when to look directly at the person, when to use peripheral vision, and when to sweep the total scene. It is also most helpful to "develop eyes in the back of the head."

Observing gestures is important. How a person complements his spoken word with actions often reveals mood and temperament. Some gestures are *symbolic* (they relate to a conventional sign such as the index and third finger's forming a "V" for peace). Head nodding and finger pointing are *emphatic* gestures that are often used for clarification in heated discussions and arguments. People try to win others over to their sides by using emphatic gestures.

Ears imply *hearing* what is going on in the room and beyond it. One should try to hear all sounds and noises regardless of what extra traffic is introduced.

The sense of *smell* has deteriorated in humans because of our social orientation, but the ability to note various odors is important. Olfactory sensitivity may detect scents and aromas as well as stenches.

The technique of *touch* has generally been less emphasized as a technique in the psychiatric care of adults. Touch as a technique is important in child psychiatric nursing in which the care and therapy of children require much physical contact. Touch does remain a central technique in general nursing practice and the "laying on of hands" is historical practice in both nursing and medicine. Handshakes may yield useful information about a person and how he feels about himself.

The sense of *taste* is not popular as a clinical instrument unless the patients' cooking club invites the staff to lunch. Nursing students often get involved in these activities and what the patients choose to serve may reveal some insights into their current moods.

Setting goals

The task of setting goals in any therapeutic situation is essential to the anticipated gains for the individual. From the team standpoint, goals may be separated into the overall goal (long-term) and the subgoal (short-term). The overall goal tends to reflect the philosophy of the hospital or clinic, for example, determining when the patient may be out of treatment and return to family and community. The subgoals are indicative of the intervening steps necessary to be taken in reaching the overall goal.

A necessary component in the task of setting goals is the inclusion of the goals the patient has for himself. Hopefully, the goals of the treatment team match the goals of the patient. When they do not, negotiation must take place.

The analogy may be made to the nursing student and the nursing education program. Generally, the overall goal for the student is to complete the program requirements of the school and to achieve the registered nurse license. The various courses taken during the educational experience, such as liberal arts and science courses and the clinical nursing specialty courses, represent the subgoals necessary to reach the overall goal of the registered nurse license. The nursing students, however, also have personal subgoals related to personal fulfillment, family, and community that are necessary in order to complete the overall picture. A nursing program that fails to combine the goals of the student with the educational goals of the program will have as much difficulty in graduating students as the hospital will have in discharging patients when it fails to combine the psycho-social-economical-spiritual goals of the patient with the goals of the treatment team.

In the general hospital the task of setting nursing goals is often straightforward and possibly routine. For the patient suffering from pneumonia, specific nursing skills, such as treatments, positioning, and medicating, are required and necessary in order to aid in the healing process. When the patient is admitted solely for diagnostic tests, the situation becomes more complicated. For example, when the patient is having diagnostic tests for abdominal pain, one of the doctor's goals may be to rule out certain diseases, such as pancreatitis, appendicitis, or gastric ulcer. The nurse's goal lies in talking with the patient and listening to his anxiety resulting from the fear of the tests, from the uncertainty inherent in the situation, and from the possible physical discomfort. Regardless of the physician's diagnostic conclusions, this nursing goal will psychologically help the patient.

In the psychiatric setting, formulating goals begins with knowing exactly why the patient comes for treatment. For example, the patient may be hospitalized for an acute short-term crisis of possibly one or two months' duration. It is important to know that the overall goal is to help the patient to return to the community and to prevent him from becoming a chronic patient. It is not necessary to announce this goal to the patient, but it should be uppermost in the mind of the nurse. Or if the patient is in a psychiatric hospital where the major treatment modality is long-term psychotherapy, the treatment goal might be confinement to the hospital for a year of intensive analysis.

Establishing a goal protects the nurse from trying to be everything to the patient. Goals are the reminders and limits to the reality within which one must work. The nurse does not have vague or unrealistic plans for the patient when the purpose or goal for being with the patient is clearly defined.

Some goals stated by patients may be misleading. Patients will say, "I want to establish meaningful relationships; I want to relate better to people; I want to understand myself better; I want to increase my socialization." These tend to be psychiatric clichés and the nurse should be alert to recognize them and to help the patient more clearly state what his expectations for therapy are.

Well-meaning as these goals may be, they are almost impossible to put into practice effectively. They are difficult to achieve and only serve to make both patient and therapist overwhelmed or confused. Well thought through, achievable short-term goals are more useful in a therapeutic program.

Goals may be stated in terms of activities of daily living. Standard V defines this goal setting as follows.[2]

STANDARD V

THE ACTIVITIES OF DAILY LIVING ARE UTILIZED IN A GOAL DIRECTED WAY IN WORK WITH CLIENTS

RATIONALE: A major portion of one's daily life is spent in some form of activity related to health and well-being. An individual's development and intellectual level, emotional state and physical limitations may be reflected in these activities. Therefore, nursing has a unique opportunity to assess and intervene in these processes in order to encourage constructive changes in the client's behavior so that each person may realize his full potential for growth.

Assessment Factors:
1. An appraisal is made of the client's capacities to participate in activities of daily living based on needs, strengths and levels of functioning.
2. Clients are encouraged toward independence and self-direction by various skills such as motivating, limit setting, persuading, guiding and comforting.
3. Each person's rights are appreciated and respected.
4. Methods of communicating are devised which assure consistency in approach.

[2]Congress for Nursing Practice, *Standards of Psychiatric-Mental Health Nursing Practice* (Kansas City, Mo.: American Nurses Association, 1973), p. 4.

What are realistic goals? What should be established with a patient as to the psychiatric accomplishment desired for a short-term setting? Depending on the behavior of the patient, some suggestions are:

Talking about daily ward activities.

Performing a structured task, such as getting up for breakfast, or getting to school or work on time, or staying at school or work for the full time.

Discussing a particular incident that occurred at the unit that was upsetting or successful for the patient.

Looking at the manner in which his behavior leads to favorable or unfavorable reactions from other people.

Looking at his anxiety about specific situations and the reaction it has on him and others.

Determining if the patient is harmful to himself, for example, is suicidal.

Talking in order to clarify the patient's wishes and expectations in life and how he intends to obtain them.

Deciding if a doctor or another staff member should see the patient.

The covert agenda of the patient is often overlooked. Although the nurses' goals are to help the patient, the patient may have totally different goals. It is necessary to keep this in mind because unless there is some merging of the goals, very little can develop. If the nurse's goal is to be a helpful listener and the patient feels like being helpfully listened to, the conversation usually goes well. If his goal, however, is to get the nurse to get him a glass of water because the other nurse has not been around to get him one, the nurse is going to have trouble. If the patient's primary goal is to leave the hospital and the nurse's goal is to merely help him understand his feelings, there will be little interchange.

The nurse might say, "What are you hoping or wishing for yourself? You look preoccupied." The patient might respond, "I'm being discharged in an hour and I am wondering if my husband is going to be his old self and start shouting and screaming at me." If the nurse's goal is only to listen, the approach will be irrelevant to the patient's goals. The patient will want and expect a more direct involvement on the nurse's part on how to deal with the potential situation that she dreads facing at home. Alternatives might be explored, for example, "Are you that fearful of your welcome at home?"

The role of the therapeutic person is to either convince the patient that staff goals are the right goals or to change staff goals to patient goals. If staff is at an impasse with the patient, then there must be a reevaluation of the situation with the staff team.

Find out what the patient wants. For example, "It seems as though many things are on your mind. What are the hopes and wishes you are experiencing and let's look at them." This will give a whole new area for discussion.

A final consideration of the task of setting goals is relevant to the teaching situation. A third goal, along with the staff and patient goals, is identifying learning goals for the student. One learning goal may be learning to look for and to observe psychiatric symptoms, for example, schizophrenia as part of the psychiatric nursing experience.

Learning goals such as these does not specifically aim at helping the patient. Nevertheless, it has been our experience that these learning goals do turn out to be therapeutic for the patient even though the primary aim is teaching. The teaching staff generally takes responsibility that the learning activity, such as teaching interview conferences, is not harmful to the patient.

In summary, helping the patient to be discharged from the hospital and return to his family and community is usually the overall goal. This goal implies determining his ability to cope and manage his life. The patient's wishes and expectations must be considered concurrently with the treatment team's goals. Otherwise, an impasse arises. In the psychiatric setting the patient may say that he never wishes to leave the hospital and return home. In the medical setting the patient with pneumonia refuses to take his penicillin because he wants to die. Careful goal planning between staff and patient sets the stage for therapeutic progress.

Encouraging the patient to talk

Talking helps people feel better. The free expression of emotions is fostered and encouraged in psychiatry because emotions give importance to an experience and communicate their importance to other people. If a student does not talk about her academic and clinical experiences to family and friends, the importance of her education is not transmitted to others, but if she does tell them of her nursing encounters, she finds that they react favorably or unfavorably to what she says. Their behavior adds a definite dimension to the meaning of the experience for herself.

Talking brings one's emotions to the surface, often displaying to the patient what he has not realized before. By identifying his feelings, he has better control over them. For example, a patient fears a job interview after a hospitalization for a depression. Brooding over the problem by himself magnifies the fear. Talking about it to a therapeutic person puts the problem into proper perspective and helps him view the pending interview more realistically.

People are often frightened by intense feelings and emotions, their own as well as those of others. This often accounts for the statement by some that it is better not to express how one feels. Part of this reasoning results from the fear that the other person will not be able to tolerate or be receptive to the feelings. This may occur especially if the other person suffers from the same anxiety. An example of this is the nursing student who fears failing state board examinations. When this is discussed among nursing classmates,

anxiety can run high and some students prefer to avoid this trauma altogether. When the fear is expressed to a truly supportive person who understands the situation, the anxiety can be more realistically viewed and the
feelings can then be expressed, shared, and resolved.

It is important to consider cultural influences and the individual's
upbringing as to how free people feel to express feelings. For some people
who have difficulty talking, this may be a totally new experience. They may
never be spontaneously verbal, but the difference evident in previous verbal
behavior and current verbal behavior can be quite dramatic.

Listening

Encouraging a person to talk and to express himself will not be helpful if the
person feels that he is not being listened to.

Listening is a highly valued art that requires understanding, patience,
skill, and perseverance. It is a grossly underrated art. It is often much easier
to not listen than to listen. Almost all the discussion on the mechanics of
listening may take a few paragraphs, but the pitfalls to be encountered and
overcome in listening will fill many pages.

The concept of listening has major implications in the talking therapy
of patient care. Listening implies a voluntary effort to understand what is
being said. Hearing, as distinguished from listening, is the audible reception
of the spoken word or noise.

Listening is most successful when there is a definite goal. Being in a
crowd with many people talking at the same time shows the difficulty in
knowing to what or whom to direct attention. If there is no purpose, the
attention will wander when someone is talking or the mind will wander when
one reads a textbook. Reading implies listening with your eyes. And mama
cat said, "Which of you kittens has lost your mittens?" If you are listening
here, that sentence will not make sense.

Perhaps you have had the experience of being with a person who is
talking yet you are trying to hear the conversation of the person behind you.
Or you have been in a class and found to your discomfort that you were not
listening when a question was specifically directed toward you.

By having the purpose of listening in mind, as you listen, what is heard
captures your attention. If this happens, you will start to actively think about
the subject. The dialogue then becomes meaningful and important. When the
speaker engages your interest, your voice and manner reflect enthusiasm
and you respond to the speaker. The conversation then takes on meaning.

In talking face-to-face, the response the nurse gives, such as leaning
forward when the patient says something important or nodding her head in
agreement, is the nonverbal message to continue. In telephone conversations the tone and pitch of the voice are clues that you are listening.

If the nurse's listening behavior has been successful, the feeling of satisfaction is inherent in the dialogue. To feel that one has been successfully
listened to is a therapeutic gain for anyone. It makes people feel important
and respected.

Understanding

Although nurses may be successful in encouraging the patient to talk and they may be successful with their listening behavior and in their ability to show the patient that they are interested and care about his welfare, the entire purpose of the interchange will be missing unless they understand the patient and unless the patient realizes that they understand.

How do you show that you understand? If in talking the patient expresses sadness, to listen is therapeutic but to acknowledge your understanding of his distress in your own words indicates understanding. For example, to say to the patient, "Everything I hear you talk about speaks of sadness. Your heart must be aching today," is to communicate that you do indeed understand. It is therapeutic to offer statements expressing understanding with such remarks as, "I can see how hard that was for you to say" or "That must have made you feel better." Statements of this kind should indicate understanding of what the patient has endeavored to express.

Be precise with a message. Try to say exactly what you mean and be certain that the patient understands completely. If a goal is stated to the patient as, "It is important to work through problems in order to develop meaningful relationships," the patient may not understand what is expected of him. This expression may be far over his head and entirely incomprehensible to him.

When one is understood, one is no longer so alone. When a person can verbalize what is on his mind, he feels more in control of the situation. He preserves his dignity and quality as a human being. The display of understanding and interest takes a person out of his loneliness and isolation. People who are about to die are often abandoned by being placed in a room and left alone. People are grateful when someone does not abandon them and does come to talk with them. To listen is therapeutic, but to understand still goes far above and beyond listening.

Bearing painful feelings

A special dimension of listening and understanding is to help bear the feelings that the patient is trying to express. When a family approaches the nurse in the ward or on the medical floor after a family member has died, it is reaching out for a human presence to help it bear that which is unbearable alone. It needs someone to help share a part of the pain and grief.

Nurses may find this a difficult skill to master. It is extremely difficult for some nurses to sit with a depressed or sobbing patient. Experience helps condition one to be able to sit for longer periods of time with someone in psychic pain. Often, for example, families will say after a death, "Don't talk about it; it is better to say nothing." This position is not therapeutic. The feeling must be expressed and someone should be supportive and help by listening to the suffering person. The nurse should try to be able to help bear the sadness with the patient during stressful times.

If patients cannot bear painful feelings, they will deal with them in unhealthy ways. Some patients will develop psychotic thoughts; others will develop depressions or antisocial behaviors in response to the feelings. These reactions can be warded off or lessened by helping the person to cope and bear the feeling.

It takes practice in order to be helpful; and even having had considerable experience, the therapeutic person often feels uncomfortable when helping another person bear the painful feelings. It is a learning process that takes many and varied encounters of these situations. For example, being able to sit with a crying patient in the general hospital is a skill that is learned and developed over a period of time and only after several of these experiences of sitting and listening to the pain of the person. Let us use an example from child-rearing: When the child wants something immediately, you attempt to help the child bear the tension. You do not give the child a pacifier or piece of candy every time he cries.

A clinical example of a situation in which grief feelings were not adequately resolved follows:

> A 55-year-old woman was referred from the medical unit of a hospital to the psychiatric unit because she "refused to have a myelogram" to determine a cause for her back pain of 15-months duration. The symptom went back to her hospitalization following a car accident. The patient related the following: "We were returning from my son's home after a weekend. I was in the back seat of the car with my two grandchildren; my son-in-law was driving. He said I interfered too much and complained too much about his drinking. I wanted to drive because he was intoxicated but decided to say nothing. The car was swerving back and forth and suddenly missed a curve in the road. We went over the embankment. My daughter was killed in the accident."

> The question was asked during the interview what other deaths the patient had experienced in her life and with considerable crying and sadness she said, "When I was 11, we were all summoned into my mother's room as she was dying giving birth to my sister . . . . When I was 30-years old, I had 3 children; the boys were 7 and 5 and one daughter 3 weeks old. I went in to get her up from a nap and she was dead in her crib . . . . 18 months ago my husband was getting into his car and dropped over dead with a CVA . . . . 15 months ago my daughter was killed . . . ."

Death and human loss are predominant issues with this woman. The main therapeutic task in the psychiatric setting is to sit and listen to her as she recounts her feelings of grief. This demands much from the nurse, but until the patient can make peace with the agonizing tragedies in her past, she will be unable to be free to live in the present.

Setting limits

If emphasis is placed on the open expression of thoughts and feelings, it may seem surprising that setting limits on a patient's behavior can be an important part of the therapy.

It may be easier to understand if we begin with the normal child. A child left to himself will behave in ways that are self-destructive. He might eat paint, walk in the middle of a busy street, or destroy the possessions of others. The child possesses neither the intelligence nor the inner controls to cope with the complexities of the outer world or the tensions of his inner world. The adult does it for him in order that he may remain alive. He can thus be free to gradually learn inner controls and then he can learn to channel his drives into constructive outlets.

The medical–surgical patient has limits set on him by the physician's orders that the nurse implements. Limits are usually placed on his physical activities (getting out of bed, going to the bathroom), his diet, or even his visitors. Some patients, like young children, are often reluctant to accept these limits even when their very survival is at stake. The patient may want so badly to deny being weak, sick, or dependent that he insists on behaving as if he were healthy.

In psychiatric units, where behavior is the very basic material one works with from moment to moment, limit setting takes on special importance. Nurses must decide if a hyperactive patient (mania, for example) is being overstimulated and needs to be controlled. They must decide whether or not suicidal patients must be restricted for their own protection. They must also decide when the adolescent patient needs to have someone say "no" in order for him to know someone cares. For example:

> A 16-year-old female patient asked an aide if she would intercede for her and ask the physician to let her stay out until midnight. The aide asked the patient how she would feel if the response was "yes." She replied, "Scared! If he let me out, it would mean he really doesn't understand me."

The nurse learns when limits are necessary from several cues: (1) if the patient's behavior is disturbing to everyone else; (2) if the patient seems to be upsetting himself by his own behavior; (3) if the nurse worries excessively about a suicidal patient; (4) if the nurse feels the patient is saying, "Please take over." When the nurse discusses concerns about setting limits with the patient, frequently the patient will give a clue that helps the nurse to make a decision. For example, the nurse says to a suicidal patient, "I am especially worried about you today and am trying to decide whether you should stay on the ward." The patient may respond with relief, "You should be worried about me. I intended to walk right in front of a car."

The nurse first tries to set limits with a supportive verbal interchange. For example:

> A patient was loudly banging on the piano much to the annoyance of other patients and visitors. The nurse went over and asked the patient to please stop or to play softly as it was disturbing. The patient said, "You're not big enough to make me stop. Want to try?" The nurse said, "I'd be a fool to try that. I can't make you do anything, but I can talk with you for a while."

In this situation the nurse avoids a physical confrontation. She gently offers an alternative behavior that will be socially appropriate. There are times, however, when setting limits by using medication or by actual physical restraint may be necessary.

Setting limits on a medical or psychiatric ward is always necessary. The need for limits will be kept at a minimum when all the members of the team agree on a plan of care and keep the channels of communication open. When the staff disagrees—just as when mother and father disagree on the rules for their children—the patient will become anxious and will then begin to test the limits.

Providing support

All the therapeutic tasks are provided in the physical presence of the nurse who defines the goals and encourages the patient to talk. The nurse also listens, understands, helps bear painful feelings, and sets limits. All these tasks are embodied in the truly supportive person. Providing support is the strength one person gives to another and anyone in a therapeutic situation must be supportive.

Support helps people grow and become independent themselves. In the process of psychic development, support is necessary in order to sustain the individual through the pain of learning. Support provides trust and strength in the event of faltering during the experience. Being a part of the achievement reached is the only satisfaction needed by the supportive person. Understanding of what is truly supportive and truly helpful gets to the love and positive caring forces inside the other person that needs to be brought out and developed.

Providing a corrective emotional experience

The therapeutic process may be perceived as a corrective emotional experience. When the nurse responds to the patient in a healthy, direct, accepting, yet limit-setting fashion, the patient may be experiencing something quite new in his life. The patient, not convinced that the nurse "means business," may withdraw or express hostility toward her. The nurse persists, however, in her therapeutic attempts.

After a period of time the patient may alter his behavior, possibly because of his corrective experience with the nurse, and if the nurse respects and accepts him, he then begins to believe he is worthy of respect and acceptance. He may reciprocate these feelings to the nurse and if the therapy succeeds, he may begin to generalize the healthy behavior to others.

For example, a 17-year-old male said:

"A year ago things really started getting bad. I'd get so depressed I thought a great deal about killing myself. I seriously wanted to die. I began drinking a lot at that time. When my parents would go out, I'd drink all my father's liquor. He was pretty disgusted I guess and my mother was angry too, but they never said anything."

The point here is the parents' indifference to the boy's behavior. In order to provide a corrective experience, the nurse must show she is not indifferent to him, and by seeing him daily to talk over his experiences of the day she can then set limits on him when his behavior is not appropriate to the situation. This physical intervention action shows that she cares about his well-being and her presence each day indicates her concern and interest in him as an individual.

Aiding the healing process of the mind

Nurses and physicians do not cure. The mind and body cure themselves while the professionals help the normal healing process. We find this perspective a useful one, as we will attempt to illustrate.

A patient comes to the emergency ward with a knife wound. The surgeon cleans the incision, sterilizes the area, and stitches the skin. The wound then heals. Without the surgeon the wound would still heal, but there would be considerable scarring.

In an acute psychiatric illness the mind has suffered a wound that may be called schizophrenia or depression. It is a wound nevertheless. The mind will heal, for it will not remain in its tormented state for long. How the mind will heal remains uncertain. If the healing process is not assisted and protected, scarring may occur. In psychiatry, scarring is chronicity. The patient, no longer acutely pained, is resigned, apathetic, and withdrawn. Many chronic schizophrenic patients who have been hospitalized for years have made this "peace" for themselves.

When the healing process is assisted, the mind is less likely to be subjected to scarring. In other words, with proper treatment, chronicity can be avoided.

> A patient who is overwhelmed by his insignificance and impotence develops the delusion that he is king of the universe. If he is neglected and treated as if he were insignificant, he might "decide" that his delusion is worth keeping. If he feels respected, supported, and important to someone, the patient will be more willing to give up the delusion of being king and return to being a normal human being.

The hospital provides a nutrient environment for the patient who is psychologically depleted. He can rest from the stress and strain of his home environment and have his inner resources replenished.

Listen well when the patient says that he has come to the psychiatric hospital because his "nerves are shot" and he needs a good rest. Or the housewife who says that the children are "driving her crazy and she just had to get away from them." There is a great deal of truth in what they say. The people expect the hospital to be the nutrient climate to enable the mind to heal properly.

Health teaching

Health teaching is one kind of direct nursing service in which the nurse is able to provide information about physical and mental health issues. Standard IV further emphasizes this skill.[3]

[3]Congress for Nursing Practice, *Standards of Psychiatric-Mental Health Nursing Practice* (Kansas City, Mo.: American Nurses' Association, 1973), p. 4.

STANDARD IV

INDIVIDUALS, FAMILIES AND COMMUNITY GROUPS ARE ASSISTED TO ACHIEVE SATISFYING AND PRODUCTIVE PATTERNS OF LIVING THROUGH HEALTH TEACHING.

RATIONALE: Health teaching is an essential part of the nurse's role in work with those who have mental health problems. Every interaction can be utilized as a teaching–learning situation. Formal and informal teaching methods can be used in working with individuals, families, the community and other personnel. Emphasis is on understanding mental health problems as well as on developing ways of coping with them.

Assessment Factors:

1. The needs of individual, family and community groups for health teaching are identified and appropriate techniques are used in meeting these needs.
2. The principles of learning and teaching are employed.
3. The basic principles of physical and mental health and interpersonal and social skills are taught.
4. Experiential learning opportunities are made available.
5. Opportunities with community groups to further their knowledge and understanding of mental health problems are identified.

Nursing management of the milieu

There are several aspects to the nurse's increasing responsibility for patient care that have implications for the nursing management of the milieu. The nursing staff sets the ward tone and climate—whether it is to be a permissive or strict atmosphere, a cooperative or competitive atmosphere, or a caring or rigid atmosphere.

The nurse also is the one who sets the pace and adjusts the climate of the hospital unit. This responsibility involves judging with whom to spend time and in what capacity; with whom to sit in silence; whom to scold; whom to support; with whom to avoid a harmful dependent relationship. In this hospital discipline the responsibilities of the nurse have steadily increased to the point where she usually makes the final decisions on the ward milieu.

This broadened responsibility has moved the psychiatric nurse from the subordinated position of asking that the doctor do something for the patient to sitting with the patient and their later collaborating with the treatment team to determine what the patient's problem is and to decide what the patient care plan should be. In other words, when Mrs. Smith comes to the nursing station and says that she is feeling anxious and needs medication, the nurse does not immediately call the doctor for the medication order. Instead, the nurse takes time to sit and talk with Mrs. Smith to find out why she is anxious. It may be learned that the patient is overly concerned because her husband is coming to visit that evening. Defining the issue as the patient's ambivalence toward the anticipated visit of her husband gives the

126

team considerably more information so that it can consider what therapeutic plan should be used.

Standard VII specifically deals with the milieu concept as follows:[4]

STANDARD VII

THE ENVIRONMENT IS STRUCTURED TO ESTABLISH AND MAINTAIN A THERAPEUTIC MILIEU.

RATIONALE: Any environment is composed of both human and nonhuman resources which may work for or against the person's well-being. The nurse works with people in a variety of environmental settings, e.g. hospital, home, etc. The milieu is structured and/or altered so that it serves the client's best interests as an inherent part of the overall therapeutic plan.

Assessment Factors:
1. The effects of environmental forces on individuals are observed, analyzed and interpreted.
2. Psychological, physiological, social, economical and cultural concepts are understood and utilized in developing and maintaining a therapeutic milieu.
3. Communications within the environment are congruent with therapeutic goals.
4. All available resources in the environment are utilized when appropriate in the therapeutic efforts.
5. Nursing participation and its effectiveness in establishing and maintaining a therapeutic milieu are evaluated.

SUMMARY This chapter described those human qualities and therapeutic tasks that help patients to recover. The nurse as an individual is a primary asset in the therapeutic situation.

Being therapeutic requires a feeling of professional ease and an understanding of talents, feelings, and reactions. When people are able and competent, it is evident to all that they are their natural selves. Therapeutic style is developed from understanding the self, from observing other people, and by making identifications with many people to see what feels right and comfortable.

The practice of being therapeutic requires using one's behavioral style, encouraging the patient to talk, listening, understanding, bearing painful feelings, setting limits, providing support, providing a corrective emotional experience, and aiding in the normal healing process of the mind. These factors, coupled with the setting of goals for treatment purposes and the use of therapeutic concepts for practice, convey our real concern for the patient who is in distress and is suffering. Every aspect of contact with the patient

[4]Congress for Nursing Practice, *Standards of Psychiatric-Mental Health Nursing* (Kansas City, Mo.: American Nurses' Association, 1973), p. 5.

should demonstrate that he is respected, that he is a responsible human being, and that he will be dealt with in a consistent and straightforward, honest manner.

The patient is looking for the real and honest quality within the nurse, and this quality must be allowed to be revealed. The therapeutic goal is to allow the very best of one's humanness to be brought into the situation.

Standards V, IV, and VII of *Psychiatric-Mental Health Nursing Practice* are included in this chapter.

**REFERENCES
AND SUGGESTED
READINGS**

Baumgartner, Margaret (1970). "Empathy," in *Behavioral Concepts and Nursing,* coordinator Carolyn Carson. Philadelphia: Lippincott.

Brinling, Trudy (1971). "Tearing Down a Wall," *American Journal of Nursing,* **71,** No. 7, 1406–9.

Burkhardt, Marti (1969). "Response to Anxiety," *American Journal of Nursing,* **69,** No. 10, 2153–54.

Lenarz, Dorothea M. (1971). "Caring Is the Essence of Practice," *American Journal of Nursing,* **71,** No. 4, 704–7.

Ludemann, Ruth S. (1968). "Empathy: A Component of Therapeutic Nursing," *Nursing Forum,* **7,** No. 3, 275–87.

Sinkler, Gail H. (1970). "Identity and Role," *Nursing Outlook,* **18,** No. 10, 22–24.

STALLS IN THE
THERAPEUTIC PROCESS

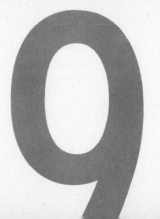

An analogy may be made here to aerodynamics and a student pilot learning to fly an airplane right side up and safely. In Chapter 8 the practice of being therapeutic was discussed as a guide to effective interaction with people. Student pilots also identify their assets and reactions and learn the dynamics and mechanics of flying. With this knowledge they then get into the cockpit of the plane and put theory into practice.

THE STALL CONCEPT It is not until the student starts flying the plane that an actual stall is experienced. A stall means that the airplane has lost the lift that it needs to stay in the air. A variety of conditions can cause a stall and a stall will not necessarily put the plane out of control. It does mean that a corrective measure is necessary to help the plane resume its path of flight. A red light or buzzer in the plane alerts the pilot of a potential stall position in case he has not "felt" that the lift is gone. At this point the pilot must then consider his alternatives if he wants to stay aloft.

The psychiatric nursing student is now at the point of having some concepts of therapeutic meetings with patients. The next step is to test what has been learned in the psychiatric setting. Here it is helpful to know the common stalls that impede the therapeutic process.

There are many situations that lead to a stall, and we will attempt to describe some of them. In addition, we will attempt to describe the warnings that signal a stall is imminent.

The stall warning occurs when you feel that something is wrong before the patient reacts unfavorably to the situation and you are into the stall. Ideally, you try to remedy the situation before the stall occurs. You will, however, feel that the stall is imminent because you will receive warnings such as a vague feeling of discomfort within yourself, the realization that the therapy is getting nowhere, the patient's sudden change in attitude toward you, his expression of hostility, your autodiagnosis of your own withdrawal, or a feedback from the staff of the patient's reactions.

In this chapter we will mention some specific stalls and the general warnings of other potential stall situations. The corrective mechanism to "right the flight" or remedy the stall will also be given.

Behavioral style

STALLS IN HUMAN QUALITIES People beginning their training in the psychiatric–mental health field often seem to have a pseudoprofessional approach characterized by their looking and acting stilted and rigid. This may result from their trying too hard to follow the book and the prescribed rules. By the time their training has ended, however, they act far more natural, for they have learned to be themselves and are thus able to reveal their humanness and genuine concern for their patients.

When a nurse behaves in a pseudoprofessional way, the patient feels uncomfortable and wonders what is happening to this person who is supposed to know what she is doing. When the patient feels no confidence in the helping person, there is a stall.

In this situation, the stall warning occurs when you notice yourself becoming tense, rigid, and stilted and wishing that you felt more professional.

In order to correct the stall, you should try to worry less about the rules concerning methods of listening and talking with people. Strict adherence to rules can prove burdensome and may hinder the development of the naturalness of one's skills. It is important not to abandon one's common sense approach for the pretense of the professional approach. Being natural can impart the feeling of security and competence as a therapeutic person.

Judgmental feelings

STALLS IN FEELINGS Judgmental feelings surface when the nurse arrives at a clinical situation with an already formed judgment or prejudice. The word *prejudice* has a similar root as the word *judgment*. Prejudice is prejudging without having any actual data or experience. It is often opinion based on cultural values or upbringing.

The patient generally can tell when a person has negative feelings toward him. The patient feels isolated, ignored, or dealt with in an abrupt manner. The therapeutic progress stalls because the helping person unconsciously rejects him because of strong negative feelings.

The stall warning occurs when nurses realize that they have strong negative opinions of the person before even meeting him. In the staff report you may hear the patient described in highly negative judgmental terms or perhaps the history of the patient may give you an uncomfortable feeling. You have a strong negative visceral reaction and you know that it comes from a previous unpleasant experience in your life.

A negative feeling triggers a strong reaction through the sensory system and adversely reflects the way one person looks, sounds, smells, or responds physically to another person.

In order to remedy this stall, nurses must realize the scope of their judgmental feelings and be able to keep them in check so that they do not interfere with the therapeutic process. If they cannot stand a geriatric patient, they should be aware of it so that they can be therapeutic and polite. If they acknowledge this, they will not have to say at nursing report, "That old lady in 356 — I wonder what she is ringing her bell for this time?"

The nurse brings all her feelings to any new situation and everything proceeds smoothly as long as the feelings are positive. For example, if the nurse says, "That patient reminds me of my grandmother. I really like her and want to help her," she probably will be therapeutic because of the positive feelings.

Judgmental feelings can help or stall the therapeutic process. What we are concerned about in this section are those judgmental feelings that hinder and stall.

The stall in the judgmental situation may be more easily detected by impartial staff members rather than by the nurse herself. The objective person may hear the stall as a labeling of the patient, such as "the lady is just an alcoholic" or "we had another drug abuse patient admitted last night."

For example, a student says, "I really dread going to the psychiatric nursing experience." The student probably has formed an opinion of the experience from past remarks made by relatives and friends regarding psychiatric patients or even from hearing other professionals talking about the clinical specialty areas. This is a judgmental feeling because the student has never experienced the situation personally, and thus the entire discipline is condemned beforehand.

The judgmental attitudes we all develop because of our upbringing become a pattern for searching inquiry when working with people with emotional illness. The ideal is to proceed above and beyond the judgmental attitude. This helps to understand the patient as a human being in his own right rather than to see him as someone with unacceptable behavior. When two people talk together, what they say depends not only on what they want to tell each other, but also on what they think of each other. Patients will be reluctant to reveal themselves to people who they feel will judge them critically.

There is no doubt that even nurses with considerable experience will at times find themselves automatically judging a patient. When they realize how nontherapeutic this is, they will then reassess their attitude. For example, nurses may find themselves reacting unfavorably to girls hospitalized for abortions, venereal disease, and illegitimate babies. This is not just a problem for beginning nurses, it is also a problem for the entire medical and nursing professions. Behavior that deviates from society's norms is difficult for people to accept. Two cases in point that illustrate this are drug abuse and alcohol consumption. These problems of society are compounded greatly when the medical–clinical professions tend to use judgmental terms in prescribing treatment. For example, the physician says, "It's all in his head — just give him a tranquilizer. He is always complaining." Nurses may assume judgmental attitudes from what the physician has to say about a patient. This approach, in itself, is far from helpful in dealing with or attempting to understand the problem.

No one is without bias and no one is without judgmental feelings. Our feelings and opinions about people and situations derive from our experiences and interactions in life. The question is how to facilitate the process of becoming more objective and less judgmental. How is one able to step back and look at the situation objectively and thereby prevent a stall in the therapeutic process?

The process of becoming objective is twofold and involves (1) auto-diagnosis of feelings and (2) accepting the feelings and realizing it is not excessively harmful to have negative feelings about someone. It is harmful if the judgmental feelings are suppressed and then unconsciously acted upon. The patient will be rejected, ignored, and relegated to a powerless position.

The nurse has the right to be human, which implies the right to have judgmental feelings. There is, however, the ideal to which one can aspire. Even when you cannot give up your judgmental feelings, you can recognize them as such. You can rise above the feelings and not let them interfere with the therapeutic process.

Ambivalent feelings

The term *ambivalence* implies having both positive and negative feelings toward an object, a person, or an action. We have all experienced feelings of ambivalence.

The stall in the therapeutic process comes from denying ambivalent feelings, especially the negative aspects of the ambivalence. As a result the staff becomes overly solicitous. It may be the nurse acting as "Suzy Goodshoes." Alternatively, the staff may handle the negative ambivalence by displaced anger.

The stall occurs when nurses simultaneously like and do not like the patient. They then feel guilty for the negative feelings. The anger does not come through because they are unwilling to be open and honest with their feelings. They may not dare be angry because nurses are supposed to like and relate to all their patients. If they cannot deal with their ambivalence, the anger comes through in covert ways and the patient then senses something is wrong. There is a stall.

The stall warning occurs when nurses notice themselves being overly nice to a patient or they have either all positive or all negative feelings toward the patient.

Ambivalence is part of all human relationships. People who are in the health fields generally are there because they sincerely like people and wish to help them in stressful times. Too often it is assumed that one must have positive feelings for the patient at all times. Assumptions like this will only put a student or practitioner in direct conflict because ambivalence is a natural feeling in any relationship.

The nurse must realize that ambivalence is a normal feeling. If you dislike the patient a great deal, chances are there are positive feelings too and you can still work with the patient even though you have negative feelings.

If you look closely at your own personal relationships, you will find that even with those you love, you can also be furious at times. For example, when you are shopping in a store, a child begins to fuss and cry, and all attempts to pacify him only distract and upset you further. If you have not had such an experience, we suggest you spend an hour observing mothers shopping in the supermarket with their children. The ambivalent feelings are most evident when we are tired, upset, under pressure, or generally unhappy.

Despite the pain of ambivalent feelings, it is still preferable to having no feelings at all.

Ambivalence shows that you are real, and by acknowledging and dealing with your positive as well as your negative feelings, a stall will not occur and the therapeutic process will be facilitated.

A well-established psychiatric nursing principle states that patients need to be accepted exactly as they are. This means that the patient is seen as a person, but it does not mean that the nurse necessarily approves of his behavior. Accepting the patient "as is," although not necessarily approving the behavior, sets the scene for judgmental and ambivalent feelings. It may be that the nurse does not like the person or what he has done. If the patient has committed a crime, such as robbery or murder, this behavior will produce a negative bias or will induce prejudiced feelings in the nurse. It is difficult to acknowledge these feelings and still remain therapeutic in dealing with the patient. A clinical example shows a staff reaction to a patient who did have trouble staying within the limits of the laws of society.

> A 17-year-old girl was referred to a Halfway House residence by her social worker. Her presenting behavior pattern showed frequent environmental moves since age 11 when the total family was broken up because of the mother's psychiatric hospitalizations and the father's desertion of the family. In the last 6 years Susan had lived in 14 different foster homes. Her typical pattern was to become increasingly unmanageable after a 3- or 4-month period. She would refuse to meet the expectations of the home by coming in at odd hours, being truant from school, and ignoring her household duties. She would become verbally aggressive with the mother in the home and this would inevitably lead to her referral back to the social worker. Her life-style made her a target for the drug culture, for her boyfriend was a pusher and her promiscuity made her vulnerable to pregnancy and venereal disease.

> In the new situation at Halfway House, Susan was pleasant, attractive, and bluntly honest regarding her pseudoinvolvement with people and her negative regard for the "establishment."

Susan first induced the staff to help her by appealing to their rescue feelings and by making them feel guilty. Staff felt that they could help Susan by being supportive and understanding. She responded by making staff feel helpless and by behaving in her natural style. She did not abide by the House rules but instead brought drugs and alcohol into the House. She initiated some younger and more inexperienced patients to the world of drugs. This behavior provoked guilt feelings in the staff. When staff finally said that they could not tolerate this deviant behavior, she burst forth with positive behaviors of cooking, cleaning, being pleasant, going to school, and promising to avoid all drugs. The staff again felt guilty after talking with the social worker and learning that Susan had no place to go for everyone had "kicked" her out.

Staff was ambivalent over discharging Susan because she was appealing as a human being in distress, but her behavior was not appropriate for the House. Ambivalence creates and perpetuates uncomfortable feelings that people find hard to compromise. Here staff needed repeated conferences to talk out their feelings and to recognize that their treatment model was not therapeutic for Susan with her manipulative abilities.

To be able to accept and possibly understand Susan's behavioral style helps one to avoid the conflict in feelings resulting from expecting behavior that Susan simply could not manage. Staff had to realize and to expect that initially this patient would lie, cheat, and manipulate because this is her lifestyle and she is accustomed to behaving in that manner. Expecting people to behave as society dictates when it is not their style sets the stage for judgmental and ambivalent feelings. It is comparable to expecting the alcoholic to give up alcohol because he is told it is harmful to his body.

The problem with ambivalence is that some people find it difficult to accept ambivalence in themselves. They suppress unpleasant feelings and try to counteract the negative feelings by being generous and altruistic, which only displaces their negative feelings. Therapy thereby stalls rather than progresses.

Rescue feelings

Rescue feelings occur when the helping professional believes that he can do for the patient what no one else can do. The feeling is that one possesses the magic cure and will help the patient get better when everyone else has failed. Even though this is unrealistic, it can be helpful in small doses; this is the therapeutic side of the double-edged sword of rescue feelings.

Rescue feelings lead people to believe that there is some magical quality about them that can change a secluded, regressed psychotic person into an outpatient neurotic person. During the painful descent into reality, the nurse often becomes preoccupied with what can or cannot be done for the patient. This frequently prevents the nurse from seeing the patient as he really is.

The therapeutic process stalls when nurses ally themselves against the family or when they promise the patient more than they can reasonably deliver. The patient's hopes are raised sky high and when the nurse does not deliver, the patient feels hopelessly let down. The stall warning is there when you feel that you are clinically better than anyone else or when you feel the family has done everything wrong.

For example, a psychiatric resident physician allied himself with his patient against the family during the therapy. He advised the patient to get an apartment of his own, continue going to school, and everything would be fine. The patient agreed that this sounded like a fine idea and a family conference was arranged to tell the parents of this decision. At the conference the patient said to his parents, "I want to move out and get my own apartment. What do you think?" The parents replied, "Fine. Go ahead." The patient then said, "I think I am going to commit suicide."

This example shows that the patient was not prepared for such a major decision in his life and he had to be hospitalized for a short period to help him recover and learn to deal with his feelings about this situation. This situation illustrates the potential for a permanent stall to the therapeutic situation. One must avoid making secret alliances with the patient. The patient often contributes to this by saying, "You are the only one who understands me." This statement should be a warning signal, and the nurse should then realize that she may be in for a problematic and difficult situation.

The stall warning occurs when the patient plays up to the nurse's omnipotence and she thinks that perhaps what he is saying is true. Possibly she feels that she is the only one who understands him.

In order to remedy the stall, the nurse will have to consider what is going to happen to the patient when he is discharged and when she is not going to be there. This will help her put other relationships into proper perspective.

Sharing the responsibility with other staff members in order to accomplish treatment goals will usually be more rewarding and successful than feeling that the nurse and patient will solve the problem alone.

Feelings of pessimism

At times beginning nurses will have a difficult time understanding why the patient cannot comprehend his problem and why he cannot seem to be helped. This leads to feelings of pessimism about the patient's recovery. They have listened to people say, "You can't teach an old dog new tricks." "He has always behaved that way, he will never change." With this negative expectation about the potential of people to change and to be helped, any dialogue with the patient is likely to be antitherapeutic.

The stall here occurs when the patient realizes that the nurse feels that his situation is hopeless. The warning sounds when the nurse is feeling desperate and helpless in dealings with the patient.

The remedy for this stall is for the nurse to talk over such feelings with a staff member, supervisor, or instructor to try to get a therapeutic approach to the situation.

It is difficult for beginning nurses to grasp a person's potential for change, especially in psychiatric situations. Often the person is seen in terms of what he has achieved rather than in terms of what he could achieve. The positive adage, "Today is the first day of the rest of my life," should be reexamined in terms of individual potential.

If one looks for the negative side, the therapeutic leverage loses its reason for being. We all know people who have made slighting remarks about prominent people as if they were comparing them with the ideal. The human element of a person is lost in these remarks. What does stand out, however, is the unforgiving quality of the remark. In that context, who can be expected to change or grow and who can be helped?

Feelings about an individual's ability to change may be evaluated by looking at one's own capacity to change. Frequently, a low achiever in high school will do an about face and become a high achiever in college once he identifies with what it is he wants.

In American politics there are examples of senators, governors, and presidents who were known to suffer from specific behavior disorders. Chronic alcoholics have withdrawn from alcohol and achieved much in public office. People do recover and go on to other important aspects of living.

People who know themselves well say that when teachers or parents had confidence in their ability to develop and grow, they did grow. Those who were unfortunate in having teachers or parents who thought they would not make it usually were the ones who did fail. The expectation and positive attitude of the senior helping person determine in large part what the child or patient will do. Supportive encouragement by a person important to the patient, coupled with an optimistic expectation for the individual, will be effective in helping the patient develop and grow.

Feelings of omnipotence and omniscience

Nurses and others in the helping professions sometimes feel that they are all powerful and all knowing. The patient's ideas and feelings tend to be regarded as irrelevant because the professional thinks he can be a better judge of the situation.

The stall occurs when the patient becomes furious with the nurse for not listening to him and for thinking that she knows all the answers. The patient may respond by withdrawing and saying, "Everything is fine with me. I need nothing." Nurses sometimes misinterpret this as "the good patient who has no complaints." The nurse may have the feelings of omniscience that the nursing care is excellent and all patient needs have been met.

The correction of the stall implies that the nurse takes the time to listen to the patient's requests and to his perceptions of the situation. This information is essential in planning the patient care. If the request is unreasonable or the nurse feels that she cannot meet it, this information should be conveyed to the patient so that he knows it was considered. For example, if the patient asks whether or not he may telephone his family, and the staff feels that it would not be helpful to the patient at that time, the patient should be told why he cannot do as he requested. Then this request may be negotiated, thus giving the patient a part in the planning of his care.

Two examples involving a doctor and nurse, who were hospitalized medical and surgical patients themselves, are cited in order to illustrate feelings of omniscience displayed by nurses regarding the administration of pain medication.

Situation 1

A doctor required emergency surgery when he was visiting in a strange town. He did not initially tell them he was a doctor because he felt that it was irrelevant to the situation. Less than 24 hours following his appendectomy he was requesting pain medication every three hours, although he was not wearing a watch and did not know this. A nursing supervisor appeared at his bedside and asked him whether he knew he could become a drug addict the way he was requesting pain medication. He finally could not tolerate this and had to tell the supervisor that drug addiction usually needed a three-week period to develop and not a 24-hour period, and that the pain following surgery does justify medication around the clock.

Situation 2

A nurse was hospitalized for back surgery. The pain was considerable and she requested her medication as frequently as she could but within the "proper" limits. The nurses presented her with such a suspicious attitude that she found herself going through "games" so that the nurses wouldn't think she was a drug addict. In desperation she told her physician who finally decided to handle the situation by allowing her to keep her medication at her bedside.

Part of the problem in these two situations is that nurses somehow feel that they are in a position to judge how much pain a patient is having. Nurses are usually the first ones informed of the patient's pain and are instrumental in determining what and how much medication a patient receives. The nurse will say such things as, "He is getting too much medicine," or "He is not getting enough," or "He needs a weaker dose," or "He needs a sleeping medication."

Nurses should not be placed in the position of judging whether or not the patient is having pain. That is where the problem lies. The only real indicator as to whether or not the patient has pain is to listen to the patient. If he says he has pain, he has pain. All pain hurts. There is no all embracing and infallible measure of pain. You simply cannot prove your pain threshold to someone else; you can only tell them. Nurses somehow feel that they should be able to sense or measure pain as indicated by how much the patient fidgets, is restless, or is contorted and doubled over. If the patient asks in a normal or even off-hand manner for pain medication, the nurse may feel the need to justify this request. She may become annoyed with the patient if she does not feel that he is having enough pain. The annoyance may be reflected onto the patient by making him wait for the medication or saying that the doctor must be consulted first.

When a patient says he has pain, the nurse should first determine what measures are available to relieve the pain. Trying to relieve the pain is being therapeutic; trying to prove whether he does or does not have pain is psychonoxious. The nurse might assess: Has the patient complained recently of pain? Does he complain after he has had visitors or when he does not have visitors? Does he have more pain at night than during the day? What circumstances surround the pain?

In contrast to feelings of omnipotence and omniscience are the feelings of humility and respect — humility in that perhaps the nurse does not have all the answers and respect in that possibly patients can help out by stating requests and needs.

No human being knows all the answers, and certainly no nurse has all the answers to patient situations. There are times when no one is able to provide the answers to a given situation. Very often consultation with colleagues and supervisors is necessary to deal with clinical situations. The important point in correcting this stall is to realize that humility and respect go a long way in facilitating the therapeutic process.

Setting goals

STALLS IN THERAPEUTIC TASKS

The failure to set goals leads to confusion in the treatment triad of patient, physician, and nurse. The stall occurs when one member of the triad does not know all the facts. For example, the patient or the physician or the nurse says, "What is the patient here for?" or "I wonder why the patient has not been discharged?" The therapy is not progressing satisfactorily when these questions are asked. It means that goals have not been clearly defined and communicated. The treatment is then stalled.

The remedy to be used in correcting this stall is for each one to begin communicating with the others to know what is occurring. The negotiation of goals implies that everyone is aware of what is going on in the therapeutic process.

For example, when the overall goal is interfered with, the patient may say, "I don't want to go home." This means that the patient has not cognitively agreed to the overall goal that he is to return to family and community when he has recovered.

When physician and nurse know what the treatment goal is and the patient does not, the patient says, "I don't know what I am doing here. Nothing gets done. No one tells me anything. The nurse says to ask the doctor and the doctor is in and out so fast and he won't give me a straight answer anyway. I might as well leave and go somewhere else if I want an answer."

The patient feels ignored. This behavior disregards the needs of the patient. The patient can share remotely in the therapeutic goal by being verbally passive and doing what he is told or he can be pleasant and uncomplaining, for example, asking only for such minor things as a wash cloth in order to help himself. On the other hand, the patient may absolutely refuse to cooperate. The patient who is uncooperative may receive the label of a rebellious patient and may discharge himself against medical advice. This kind of stall in the therapeutic process tends to be irrevocable.

In order to avoid the stall situation described above, it is necessary that interdependent relationships be established. For the whole to function smoothly, the parts must be synchronized and all must relate to the direction of the goal. The overall goal should include all team members. Each member may then have contributing aims or goals specific to his role.

When the treatment goals are not stated to the patient either before admission to the hospital or within the diagnostic and assessment period, this approach shows inconsideration for the needs of the patient. This method could imply that treatment may be forever and that the patient may never leave.

Beginning staff, not yet aware of what is therapeutic, may tend to compensate for this lack of setting goals by giving the patient that which he can either manage for himself or do without: a pat on the back, several different medications, extra appointment times, or a lecture to the patient's family. As the psychiatric staff member becomes more comfortable with the role and learns the therapeutic tasks, the patient is then seen as a distinct individual with requests and needs of his own.

Being reassuring

Reassurance may be therapeutic when it is based on fact. The surgeon says, "I am reassuring you that you do not have cancer. I have done a biopsy." He has the proof. This is also a supportive statement. If the reassurance is based on truth and concrete evidence, then it is supportive. If the reassurance is not based on truth, the patient senses that it is insincere and this is false reassurance.

The stall occurs when nurses reassure a patient and the patient is smart enough to know that they are unable to really predict or prove the truth of the statement. For example, the patient has had a kidney transplant and the nurse says, "Don't worry, you have the best surgeon and you will be fine in a few weeks." The patient knows that the nurse does not have a solid basis for that information and thus sees her as one who no longer has anything of value to offer. The patient will not find the nurse a useful, supportive, or helpful person. He will probably withdraw and get angry.

Other stall situations that can be called false reassurance are as follows:

Reassurance is sometimes used under the guise of protecting the patient. A patient who has a diagnosis of a terminal illness and has not been told is often the recipient of this kind of reassurance. The patient may say, "I am feeling worse today. I wonder why I still have that pain?" The nurse with good intentions may say, "It should go away. Don't think about it; put your mind on other things." What actually happens is that the response protects the nurse's feelings. This answer to the patient avoids any further discussion. A better response might be, "The pain is making you uncomfortable and is worrying you. What are you thinking?"

False reassurance is commonly observed in dealing with children in pediatric nursing. The goal tends to be to complete as quickly as possible the nursing procedure, for example, when giving an injection or changing a dressing regardless of the patient's feelings. In this service, statements are made such as, "Just a little medicine to make you feel better." The child's concept is here-and-now, not future oriented. Feeling better later does not make sense to him when at present the medicine feels painful. It is best to tell the patient that it will hurt or taste bad and that it is perfectly all right to cry. It is cruel to expect stoic behavior from children or adults. It is therapeutic to encourage genuine feelings.

In another case the nurse says to the patient pre-operatively, "Don't worry, a herniorrhaphy is a very ordinary operation today and you will be up and about within a few days." The nurse's goal is to be supportive to the patient pre-operatively. She feels that her statement is reassuring to the patient. Undoubtedly, the patient will have an uneventful postoperative course. The statistics are heavily in his favor. Nevertheless, the statement is actually denying the patient's concerned feelings regarding surgery. All the patient's real fears and anxieties are allowed to remain untold. Further exploration of the patient's concern is abruptly denied. Verbal reassurance is not supportive when it does not allow the patient to first express feelings of concern.

The nurse in the community talks with a patient who says, "I think I am going crazy." The nurse may then say, "But you don't have any of the symptoms and I don't think you are going crazy." This is nonsupportive reassurance. It is more useful to ask what "crazy" means to the person or what factors are leading him to feel as he does. Nurses should seek out and explore the anxious thoughts if they want to be helpful. This action shows the patient that he is being taken seriously and that the nurse can stand to hear what is going on in his mind. By allowing the patient to express himself, the powerful aspect of the anxiety is reduced to more tolerable limits.

Sometimes well-meaning reassurance can inhibit the patient. For example, if the patient says, "I need love and I can't get it," one response might be, "That is a basic human need and you are not alone in that feeling." This is going from a specific issue (the patient and his feeling) to a general issue (the feeling and everyone's need). This response will put the conversation in more general terms and inhibit the patient from further talking about himself. A more useful remark would be, "What seems to prevent you from getting love?" The second response still supports the patient because he needs to be cared for and it allows him to talk further about his feelings.

Another false reassurance situation is present when the nurse tells the patient he can trust her. This is not particularly effective or reassuring to the patient. The nurse must demonstrate trust and be prepared to have the patient test this before he will accept and agree that she is sincere about him as a human being and in helping him. The patient may ask, "Can I trust you?" The best response in this situation is to tell the patient that he will have to decide that for himself. That response is honest and allows the patient the option to make his own decision.

The stall warning is sounded when the nurse thinks that she is giving reassurance and the patient does not respond. This may be one sign that the reassurance is felt to be false. Some examples of this are:

"Don't worry about your illness. Think about going home."

"You will feel better tomorrow."

"Don't worry about it; everything will be fine."

"Your doctor is very good."

"Lots of people lead productive lives after such an operation."

Other warning lights flash on when you feel a strong urge to leave the room when talking with the patient, or when you hear your own words echoing as you talk, or when you hear yourself saying something that you would not want said to you.

It is normal to attempt to reduce human suffering. When a patient expresses his anxiety, the nurse will often automatically think of reassuring him. The nurse feels uncomfortable in helping the patient bear his anxieties and fears. For example, the patient says, "I am depressed. I don't want to live." At such a time it seems easier to say, "But you shouldn't feel that way. You have much to live for." The stall is corrected by being supportive rather than reassuring. The nurse rectifies the situation by trying to understand the concept of support rather than by giving a reassuring statement.

Confrontation and misuse of the analytical approach

To attempt to treat all dialogue as containing significant psychological messages having deep interpretations is not being therapeutic. People resent this intrusion and sometimes freely say, "Don't psyche me out."

One reason why confronting the patient with a psychological interpretation of his behavior will lead to a stall is because it is inappropriate. For example, a patient is late for an appointment with the nurse and says, "I overslept and I am sorry I am late." The nurse then says, "You must be angry with me and not want to see me or you would have been here on time." The feeling the patient is left with is either total bewilderment or intimidation. That statement is not appropriate or germane to the situation. It is an interpretation of the patient's behavior that may or may not be correct. The correctness of the interpretation, however, is not the issue. These interpretations can stall the therapeutic process.

The interpretation of a patient's behavior depends on the role assumed by the helping person. If this were a psychotherapy hour and the therapist felt the timing of such an interpretation were appropriate, then it might aid in the therapeutic process.

In a role assumed by a staff nurse there are more helpful ways of ensuring that the situation does not stall and yet the patient begins to understand what his behavior means. For example, in the above example a more exploratory approach to the details of the "oversleep" behavior might bring about the patient's understanding that his behavior was based on feelings about the appointment. The nurse might have responded, "Maybe it was easier to sleep through the alarm than to have to get up and come all the way over here for an appointment?" This might lead the patient in a less psychologically exposed way to be able to say that it is indeed difficult to talk to someone about painful issues.

Interpretations of behavior often are given for the shock value they impart. The manner in which they are offered may be and usually is nontherapeutic, For example, a patient is hallucinating and responding to the voices he hears by running up and down the corridor. To confront the patient with an interpretation such as, "That is crazy behavior. We don't want you to act crazy. You must stop," offers no support, understanding, or alternatives for the patient. A more helpful response might be, "I do not understand why you are running up and down. Something must be happening inside you that we do not know about. I will walk with you and see if it helps you feel better so that you can tell me what is upsetting you."

The analytical approach and use of interpretations are very important to seminar and class or staff discussion of patient behavior in trying to understand the patient. It is used mainly for teaching purposes and for understanding behavior—it is not to be conveyed back in an unsettling way to the patient. If interpretation technique is used during a therapy interview, it is done only after careful supervision and is generally not required as an initial nursing approach.

Currently, a large percentage of the people seeking psychotherapy are trying to understand and correlate their current day-to-day methods of either adapting and relating to people or not adapting and keeping people at a distance by using defense mechanisms. These ways of adapting may have less to do with early trauma than with ongoing styles of interacting. In therapy, styles have to be worked through in order to help the patient change and become more adaptive.

Often therapists will think that if the patient has an insight into his problem, he will be able to change. The insight concept, however, often works in reverse with the therapist saying, "Now I understand why the patient does such and such," but the patient does not understand. Therefore, there is no change in the way the patient behaves.

The nursing student is more helpful to the patient by staying with the here-and-now issues rather than trying to explore past history and attempting to make profound interpretations. There is no one simple reason for the illness. The patient's difficulty in living within his present existence is the issue.

Misjudging the patient's independence

The nurse needs to assess and evaluate how much to do for the patient and how much he should do for himself. The stall developing from infantilizing a patient occurs when he tries to exert his freedom and prove to you he can do it. He says, "See, I can go to the bathroom by myself. I don't need the bed-pan." He gets out of bed when he is supposed to remain on bed rest. This behavior is a stall in the therapeutic process.

The patient may try to prove his point by leaving the hospital without permission simply because he was not allowed to go home for the weekend and is angry about the restriction since he felt he could handle the visit. It may be antitherapeutic to punish the patient for this behavior and a better solution would be to reconsider the patient's request and re-evaluate his independence.

The corrective measure is to try not to be oppressive in dealing with the patient when he has overridden the restriction placed on him. The nurse may have to acknowledge that the situation was misjudged and ask the patient what he can do for himself. Or it may be the reverse. The patient tries to go beyond his limits and finds he still needs help from the nurse. For example, a patient may try walking after surgery, feeling he does not need the nurse, but may find after ten steps that he has to sit down. He has over-estimated his capacities.

The stall warning is present when the nurse fails to ask the patient what he can do for himself and she assumes that she knows his limitations. This kind of clinical judgment is not helpful to the patient.

Similarly, as the nurse assesses what the patient can do, the issue of assessing how the family can deal with its own problems is important. For example, the patient may ask to have a phone call made for him or request the staff to tell his wife something. A member of the family may call the nurse's station to say that an uncle has died and will someone please tell the patient. The nurse must remember that these are family matters and that it is the family and the patient's responsibility, not hers. The family should tell the patient unless it has been decided that the family is unable to handle that responsibility.

Doing anything more for the patient than he could do for himself is infantilizing and anything less is withholding. For example, if the child wants to walk and if he is carried, the child resents it. If the child has walked some distance and he is forced to keep walking, that is cruel and negative to his development. A good rule to follow is to do for the patient and family only what they cannot do for themselves. This protects against infantilizing.

Labeling the patient

Labeling the patient instead of describing him or his behavior dehumanizes the person. It is a singular way of not wanting to see the patient as a real suffering person. To label a patient usually implies that the patient bothers the nurse and she has not autodiagnosed her own feelings.

Labeling may be a result of patient requests; for example, "That cranky old man in room 407 who is always complaining now wants another cup of coffee." Or the labeling may refer to the patient's illness; for example, "The appendectomy wants to get out of bed today."

In psychiatric nursing the problem of labeling may be a troublesome area even for seasoned staff. This involves talking about people in terms of their ego control, their delusions, or their schizophrenia. The staff may say, "He is just a manipulator" or "He is just acting out" or "She is just an hysteric." Almost all labeling is preceded by the cliché, "He is just a. . . . This does not describe the patient as an individual who happens to be dealing with an episode of mental illness in his life.

Another stall involving labeling occurs when the statement is made, "The patient is not motivated for therapy." This may often be a way for the therapist to justify his failure to elicit a therapeutic response in the patient. Instead of saying that he is partly responsible for the failure, the patient is blamed for not "being motivated."

Labeling may be viewed as a defense for the nurse. The labeling may occur when it is too difficult to see the person as a human being because his suffering is so great. For example, the nurse may think, "I don't want to think of Mrs. Jones as a person because she is about to die. It is easier to call her the cancer patient in room 389."

The corrective measure to the stall would be for the nurse to acknowledge her feelings and be painfully honest in her reaction. If the nurse does not like a patient, she should admit it to herself, and she should not call the patient a name. She has to admit to herself, at least, that the patient makes her uneasy.

Labeling is sometimes done in the service of diagnosis. It is important to remember that a psychiatric diagnosis accounts for a small percentage of the patient's behavior. Labeling sometimes seems to convince people that they know more about the patient than they really do. Labeling seems to make the professional feel better, as though he understands the situation better. If nurses do not have to label a patient, they are then free to see the patient as a real human being in distress. This view facilitates the therapeutic process.

Overidentification with the problem

Overidentification with the patient and his problems is another human reaction of staff and beginning students that brings about a stall. For example, the patient will tell about his belligerent wife and the student agrees with him and says, "I know how mean she can be." The student continues to see the patient as the victim of his unsatisfactory marriage. The student fails to see that the patient chose the wife in the first place and that the cruelty displayed in the marriage may be equally shared. One often hears a similiar story when listening to a family complain about an alcoholic father. The family says, "Everything is his fault and is his problem. If he didn't drink, things would be just fine." They fail to realize the importance of their role in the situation. A patient simply does not live in a vacuum.

Overidentification with the patient's problem leads to a stall because the therapist says, "I understand your problem" or "that's not really a problem" or "I know what it is like." When you say, or even imply, these things the nurse then becomes a sympathetic person and stops being a nurse. The patient feels that although it is nice to have someone sympathetic, he also needs someone who can provide a different perspective to the problem. If you cannot give him a new perspective, you have nothing to offer. Once you tell the patient that you agree with him, he may like you, but he is then convinced that there is nothing new to be learned and there is no more therapy taking place. Here there will be a stall.

The warning light is on when nurses cannot understand why a patient is in the hospital or they do not see that the patient has any problems or when they feel so much akin to what the patient is describing.

To remedy the stall, the nurse must talk over the patient's vital part of his problem. The nurse can be therapeutic only by helping the patient look at the problem from all sides and view it from different perspectives.

Nontherapeutic involvement

Negative involvement means becoming involved with the patient in a non-nurse way. To feel that one can be the patient's mother, father, sister, brother, lover, or friend is nontherapeutic. Beginning students often face this dilemma and say to the patient that they want to be a friend. This statement presents multitudinous problems.

It is often easier to assume a role one already knows than to work at learning a new one. The beginners in psychiatric nursing may not be convinced that they can be therapeutic. They feel that at least they can offer friendship. It is one thing to be friendly and another to be a friend. Nurses may want to be friends because they feel they cannot be therapeutic in any other way. As one develops therapeutic skills and more expertise, one learns how to put limits on friendships in order to be a therapeutic person.

The stall occurs when the nurse is the friend or buddy of the patient because she is no longer the nurse. If the patient does not have a nurse, he no longer has anyone to help him. By definition, the nurse ceases to be the professional. The patient may need a friend and he may ask the nurse to be his friend. He can, however, find a friend more easily than he can find someone who can offer professional help. That is why he is in the hospital or has come to the clinic.

A friend is someone with whom you maintain contact and to whom you may turn at any given time. The feeling of mutual reliance and comradeship is usually present and evident. To talk with the patient about one's personal life and its vicissitudes is not therapeutic for the patient and is strictly within the realm of social conversation. This is what one does with friends and acquaintances. This limit to the relationship does not mean that the patient should know nothing about the nurse for this would be equally unreal to the relationship. The same phenomenon may occur in the parent-child relationship in which the mother feels that it is modern and beneficial to be a friend as well as a parent to her child. Almost all children find it difficult to listen to parents' problems or to know how to relate to them. Children want parents to be parents. Patients want professionals to be professionals.

An example of this was evident at one mental-health clinic where many hippies came for help. The doctor felt that he should be like them in order to relate to them better. He removed his tie, grew long hair, and used the language of this group. The hippies became angry because they wanted the professional to be professional and they did not want someone resembling their own group. That is why they came to the clinic.

Once the helping person abdicates the therapeutic role, therapy stalls. Correcting the stall means developing therapeutic skills so that the nurse realizes the actual power she has as a nurse and as a therapeutic person.

A good rule of thumb to follow is to discuss with the patient only those facts regarding one's personal life that are public knowledge. To discuss a situation that is relevant to a friendship tends to be non-nurse oriented. Nurses who tell a patient they want to be a friend promise many things that they will be unable to fulfill. Do not try to provide something that the person can find elsewhere.

There are other nontherapeutic involvements. To call the patient at home about something that is not concerned with a goal-oriented issue or to accept a patient's invitation for a social evening is to develop a personal social relationship that is a non-nurse one.

Being honest and telling it straight are important therapeutic techniques especially concerning role appropriate attitudes and behavior. For example, it is natural for some patients to want to relate to the nurse in a nonrole appropriate manner and they will ask such questions as, "Would you date me?" or "Could I have your phone number?" This frequently happens with young people and should be dealt with as a therapeutic issue, not as a social request.

Patients will deny the reality of the hospital setting and blurt out this feeling during their interaction with staff. To go along with this denial is not therapeutic.

It is important to make it clear that it is a nurse-patient relationship and to define the limits of the relationship. When the patient makes such requests as wanting to see the nurse on off-duty time or after the psychiatric nursing experience ends, one sometimes has to say that there are some difficult feelings to bear when relationships end.

Dealing with the patient's wishes to have a nonprofessional relationship by saying to the patient, "If you weren't a patient, I would give you my phone number" is another stall to avoid, for a week later the patient may be discharged from the hospital and he may then phone for a date. By not dealing with the reality initially, a more complicated scene now develops. The question becomes What can the nurse now deliver to the patient and what has she promised? A better solution to that original situation would have been to have autodiagnosed one's reaction initially and have brought it up for discussion with staff members, the instructor, or supervisor. If one is unable to step back to view the situation clearly, others may be able to help.

The patient is in the hospital because he is genuinely ill. His illness is serious and the nurse must be serious about therapeutic involvement. As long as one's actions and words make clinical sense, the involvement is therapeutic.

Bearing painful feelings

The inability to help bear the painful feelings of another person can lead to a stall. Nurses may feel so helpless or angry or incompetent that they wonder if they can be of help. They feel drained, as though they have nothing more to give, and consequently they withdraw. The warning of the potential stall comes when they feel that they want to withdraw.

The corrective approach to this stall is for the nurse to autodiagnose the feelings of anger and helplessness and then to look calmly at how the patient's pathology fits into the situation.

In the general hospital setting this stall in patient care is often seen when one is nursing the dying patient. The staff feel so uncomfortable and inadequate in helping the patient with the dying process that they isolate the patient and withdraw to allow him to die alone.

An example in the psychiatric setting illustrates how difficult it is to tolerate the feelings of anger that a patient expresses as she yells and screams at a nursing student.

> A nursing student was assigned to talk with April, a 29-year-old airline hostess who had been hospitalized for a three-month history of drug abuse and depression. The student entered her room and immediately had the impression of being backstage in an actress' dressing room. Perfume hung in the air; clothes and make-up were strewn everywhere. The student introduced herself and asked to talk with April about her hospitalization. April carefully looked the student over, threw her head back, and laughing loudly said, "Now I've heard everything. I'm assigned to a little student nurse who looks 12 years old and wet behind the ears. I'm supposed to tell you my problems. That is ridiculous. Get out of here, little Miss Nightingale." With that, April started to yell, grabbed a book, and threw it at the student.

Needless to say, this patient's behavior is not the kind that produces a cordial therapeutic nurse-patient relationship. The important step to be taken here is to learn how to accept and adjust one's own feelings when the patient's behavior is so upsetting and obnoxious.

An alternative is to talk out these feelings with other people. This particular situation would be best handled at a staff or nursing report meeting to see what reaction other staff members were receiving. This collaboration will indicate how much of a pattern there is to this woman's behavior.

Bearing painful feelings is a difficult task, but it can be one of the strongest aspects of facilitating the therapeutic process.

Misuse of honesty

Being dishonest with the patient is a subtle and often unintentional act by the staff. Insufficient regard for this concept of honesty in a relationship may stall the therapeutic process.

If the patient feels that the nurse is not being honest with him, he simply will not trust her, and without trust there is no therapy. This is the stall. In order to correct the stall, the nurse may have to discuss the situation with the patient again and admit that she was wrong. If the nurse knows that she has done something dishonest to the patient and the patient withdraws, she should then assume that she has stalled.

Situations having stall potential of this kind are the following:

1. The nurse promises something to the patient and fails to meet the promise. Setting an appointment hour and not being punctual or saying that you will get a certain medication and then not coming back with it may imply to the patient that you are untrustworthy. Such responses as telling the patient that everything will be all right when it won't be or telling him that he will be better in a certain length of time are dishonest.

2. The nurse does not answer a simple, direct question truthfully. The patient may ask if you are angry or upset. He is asking directly and openly about a feeling he thinks you have. If you immediately deny this when you are really angry, this may tell the patient that you are not always truthful. This may also confuse him and increase his anxiety about his judgment of people's emotions. Do not forget that facial expression, tone of voice, and gestures may say more than words, and they can be interpreted by the patient as accurately as by anyone else.

If the patient asks you if you are bored, you may feel you do not want to answer directly that you are. You might say, "Sometimes I feel you are trying to bore me." There are subtle yet effective ways of dealing with the honest answers to patients.

The various responses that can be made are more thoroughly discussed in Chapter 10. If students are to be at all adept in human relationships, they must treat patients with as much respect as family and friends are treated. In other words, one simply does not blurt out to friends such immediate responses as "I don't like you when you stay in your room all day" or "You make me angry when you pout like that." Children are prone to telling friends they are "stupid" or "dumb" when the friends have hurt them or made them angry. This is a defensive purpose with the child. It is neither kind nor respectful. If negative comments are felt appropriate, they are usually best stated in terms of the behavior that is annoying. Here, tact, common sense, and diplomacy are needed and bluntness and dishonesty should be avoided. Treat your patient as you would want to be treated at all times.

3. The nurse is dishonest by omission. Neglecting to tell a patient of a conversation that you had with his family may prove difficult to handle when the patient finds out about it. And the patient inevitably does. This situation may be compared to the academic situation in which a previous instructor talks with a current instructor about a student's performance. The student usually finds out and inevitably has feelings about it.

Pitfalls in listening

After one has attempted to listen, it should be helpful to review the following pitfalls involved in listening that may lead to a stall situation:

1. The nurse becomes so verbal during the interview that she forgets to listen. The patient begins to think that the nurse is thinking ahead about what should be said next, rather than listening to his present thoughts. The nurse would rather hear herself talk and thus the therapy stalls.

In psychiatric nursing one needs to understand and distinguish between being therapeutically active and therapeutically passive. The nursing student often has difficulty in developing the skill of becoming therapeutically passive in the interview situation. Passive in this case does not mean to imply simply "doing nothing," but rather denotes being mentally alert and active. This process implies having an open mind and being able to absorb verbal meaning by listening attentively and with eager understanding.

2. A second pitfall to avoid in listening is that you may become involved in making decisions or giving advice to the patient. Not all advice leads to making decisions for patients, but some does.

The stall in the therapeutic process is that once you give advice or make a decision for a patient, you are taking away the patient's opportunity to do something for himself. You are taking away the therapeutic process.

The potential for the stall to lead to a permanent block in the therapy is there if you give the advice or make the decision. There isn't much that you can do to correct the stall at this point except hope that the patient is similar to most people and will not take your advice. For example, a nursing student wonders about her decision to become a nurse and says to a friend, "I don't know if I want to continue studying to be a nurse." It would be defeating to have her friend respond with, "Of course you do. It is helping people. You should not change your mind." This does not at all agree with the student's feelings at the time. She is seeking help in thinking through her own thoughts in order to work out the problem. She does not want someone else to tell her what she should do.

Another situation illustrates how giving advice can be antitherapeutic: Almost all people have felt troubled or upset and have tried to seek out a friend for solace and understanding. When the friend interrupts what he is being told and prematurely gives advice, the person probably becomes annoyed, for what he really means is, "Be quiet and listen to me. I have something to tell you and please be a good listener." This wanting to be listened to is what the person in distress is attempting to tell the friend. Dominating the conversation rather than encouraging the dialogue is not helpful. People will often say, "Give us some advice," but what they really want to hear is what the other person thinks about the situation. Too often people get caught saying, "Why don't you do this and this" or "Shouldn't you have tried such and such?"

For example, a student fails a test and thinks that she may not pass the course because of this. She seeks out a friend with whom to express her distress. When the student says, "I feel like I'll never get my R.N.," the friend says, "You shouldn't feel that way." In reading this, one might note his own subjective response to the "supportive and reassuring" statement. The student may feel angry because she wanted to be listened to and not told what to feel. She really does not want advice because people do not generally take advice. The helping person provides the suggestions, but the student will make the decision and feel that it was a positive step for her rather than feeling that it was someone's advice.

Giving advice may be used as a maneuver by the nurse in order to control the patient. The patient may feel that he has to please the nurse and to act out of compliance, and, of course, almost all people react negatively to this control.

3. The nurse can stall the interview by responding in an indifferent manner and by presenting a bored appearance—faking attention, avoiding eye-to-eye contact, interrupting, and frequently requesting the patient to repeat what he has said. The stall warning occurs when you find yourself becoming bored, at which point you must stop to autodiagnose in order to determine who is producing the apathetic response—you or the patient. One possible correction of this stall is for you to listen carefully to the patient in order to determine whether or not he is deliberately trying to bore you.

4. The use of emotionally charged words in the course of the dialogue may stall the interview. Introducing a word that the patient cannot tolerate can quickly induce the stall, for example,

> *Patient:* My mother is always complaining and picking at me for not getting up in time or for not cleaning my room.
>
> *Nurse:* Your mother makes you pretty angry.
>
> *Patient:* Oh no. She is a wonderful person and she always tells me how she loves me. Oh, I have to finish that letter I was writing when you came in . . . .

This example points out the sensitivity of the patient to the word angry. If the nurse had chosen a less emotionally charged word the patient might have continued expressing his feeling.

Some patients can talk about feeling uncomfortable about or displeased with their negative feelings, but others find the use of the words "anger" and "guilt" upsetting if they are used before they have said them themselves. Part of the skill in listening to the patient is in using low-keyed words such as "upsetting" or "uncomfortable" or to simply ask, "How did you feel about what she did?" When the patient feels comfortable and more familiar with his own feelings, he will choose his own words to illustrate his feelings. Once the patient has used a word, it is helpful to use that back to him.

Another example in which the patient becomes verbally angry occurred when a psychiatric resident physician was interviewing a male patient. The man said, "My wife is hallucinating and she even managed to get herself admitted to a hospital." The resident said, "How long has she been acting crazy?" The patient yelled back. "My family isn't crazy. What do you mean?"

Sometimes the stall can actually be seen developing when the patient cringes or blanches when a particular word is used. The corrective remedy is to become adept at only using words that the patient first uses.

5. If the nurse changes the subject during the interview, the patient will think that the nurse really cannot stand to hear what he wants to say. If you cannot stand to hear what he wants to say, then the therapy is in a stall because you are not talking about what is important to the patient.

The stall warning appears as the nurse observes the patient disengaging from the conversation. This phenomenon may also be observed through reviewing process recording notes or in supervision.

To correct the stall you might try to find out why you cannot bear to hear what the patient is saying. You might ask yourself what unbearable feelings you have that prompts you to change the subject. It is therapeutic to stay with the issue that the patient introduces.

6. When the patient feels he is not being understood, he will keep repeating the same complaint or request. Repetition means that he is not being understood and this creates a stall.

Correcting the stall means paying strict attention and listening carefully to what the patient is saying.

There are three kinds of understanding: First, there is the distinct understanding of what a person is really talking about. The person is clear about the issue, his feelings, and actions. What he says can be clearly understood.

Second, there is the understanding that requires discussion until there is satisfaction with the explanation. For example, a patient complained of a headache and kept requesting medication for this symptom. Repeatedly aspirin medication was utilized by the patient until the nurse finally decided to explore further the nature of the headache in order to determine why there was no relief. It turned out that the headaches were voices talking to the patient in a deprecatory manner and were causing her great distress. The medication was not effective in relieving the headaches.

Third, there is the listening between the lines for the indirectly expressed messages. The listener must try to get a clear picture from the message, for example:

> A woman called her doctor at 5 A.M. and said to him, "I have nothing to do today." The doctor was angry at her for calling at that hour and quickly terminated the conversation. Since she had never done this before nor spoken like that before, it became clear to him that another message was being given. The doctor checked into the situation and found out that her father had just died. She had devoted her days to taking care of him. She was trying to tell the doctor that her father had just died, but what came out was that she had nothing to do that day.

The point to be made here is that when a message does not seem clear, it may be helpful to keep working on what one thinks the person is really trying to say. When you feel something is not right, you are prompted to investigate further. The clearer the message from the sender, the greater the therapeutic stance that can be taken.

SUMMARY   The analogy of an airplane stall to the practice of being therapeutic was made. A stall does not mean that the airplane is going to crash or that the therapeutic process is going to be irrevocably impaired. A stall means that corrective measures are needed in order to remedy the situation so that the plane may continue its path of flight or the therapeutic process may continue to be a helpful experience to the patient.

Specific and general stall situations were described. Stall warnings, as well as the corrective maneuvers applicable to the situation, were identified. In this chapter we discussed stall situations that are relevant to behavioral style, judgmental feelings, ambivalent feelings, rescue feelings, feelings of pessimism, feelings of omnipotence and omniscience, setting goals, being reassuring, confrontation and misuse of the analytical approach, misjudging the patient's overidentification with the problem, nontherapeutic involvement, bearing painful feelings, misuse of honesty and pitfalls in listening.

REFERENCES AND SUGGESTED READINGS

Brown, Norman et al. (1971). "How Do Nurses Feel about Euthanasia and Abortion?" *American Journal of Nursing,* **71,** No. 7, 1413–16.

Cuthbert, Betty L. (1969). "Switch Off, Tune In, Turn Off," *American Journal of Nursing,* **69,** No. 6, 1206–11.

Davidites, Rosemarie (1971). "A Social Systems Approach to Deviant Behavior," *American Journal of Nursing,* **71,** No. 8, 1588–89.

Freund, Heidi (1969). "Listening with Any Ear at All," *American Journal of Nursing,* **69,** No. 8, 1650–53.

Goldsborough, Judith D. (1970). "On Becoming Nonjudgmental," *American Journal of Nursing,* **70,** No. 11, 2340–43.

Jacobs, Linda M. (1970). "Beginning Practitioner's Adjustment to a Psychiatric Unit," *Nursing Outlook,* **18,** No. 10, 28–31.

Thompson, Naida D., Martin Lakin, and Betty Sue Johnson (1965). "Sensitivity Training and Nursing Education: A Process Study," *Nursing Research,* **14,** No. 2, 132–38.

INTERVIEWING TECHNIQUES

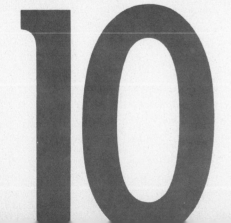

The interview is a structured, time-limited, goal-directed encounter between nurse and patient. It is also referred to as the "one-to-one" interview. Because of its structure, the interview provides the nurse with special therapeutic opportunities in just the same manner as the operating room does for the surgeon. In addition, it also plays a major teaching function in psychiatric nursing, for it is here that the nurse's response to the patient and the patient's response to the nurse can be carefully studied. We can see how goals are defined, how relationships are evolved, and how talking can be therapeutic. Having developed competence at the interview, the nurse can then enhance all contacts with patients in other nursing situations.

Therapeutic interaction between patient and nurse certainly occurs in less formal situations, for example, when eating lunch with the patient, passing out medications, or talking with patients in the corridor. These efforts should not be minimized because for some patients they provide their most meaningful experience during the hospitalization.

In this chapter we will discuss four areas of the nursing interview: the phases of the interview, interviewing techniques, recording the interview, and the interview in various nursing roles.

General considerations

PHASES OF THE INTERVIEW A word should be said about the length of the interview. Generally, the time should not exceed one hour. For patients who are acutely disturbed, severely regressed, or suffering from serious organic impairment, the interview should be informal and brief (5–10 minutes) until the patient is well enough to tolerate regular meetings of increasing periods of time.

For the interview to be optimally successful, the patient should be seen in a quiet place. It is distracting to try to talk in a busy, open ward where there are many patients walking about. Concern for privacy is vitally important. The more insistent one is upon uninterrupted interviewing, the greater

155

the possibility of concentrating on the patient's talking. This also holds true for the patient who is being seen in the setting of the general hospital, the home, or the community. Try to select a quiet, private place to talk.

One's subjective comfort during an interview is essential because you must be able to hear what the patient is saying and you must be receptive to what the patient is having difficulty in expressing. For example, it would be unwise for you to schedule an hour meeting during your lunch hour when you have already missed breakfast. When you are hungry, tired, preoccupied, or unhappy, you are not going to be a good listener.

Starting the interview

If the nurse has not yet met the patient, an introduction is necessary. The formalities of the introduction are important in order that the patient will know who the nurse is and why the interview has been planned.

The process of becoming comfortable enough and establishing a talking arrangement between nurse and patient is not easy. The nurse and patient are two strangers meeting together in a particular setting with the intent of getting acquainted. The following example describes some problems in beginning the interview:

> *Student:* Hello, Mrs. Smith (pause for the patient to acknowledge her name). I am Mrs. Susan Jones from State College and I will be here for the next three weeks as part of my psychiatric nursing experience. I would like to talk to you the days that I am here to get some understanding of your being here in the hospital.
>
> *Patient:* Where did you say you were from?
>
> *Student:* The State nursing program.
>
> *Patient:* That's in town, isn't it. Down by the square?
>
> *Student:* Yes, it is. Perhaps you could tell me about the hospital?
>
> *Patient:* Sure, the hospital is really fine. Good food and nice people. We go down to occupational therapy every afternoon. Want to go down now?
>
> *Student:* All right. (They start to leave.)
>
> *Patient:* Have you seen the ward yet?
>
> *Student:* Oh, would you show me around?
>
> *Patient:* (After walking around.) I've been so depressed. I don't know what to do with myself. I've been here three weeks.
>
> *Student:* What do you do in the hospital during the day?
>
> *Patient:* When did you say you would be back?
>
> *Student:* I'll be back Thursday at the same time to talk about something we decide on today before I leave.

Since the patient understandably wants to know a little about this "stranger," she inquires about the nursing school. The conversation then shifts to the current hospitalization and then to the ward. The discussion of subjects that are relevant but not emotionally charged and the tour of the ward help strengthen the relationship in its early phases. The walking also relieves tension for both patient and student. The patient soon feels secure enough with the nursing student that she begins to discuss her feelings of depression that led to her hospitalization. The student, not quite sure of how to handle the material and not sure that there will be enough time, moves the subject back to hospital activities. The student, given more time and more experience, might have asked the patient to continue discussing her feelings of depression.

For the relationship to develop and for the interview to proceed to the working phase, the patient has to respond positively to the issue that there is something in it for her. She must sense that this relationship, although brief, will be meaningful. She must sense that this "stranger" will respect her, help her bear some of the pain that is in her heart, be trustworthy and honest, and be empathetic. If the patient senses these at the beginning of the interview, she will know that there is something in it for her. Students may erroneously feel that they must be brilliant, insightful, knowledgeable, and full of expert advice. The patient will expect none of these. She will expect neither a trained psychiatrist nor an experienced psychiatric nurse, but rather, a responsive human being.

Many interviews begin with considerable stress and difficulty. The patient may vehemently refuse to talk, he may talk with much tension and anxiety, or he may be furious with the student. At this point Chapters 1 and 2 might be reread to give students an idea of what feelings the neophyte psychiatric nurse and the patient experience. This will help students become more empathetic by putting themselves in the patient's place in order to understand him while still remaining objective. These chapters should help students see and understand that the difficulty most often experienced is part of the clinical situation and that it is not because of any unusual inadequacy within themselves.

At the beginning of the interview the nurse should help the patient be as relaxed and comfortable as possible in order that he can talk. One might say, "It is hard for two people who do not know each other very well to start talking." It might be helpful to just talk about that.

Refraining (in the first interview) from asking the patient to discuss the upsetting details of his hospitalization may help the patient who is especially reticent. On the other hand, many patients will start talking immediately once the nurse has made the introduction. One must account and adjust to the differences in talking styles and then relate to the patient at his own pace.

Once the patient relaxes and begins to talk, the working phase of the interview begins. Again, with some patients this transition occurs immediately, but with others it may take several meetings. For this reason it is a good learning experience for the student to have several patients in order to note differences in the evolution of the interview.

A common reason for an unsuccessful interview is the failure to define the goal and the nature of the relationship at the start. For example, a student may only be able to see a patient for one interview. Unless this is made clear, the patient will be justifiably annoyed when the nurse fails to return.

The student could have avoided this by saying, "I am a nursing student. I will be here for a single hour but I would like to try to understand some of the things that brought you here." The goal and the nature of the relationship are honestly stated. The patient can either participate in the interview or she may refuse.

Working phase of the interview

The goal of the interview is developed in the working phase. To accomplish this, the nurse must continue to relate in a manner that the patient will find helpful. Only then will the patient find it worth his while to proceed to discuss important but painful matters.

Observing the patient

The unobtrusive observation of the patient is an ongoing activity throughout the interview. What is evident about the patient from his mannerisms and his style of communicating all contribute to a better understanding of him.

Generally, the nurse will focus on the patient's words, his mood, his emotions, and what he says or does not say. Observing the patient's appearance and the characteristics of his communication provide basic information. A keen power of observation is a much desired quality in nursing.

The initial observations of a patient's facial expression, manner of speaking, use of gestures, and general appearance tell us much about him. It will help us to perceive the thoughts and appraise the feelings that he has about himself. We can then assess whether he is oriented or confused, sad or happy, or in contact with us or not. We can possibly determine his social skills and determine whether or not he is regressed and withdrawn.

It is equally important to learn what the patient nonverbally implies as well as what he verbally describes. Almost all people have special ways of expressing anxiety that are often as individualistic as fingerprints. Some will rub their eyes, tap their fingers, fidget, or light cigarettes a certain way. The pitch and tone of a person's voice can express emotions as can the posture of his body and movements and gestures of his limbs. Emotions affect the autonomic system as well as the central nervous system. Changes in breathing accompanied by flushing, signs of perspiration, and evidence of tears may be noted. When observing the patient the student must beware of the pitfall of becoming so intent on listening that the patient receives no response. If the nurse just sits with the patient and appears nonresponsive, the patient will feel unsupported and alone.

A psychiatric resident physician, who was just beginning to treat patients, demonstrates this point. The resident thought psychotherapy consisted of listening passively while the patient talked. His first patient talked for ten interviews and then terminated the therapy. Shortly thereafter the resident and a senior psychiatrist became co-therapists in a group. After several group meetings the resident said to the psychiatrist, "You do a lot of talking; that must be because it is a group." The psychiatrist said, "No, I always do a lot of talking with my patients." The resident then started responding verbally with his therapy patients. One day one of his patients said, "You know, if you hadn't started talking, I wasn't going to come any more."

Being therapeutic is not just watching someone talk. That is being voyeuristic. One must be responsive in order to be therapeutic.

A common misunderstanding on how active the therapist should be stems from the confusion arising between being nondirective and being nonresponsive. To be nondirective is to help someone say what is innermost in his mind, and this may take considerable activity and responsiveness.

Helping the patient to talk

Showing sincere interest in what the patient is saying will generally tell him that he is cared about as a human being. Showing this interest is one way the nurse can help the patient to talk freely. When she does not fully understand what a particular experience or situation means to a patient, she should inquire further and tactfully point out that what he is saying is not clear to her. Where he is able to clarify and explain, the situation becomes clearer and has more meaning to both patient and nurse.

In order to help the patient put some of his difficulties in perspective, the nurse must pay careful attention to details. For example, when the patient tells her that he cannot get along with his parents, she might say, "Can you give me an example? What was the last argument like?" It is more helpful to focus on these here-and-now details of the situation rather than on general aspects.

As a rule, when the patient continues to talk and new material appears, the nurse should be nondirective and endeavor to let the patient maintain the initiative. When progress stalls, she should try to learn why the patient is having difficulty in talking; when the block is discovered, she should emphasize it to the patient as something that should be discussed. With this technique the problem is dealt with directly. For example,

> A 15-year-old patient had been talking well with his nursing student for a number of interviews. Suddenly he became withdrawn, just sat during the interview staring out the window, and responded with sarcasm to any remark of the student. She brought the problem to his attention by asking him what he was feeling that he could not say. He finally said that he thought that she was very pretty, that he liked her but felt this was wrong and bad and so he had stopped talking to her. He felt this was the best way to handle his feelings.

As soon as the feelings were openly expressed, the student helped the patient see that these were human feelings and nothing to be ashamed of. The student could then go on to discuss what the patient would do when he felt he liked a girl in school and how he would handle his feelings of caring in general. Verbalizing his difficulties with the nurse gave him the opportunity to explore and resolve his problem with females in general.

In the nondirective approach the patient takes the lead in the dialogue and the nurse encourages the talk without introducing new thoughts or topics. Techniques that indicate a wish to hear more of what the patient is saying include using such phrases as "yes," "I see," "uh-huh," or by nodding the head and leaning forward. If these techniques are not useful or are not part of one's style, we suggest repeating the last word of the patient's state-ment or saying: "I'd like to hear more about that" or "and?" or "and then what happened?"

Keeping the interview focused on the issue Once the goal has been identified, the nurse must guide the discussion toward that point. Patients will try to change to other topics or issues, espe-cially if and when the subject matter makes them uncomfortable. Patients may also talk freely yet say nothing. Here the nurse's responsibility is to limit irrelevant talk. The patient's right to say what he wants to say does not mean that he can talk aimlessly and without some structure. Therefore, the nurse has a twofold job: she must keep the subject matter strictly to the point and she must aid and support the patient in talking about what is so painful to him and what has made him want to change the subject. For example, the goal for an interview is to understand why Scott withdraws to his room when he is upset.

> *Nurse:* Tell me what happened yesterday morning, Scott.
>
> *Scott:* I was playing table pool and things weren't going right and I broke the cue stick. I decided right then that the rest of the day was going to be bad so I went to my room and went to bed.
>
> *Nurse:* Something bother you about breaking the cue stick?
>
> *Scott:* Sue said you can hammer on things in occupational therapy. Can you?
>
> *Nurse:* I guess so. (Pause of a minute.)
>
> *Scott:* I've been thinking of making a wallet for myself and . . . .
>
> *Nurse:* Scott, we were talking about yesterday morning.
>
> *Scott:* Yeah. (Pause of a minute.) It made me feel destructive.

The patient had been troubled by his feelings of destructiveness. He subsequently tried to avoid thinking about them by changing the subject. He felt enough rapport with the nurse that when she brought him back to the subject, he was able to discuss what bothered him.

In summary, during the working phase of the interview the nurse must be concerned with observing the patient, helping him to talk freely, listening carefully to what he says, and keeping to the issue.

As the time approaches to conclude the interview, the nurse should think back and mentally summarize what has been said and at an opportune time in the conversation bring some part of it to the patient's attention. For example, she could say, "We have a few minutes left and I wonder what our talking has meant and what we have accomplished?"

The conclusion of the interview

A number of methods may be used to conclude the interview. In some cases a specific length of time is designated at the beginning so that at the end of the 30 minutes (for example), the interview is concluded. In some interviews the student may wait for a natural pause in the conversation before con-cluding. This method works especially well with the unstructured interview. Sometimes the patient's ability to tolerate the conversation is the factor that determines when to close the interview. In this situation the patient will show signs of fatigue and/or the conversation will cease to be productive. Regardless of how the conversation is to be concluded, the patient must be warned that the interview is coming to a close. The student may say, "We will have to stop in a few minutes" or "Our time is almost up." This gives the patient a chance to unwind, collect his thoughts, say goodbye, and set the time of the next appointment with the student.

At the end of the interview there should always be a feeling of satisfaction that something of significance was accomplished. There should be a definite closing with both nurse and patient acknowledging that both understood what was said.

It is important to observe how the patient terminates a conversation. This often provides an understanding of how he deals with endings in general. For example, if the patient keeps talking and thereby makes the nurse feel that she can never get away, this might reflect his need to hang on to someone. If he seems angry when the conclusion of the time is mentioned, he may be telling of his anger toward people who leave him.

The final step in the interview is to promptly transcribe impressions of the material into a suitable record. The student may transcribe during the interview, recall the verbatim interaction after the interview, or summarize the data for interpretation. The method is usually determined by the instructor, and the procedure of record keeping will vary from hospital to hospital.

INTERVIEWING TECHNIQUES Helping a person to talk freely depends on how clearly questions are phrased, the kinds of verbal responses given to the patient, and the use of silence. These will be further discussed in order to help students to improve their interview skills.

Phrasing questions

How the question is phrased is most important. Asking a question that can be answered by a "yes" or "no" is least desirable because it elicits little information. Compare the question, "Do you get along with your mother?" with "Can you tell me about your mother?" The first question limits the patient to a simple yes or no response. The second question invites a discussion.

Using emotionally charged words usually yields little in return. If one says, "You know, smoking can cause lung cancer. Do you smoke?" the patient may become reluctant to admit that he does smoke.

The use of a double-edged question generally invites a certain answer, for example, "You don't mind if my classmate sits in on the interview, do you?" "You don't expectorate blood when you cough, do you?" "It doesn't hurt when you bend over, does it?"

Asking two questions at a time is referred to as a double-barreled question. Asking one question at a time is preferred. For example, "Are your children with you or not?" is a double-barreled question. If it is important to know the number of children, their ages, sex, and marital status, the nurse must ask several single questions. It would be better for her to say, "Tell me about your children." The missing information can be subsequently obtained by asking several specific questions.

Some answers to questions will tend to incriminate or embarass the patient. For example, the patient may think that his answers to such questions as, "Do you love your mother?" or "Do you beat your wife?" may be damaging to himself. The interviewer can learn much more by asking, "How do you feel about your mother?" and "What is it like between you and your wife?"

Use clear, simple words that are familiar to the patient. The patient should not be asked if he hallucinates if it is possible that he does not know the meaning of the word. Words that the patient normally uses are the words the nurse should use. For example, when the patient says, "I just sit around and feel bitchy at everyone," the nurse could ask, "What happens when you feel bitchy?" If the nurse substituted the word disagreeable or grumpy for the word bitchy, a different meaning of the word might result. Certainly some of the feeling would be lost. To help clarify confused feelings, the nurse should encourage the patient to use words of his own choosing.

Questions that needlessly increase anxiety should not be asked. This may occur when the nurse pursues a line of thought totally unrelated to the needs of the patient. For example,

> A nurse was being examined in the emergency room for a back sprain following a car accident. She began to notice more doctors coming in and asking her about a pigmented area on her foot, a condition she had always had. The attention they were giving her soon caused her to become suspicious when one doctor asked, "Has the food been tasting a little differently lately and who usually eats with you?"

> She finally asked what they were trying to find out. They told her the patch area on her foot looked like an arsenic poisoning patch. It turned out the resident had just seen a case in which the husband had been poisoning his wife with minute doses of arsenic in her food. With that case fresh in his mind, the patch on the nurse's foot reminded him of this and he wanted to rule out the possibility.

Needless to say, the patient may become alarmed when she is not told the reasons behind the questions. Tact must be used when asking pointed questions that might alarm the patient, yet but must be asked.

The nurse must always endeavor to ask relevant questions. She may ask seemingly irrelevant questions when she is unsure of what to say or how to begin a conversation. Students are instructed to make good use of their limited time with patients while they are carrying out routine nursing procedures. This is interpreted improperly when the nurse spends time on safe, noncontroversial, unimportant topics, for example, the weather. This approach goes as follows:

> *Nurse:* Good morning, isn't it a lovely (or cloudy) day today?
> *Patient:* (Looks preoccupied and mumbles something under his breath.)
> *Nurse:* I want to make your bed and help with your bath. That storm they had in the west was really something. I heard it was so serious that (on and on) . . . .

In this situation the nurse goes into the patient's room with her agenda already outlined: to talk to the patient about the weather. Usually, the last thing on a patient's mind is the weather unless he happens to be going sailing that day. Such topics as the weather, current news events, and community events are usually covered in detail by visitors and they help to keep the patient up to date on these issues. Nurses, in all good faith, feel that they should try to take the patient's mind off his worries and that they should be friendly and cheerful and talk only about pleasant topics. Unfortunately, this approach tends to protect the nurses from their own feelings of discomfort and is not therapeutic to the patient.

To be therapeutic in this situation means that the patient is encouraged to take the initiative in an unstructured conversation. If the patient initiates the topic of the weather or the world situation, that is different and may be responded to within the patient's frame of reference. The nurse should be responsible for the questions initiated and see to it that the questions make clinical sense. To avoid irrelevant and nontherapeutic questions, the nurse may simply say, "While I am making your bed, we can talk about any of the concerns you have here at the hospital or about the thoughts that are uppermost in your mind." This gives a wide enough range to enable the patient to really speak his mind if he so elects. If he does not wish to respond, he will then probably choose an unimportant and superficial topic.

The timing of questions is important. The more positive the relationship, the wider the range of questions one may ask. Talking with the patient about a painful or sensitive issue, for example, previous failures, is more likely to be fruitful during the fourth interview than during the second. The patient should have the opportunity to move at his own pace and the nurse should not bring up an issue prematurely by asking probing questions even though they seem important at the time.

A direct approach is useful when serious concern for the patient's ability to control his behavior arises. The patient may have to be asked directly whether or not he is having suicidal thoughts. The psychotic patient may have to be asked how troublesome the voices are or what the voices are saying. The impulsive patient may have to be asked how much control he has and how much freedom he can handle without getting into difficulties with drugs or with the police.

In conclusion, how questions are phrased can add considerable mileage to the freedom the patient feels as he expresses himself. The nurse should think about what important issues there are to discuss with the patient and try to have the questions phrased as clearly and as simply as possible.

Kinds of verbal responses

Certain responses to patients will elicit the therapeutic gains at which the nurse aims. Highest priority is given to responses that bring about *understanding*. We have already discussed the positive benefits that derive when one feels understood.

The attitude that contributes most to bringing out this response is empathy. The nurse's understanding and sensitive reactions to the patient are empathetic feelings. In other words, if the patient says that he feels depressed and the nurse reacts insensitively by asking, "What do you plan to do today?" her response indicates a woeful lack of understanding. If the nurse, however, says, "I can understand; look at what happened yesterday," she implies that she is aware of the reason for the depression and can help the patient to explore the feelings. If the nurse does not know why he is feeling depressed, a useful reply would be, "Let's try to understand why you are feeling depressed today."

The closer the patient can come to putting the content of what he says in proper perspective with regard to how he feels, the greater the understanding and the resultant control of the situation. For example,

Patient: My grandmother treats this new boarder just like one of us. She asks him what he wants and gives him what he likes to eat and all. We just fight the same as always.

Nurse: You speak with feeling about this.

Patient: Damn right. I can't stand her. I just want to get out of the house.

Nurse: What are the fights over?

Patient: My not working and not giving her any money.

Nurse: Sounds as though you fight hard with her?

Patient: Yeah, and we get nowhere.

Nurse: Is there any agreement between you two?

Patient: I've never thought about that.

In this situation the nurse helps the patient express his feelings. Then the patient and nurse are free to discuss the feelings the patient is struggling with.

Instead of the nurse's just repeating a phrase or expression of the patient, she should try to use a nonstressful word in order to see if the patient can relate to that feeling. For example, if the patient says, "I hate to go to school," and the nurse says, "You hate to go to school?" this is circumventive. In other words, the chance of repeating this issue over and over is highly probable. This approach may be helpful to a patient who cannot move verbally by himself and the repeating of a phrase keeps him aware that the nurse is with him, but some patients may think the nurse sounds more like a mimic or that they are not speaking clearly enough.

It may be more useful to phrase a response, "What I hear you saying are your strong, yet unpleasant feelings about going to school." This may bring out feelings other than the hate already mentioned.

A thoughtful reflection of that feeling would be a skillful maneuver by the nurse in responding in an understanding and in a helpful way to the patient.

The *probing* response is useful in trying to obtain necessary information. It is most frequently used in clinics or in doctors' offices. Almost all responses by nurses tend to be in question form in order to gain the information that they need.

The probing technique helps the nurse and the patient move from the general category to the particular. For example, the patient is describing the general chaotic situation in which he lives at home. The nurse should then try to focus attention on the particular situations that are chaotic, for example, the strained relationships in the family or with other people who are involved with the family.

Probing is used in order to help focus from the general to the more particularly sensitive areas of discussion. If the patient says he is always fighting with his wife, the nurse might try to find out the specific reasons for the discontent. Are they caused by financial, health, or in-law problems?

A response similar to the probing technique is the evaluative response. It is used when a judgment is made of the patient's feelings and the patient is then advised about what he should or should not do. For example, the patient may be told to stop smoking because it is harmful to his lungs. This approach is most often used in general nursing and in medicine. Since the patient can neither diagnose nor prescribe for himself, the doctor does so in terms pertinent to the disease and to the medical treatment. The nurse complies with the nursing measures in the care rendering services. For example,

> The patient had abdominal pain. His condition is evaluated and a diagnosis of peptic ulcer is made. Nursing measures are included in the hospital stay. Medicine is prescribed after discharge. Teaching the patient about his diet needs in rehabilitation terms and preventive aspects is part of the evaluative response the nurse will make.

It is important to differentiate between advice giving and information giving. We have previously described the pitfalls to be avoided when giving advice. Realizing that advice is so often rejected and that people feel better when they make their own decisions, we suggest information giving as the alternative to advice giving. For example, the patient says, "My boyfriend is so hard to get along with. What do you think?" A helpful response would be to evaluate by saying, "Let's see, you have already identified your main difficulty with him as a problem in talking with him and with his being insensitive to what you want. What do you want to try first? What possibilities can you think of?"

This implies that there may be other ways of dealing with the problem; here is an area in which to keep evaluating with the patient. In this way the patient can arrive at her own decision, with the nurse's help, rather than having to try out someone else's ideas. People do not mind half as much making their own mistakes as they mind making mistakes suggested by other people.

A nurse may respond to her patient in a *reassuring* manner. This technique is used when there is a concrete basis on which to reassure the patient. It is a universal feeling to want things to be ideal, but reality often denies this. Reassurance is limiting because the nurse may be unable to reach the patient's feelings about the situation.

When a group of nursing students asks the instructor if she feels that they will pass her course, the students are looking for reassurance that they will. The instructor cannot assure them of that. Part of life is learning to live with the uncertainties that exist and it is well understood that nurses try to deny these uncertainties and thereby attempt to reassure their patients because it helps to calm their own uncertainties.

Avoid offering reassuring comments to the patient that may prematurely end an issue of discussion. If a patient is telling of his destructive feelings, the nurse should not say, "Many people think such thoughts." More useful responses would be, "When do you get these feelings?" or "What do you do when you get these feelings?" These comments are also supportive to the patient.

The last response to be discussed in this chapter is the *hostile* response. It is usually imparted by the nurse when she is either exasperated or angry. When the patient causes the nurse to become angry, the nurse retaliates with hostility. This is often seen in situations involving adolescents who, because of their age, tend to be hypercritical and condemning of authoritative situations. Following is a typical scene:

> *Nurse:* You have broken restrictions twice today by leaving the unit when you were not supposed to and staying on the telephone 30 minutes when the time limit is 5 minutes. What do you have to say about it?
>
> *Patient:* This place is a dump anyway. Who do you think you are telling me what to do? Why don't you stay at home and take care of your kids so they are not shipped off to a place like this when they are my age. I'm not doing what you say.
>
> *Nurse:* An attitude like that isn't very adult. I thought you wanted to be free and independent. Isn't that why you have grown your hair long and quit school?

And on it goes. The nurse is responding to a raw nerve hit by the patient, and back and forth the hostility ball goes. Needless to say, it is not therapeutic.

Hostile remarks are often made in order to defend against feelings of inadequacy. A student may say that a certain program she was involved in was of poor quality. She states that she did not learn a thing and that she would never recommend that anyone take the program. It is clear that this student speaks with a strong and obviously negative feeling. An objective evaluation of the program has to be ruled out. It is cautioned to be wary of totally negative comments because the subjectivity and bias are so obvious.

Sometimes hostile comments may be made about patients when the nurse is at the nursing report and feels that the patient cannot hear the adverse remarks. Hearing someone talk negatively about you is neither a pleasant experience nor a therapeutic one in the hospital or out. When there are negative or hostile feelings to be verbally expressed about the patient, it is always good policy for the nurse to say openly only what she would say to the patient's face as well as behind his back.

In summary, we have discussed the responses of understanding, probing, evaluation, reassurance, and hostility. The nurse should aim for the understanding response. This goal implies that the nurse must be responsible for what she says and does.

Using silences

Silences may be awkward to handle for the beginning psychiatric nurse. Nevertheless, they may be worked with and used as an ally. It is wise to let one or two silences develop during an interview. Let the patient break the silence since what he then says spontaneously may be of special importance. If the patient seems too uncomfortable with the silence, one might say, "It is helpful to stop and think. You don't have to talk every minute" or "Just say what you are thinking."

If the patient seems obviously disturbed by the silence or loses contact with the interviewer, the nurse should try to help bring him back by asking, "What are you thinking of?" or "What is on your mind now?" or by saying, "You seem to be concerned about something specific."

When the silence indicates unexpressed feelings, such as anger or distrust, the nurse might say, "I sense that what I just said upset you."

When the silence implies a resistance to the interview, the nurse might say, "Something makes it difficult for you to tell me about that" or "Perhaps you are concerned about how I will react to what you tell me" or "We have to figure out why it is difficult for us to talk together." After saying that, there probably will still be a silence until the patient is ready to verbalize the difficulty.

Answering questions

The questions that patients directly ask nurses sometimes make nurses uncomfortable, and the nurses do not know exactly what replies should be made.

Sometimes the patient will ask directly about the nurse's personal life, for example, "Haven't you ever fought with someone?" or "How can you know what it is like to be on drugs? Have you ever tried them?" Some patients feel that they need to actually know of someone's experiences or credentials before they can trust talking with the nurse.

The nurse can respond by turning the question into a therapeutic issue. For example, the nurse can reply, "You feel that my having a similar experience will mean something to you?" or "You feel that my taking drugs would make a difference as to how we worked together?" It is more helpful to suggest talking about the issue than to give an answer. It is doubtful that patients really want an answer, but their curiosity about the nurse as an individual is uppermost in their minds. Or it may be an attempt to avoid the issue. By answering their questions or treating the content of the questions rather than seeing them as part of the developing relationship would be turning the relationship into a social exchange. Patients can talk this way with friends and acquaintances. Remember that the patient needs the nurse primarily to be a nurse, not a friend.

When a patient questions the nurse's credentials, for example, her professional background, she should be honest with him and admit her student status. Then she should try to get the patient to express his feelings about her position. Some patients will be reluctant to talk immediately with a student and perhaps will say, "I tell my doctor all my problems." On the other hand, many patients are relieved to have an enthusiastic and interested nursing student spend time listening to their difficulties. This depends on the individual patient and not necessarily on the experience of the student.

Sometimes a patient will ask a direct question about his illness, "Am I schizophrenic?" or "Will I ever get better?" In medical nursing the patient may ask if he has cancer or if he is going to die. The situations are parallel.

The issue here is what does the question really mean? What does the patient know, how much was he told or not told, and what are the communication plans of the total team?

When a patient asks a direct question about his condition, it is important to start by knowing how much information the patient has and what prompted the question in the first place. The nurse could respond with, "That was an abrupt question to ask. Can you tell me what you have been thinking of to cause you to ask that?" Telling the patient that it would help to look at and explore his thoughts and feelings about the issues defines the therapeutic role and does not place the nurse in a role in which she cannot be comfortable.

Nurses need not feel guilty over not answering specific questions that the patient asks any more than the nurse should feel she is expected to give advice. The patient will benefit greatly if he has to make his own decisions and resolve his own questions that relate to his life. The questions that nurses should answer are those asked when the questions apply to them directly, for example, "Are you angry?" or "Are you busy?" The nurse should answer questions about her own behavior that the patient observes simply and honestly.

Nursing notes in the psychiatric hospital

**RECORDING
THE INTERVIEW**

Nursing notes are invaluable for transmitting the patient's behavioral patterns to the clinical team. The considerable time and effort that go into sitting with and listening to the patient together with the nurse's consistent observation of the patient over the 24-hour period provide important clues to further understanding the patient and his mode of interacting.

How is a good nursing note written? What is important information to include? What does the reader want to see?

Writing relevant nursing notes is fundamental to the planning, implementing, and evaluating of a patient's therapeutic regime. The purpose of writing nursing reports is primarily to communicate and share information with others who are involved in the care of the patient.

As previously discussed, the paramount need is to have a goal in mind when talking with the patient. The same principle is essential when writing a nursing note. Conditions under which nursing notes should be written are as follows:

1. *The individual interview note.* If the patient is being seen in a structured nursing interview, a note should be written after each visit. Included in this note are the goal, issues discussed relevant to the goal, interpretation of the process, and the dynamics of the interview. This note should give the reader the main essence of the interview.

2. *A single situation event.* A situation might arise in which the patient's behavior calls for immediate attention and reporting. For example, the patient receives a disturbing telephone call from a relative, or the adolescent patient, upset from a therapy hour, starts banging her hand against the wall. These situations deserve special notes so that the rest of the staff will be aware. In these notes, accuracy, time, preceding events, quotes, and conciseness are all important.

3. *An overall behavior and mood evaluative note.* The patient's progress over a certain time period (as designated by ward policy) requires a note. Sometimes notes of this kind are written after each shift. In this note the time period of the observation is important.

4. *A conference report.* An admission planning conference or a teaching conference should be reported for the patient's chart. In this note, questions asked during the interview, the patient's verbal response, along with the plans and decisions made, should be included as accurately as possible.

5. *A summary report.* It may be desirable to tie specific observations together covering a 24-hour period. In this report, the highlights, generalities, and the concerns of staff usually will suffice.

6. *Special duty report.* A patient on constant observation or receiving special treatment should be checked frequently for any deviation from his normal behavior pattern. For example, if the patient has been talking incessantly and abruptly sits down and refuses to talk, his change in behavior should be reported in a brief, accurate note.

7. *Problem-oriented record.* Some hospitals use the problem method and the staff uses this format for recording.

Nursing notes in the general hospital

All the information learned about a patient should be communicated to other nurses concerned with the care of the patient. This information will help others to reach the patient. Nurses will sometimes say that since they do not have the entire story, they are reluctant to pass on bits of information. Sometimes in waiting we may never hear the whole story. In the general hospital setting nurses often do not have time to sit and listen to the patient. Therefore, medical-surgical nurses have to make the best use of the allotted time with the patient. They need to talk with the patient to try to learn what he is feeling and then share this knowledge with the rest of the nursing staff.

The patient may be going to the operating room the next day, and what the day shift learns about the patient's fear should be passed on to the evening shift, but often there just isn't time for this information to be passed on. Too often nurses do pick up important information about the patient but fail to pass it on because they do not think that it is relevant. For example, if it is learned that the patient seems to be using denial, the nurse should be sure to communicate that. If when each time the nurse enters the patient's room, the patient purposely evades talking about his illness, or if he says that he does not have the illness, or if he changes the subject, this is significant.

If the patient is complaining a great deal, this information should be passed on, along with the remark that no one knows why he is complaining or that he has not been reached yet. If the patient is upset about the food, the injection he just had, or being late for X-ray, this information should also be included. This information is very different from, "Mr. Jones has been so demanding today. He has had his light on constantly."

Importance of a relevant nursing note

The written word is often a critical test of the viability and soundness of one's ideas. All too often the nurse will feel that there are no ideas or information to put on paper and will seriously doubt that she knows anything about human behavior. This feeling will only postpone or delay the task of writing notes. Following are several suggestions to help formulate thoughts in order to write the note:

1. Be clear and precise in writing. Try to avoid lengthy notes unless describing an involved situation.
2. Use as little special and technical terminology as possible. The note is describing people, not structures and concepts. Framing one's thoughts in everyday language helps in talking with the patient and writing the report.
3. Use the patient's own words and quote whenever possible, and especially in describing psychiatric symptoms, such as delusions and hallucinations.
4. The note should answer the four W's: who, when, where, why.
5. Give specific examples instead of interpretations. Try not to say, "He was angry." Say, "He slammed the door of his room hard" or whatever the action demonstrated was. Write exactly what you observe.
6. Sign the note in order that the reader knows who is making the observation.

The mental status exam

The purpose of the mental status examination is to objectively determine and record observable aspects of the patient's psychological functioning. This contrasts with the history that is based not on observable behavior but on recollections. The performance and recording of a mental status examination have several major functions:

1. It is an agreed upon method of organizing clinical observations.
2. It provides a clinical baseline for a patient's psychological state.
3. It provides specific information that assists in establishing certain diagnoses, for example, organic brain disease.

Traditionally, the performance of the mental status examination has been the responsibility of the physician. We will outline the examination for two reasons. First, the nurses will hear discussion of the mental status examination and will see them in the patient's chart. Second, many nurses, especially those who are seeing patients in the community, are beginning to perform formal mental status examinations with an eye toward referring possible cases of organic brain disease for thorough medical examination.

The mental status examination generally includes the following categories: general appearance and attitude, speech activity, affect, content of thought, and intellectual function.

General appearance and attitude The interviewer describes grooming, dress, motor behavior, gait, posture, facial expressions, mannerisms, and attitude toward the interviewer.

Speech activity The interviewer describes pressure of speech, retardation of speech, blocking, flight of ideas, loosening of association, circumstantiality, rhyming, punning, neologisms, slurring, stuttering, peculiar use of words, tone, spontaneity, productivity, relevance, and reaction to time between questions and response.

Affect The interviewer describes whether or not the mood is appropriate to the thought content, labile, depressed, elated, apathetic, anxious, hostile, negativistic, spontaneous, or fearful.

Content of thought The patient's spontaneous thoughts are described. In addition, note is made of hallucinations, delusions, ideas of reference, obsession, compulsion, phobias, ideas of grandiosity, suicidal or psychotic ideation, and the like.

Intellectual function

1. *Orientation.* The patient's orientation as to time, place, and person. (Does the patient know the date, where he is, and who he is?)
2. *Memory.* Does the patient remember the recent and remote past? Does he have immediate recall for that which was discussed earlier in the interview?
3. *General information.* The patient is tested for a general fund of information by asking him the names of presidents or states.
4. *Judgment.* The patient is asked a question such as "What would you do if you found a stamped, addressed letter in the street?" It is noticed whether or not the patient orients himself to his environment by using good judgment.
5. *Abstract thinking.* The patient is asked to interpret simple proverbs, for example, "Don't cross your bridges until you get to them."
6. *Insight.* To what extent does the patient understand his current situation?

In Part Four (The Clinical Syndromes) it will be seen how diagnostic features of each of the syndromes are captured by the five parts of the mental status exam.

THE INTERVIEW IN VARIOUS NURSING ROLES The various roles of the nurse define the kinds of nursing interviews. Roles must be defined for the patient and if role boundaries change, they must be restated. For example, a role change occurs when a nurse makes a home visit in order to assess the home and community adjustment of a patient whom she previously treated in the hospital. The new role boundary must be defined for the patient. Some of the various roles nurses assume are the following:

1. A nursing student on a psychiatric unit has a specific role and goal. It is a learning situation and the final decisions are not made by the student alone. The patient should also know that the instructor is involved with the learning experience and that there is a dual goal of education and patient care. If a patient has further questions about the student role, he should have an opportunity to talk about the program. Specific questions could be directed to the instructor. The student uses the interview as a teaching tool and receives supervision at all times.

2. Staff nurses on a psychiatric unit have defined and specific roles to which the patient is oriented when he is admitted. The patient knows what he can talk about to the nurses, what limits they will place on him, and how they will be therapeutic with him. He knows that they are part of the clinical team and that they work within the framework of the ward milieu. Staff nurses use the structured interview in planned meetings with the patient. They work out the goal for the interview as part of the ward treatment.

3. Nurse-therapists on a psychiatric unit usually take responsibility for the direct treatment of the patient and work closely with the psychiatrist who is medical adminstrator of the case. They function as therapists and collaborate with the nursing staff in the total treatment of the patient. The nurse–therapist will define for both patient and staff the duration of the relationship, the goals of therapy, and the limits of the relationship.

4. The psychiatric nurse–clinician working within the general hospital defines her role to the ward in which she works with the nursing staff. The structured interview is used to provide staff with more information for the psychotherapeutic handling of patients. The nurse defines this role for the patient and then communicates the findings and recommendations to the staff.

5. The staff nurse working in the general hospital may do a structured interview in addition to regular nursing procedures in an attempt to further clarify specific psychological concerns. The nurse would work closely with the physician in order to maintain a consistent treatment plan.

6. The community mental health nurse is responsible not only for the patient and his present problem, but also for understanding the family and community of the patient. In the interview the nurse must listen for the many facets of the problem in order to make a comprehensive assessment and evaluation of the situation.

7. The visiting nurse or public health nurse working in the community may talk with someone who has not yet defined himself as a patient. Often the interview is used in order to find a social context for the problem. Sometimes the mother who is being seen for a medical problem begins to discuss her 15-year-old son who is frequently truant from school and who may be using drugs. The nurse uses the data from the interview to collaborate with other agencies in order to best handle the community problem, but at the same time is being helpful to the mother.

8. The clinic nurse in a psychiatric outpatient service is part of the clinic team that includes psychiatrist, social worker, psychologist, and rehabilitation counselor. Team members usually take turns conducting the initial interview with the patient, and later they discuss the patient at a team conference so that they can decide on treatment goals. The nurse conducts the initial interview in order to obtain the necessary information for the team meeting. How much time there is available for the interview determines

how direct or open-ended the technique can be. For an indirect method of interview, for example, in the drop-in center or multiservice center, a data sheet to be filled in at the time of interview or immediately following is often provided. The role in this case is to remember sequence and order of events as the patient talks to enable reconstruction of the interview later for presentation back to the team for treatment plans.

9. School nurses who works in either elementary or high school use both the structured and unstructured interview. They see students who have physical and emotional problems, and they assess the need for follow-up care. The school nurse may collaborate with family, teachers, administrators, and the community health center.

10. Nurses who work in an industrial organization are often the only health personnel in full-time attendance. Therefore, they have great responsibility for evaluating many presenting problems. They tend to know the employees who have been to the health office on other occasions. The industrial nurse may then choose to use the structured interview when a new employee arrives. In an emergency the interview is unstructured. The industrial nurse collaborates with family, administration, and community.

SUMMARY This chapter discussed four main areas relevant to the structured nursing interview. The phases of the interview include starting the interview, the working phase of the interview, and concluding the interview. Techniques inherent in the working phase are observing the patient and helping the patient to talk.

The second part of the chapter dealt with such interviewing techniques as phrasing questions, the kinds of verbal responses of understanding, probing, evaluating, reassuring, and hostility; using silences; and answering patients' questions.

The third area described recording the interview: nursing notes in the psychiatric hospital, nursing notes in the general hospital, and the importance of a relevant nursing note.

The fourth area described ten settings in which the nurse uses either the structured or unstructured interview. These are the nursing student in the psychiatric unit, the staff nurse in the psychiatric unit, the nurse-therapist, the psychiatric nurse-clinician within the general hospital, the staff nurse in the general hospital, the community mental health nurse, the visiting nurse or public health nurse in the community, the clinic nurse in a psychiatric outpatient service, the school nurse, and the nurse working in an industrial organization.

REFERENCES AND SUGGESTED READINGS

Bermosk, Loretta, and Mary Jane Mordan (1964). *Interviewing in Nursing.* New York: Macmillan.

Bernstein, Lewis, and Richard Dana (1970). *Interviewing and the Health Professions.* New York: Appleton-Century-Crofts.

Bird, Brian (1955). *Talking with Patients.* Philadelphia: Lippincott.

Field, William (1972). "Watch Your Message," *American Journal of Nursing,* **72,** No. 7, 1278–80.

Goldin, Phyllis, and Barbara Russell (1969). "Therapeutic Communication," *American Journal of Nursing,* **69,** No. 9, 1928–30.

Hardiman, Margaret A. (1971). "Interviewing? or Social Chit Chat?" *American Journal of Nursing,* **71,** No. 7, 1379–81.

Phillips, Lorraine W. (1966). "Language in Disguise: Non-Verbal Communication with Patients," *Perspective in Psychiatric Care,* **4,** No. 4, 18–21.

Reik, Theodore (1956). *Listening with the Third Ear.* New York: Grove Press.

Riley, Mildred (1968). "Nursing Interview for Psychiatric Patients," *Nursing Outlook,* **16,** No. 10, 54–57.

Ruesch, Jurgen (1961). *Therapeutic Communication.* New York: Norton.

Sene, Barbara Stankiewicz (1969). "Termination in the Student-Patient Relationship," *Perspectives in Psychiatric Care,* **7,** No. 1, 39–45.

Ujhely, Gertrude (1968). *Determinants of the Nurse-Patient Relationship.* New York: Springer.

THERAPEUTIC INTERVENTIONS

11

There are various forms of psychiatric-mental health interventions that are essential for nurses to know. Nurses may have the opportunity to directly provide various forms of interventions, for example, individual psychotherapy and family therapy. The dependent function of nursing includes assisting the physician in administering treatments such as dispensing medications and assisting in somatic therapies. Nurses must be alert to possible side effects and dangers of various treatments. Nurses who work in the community must know when they refer a patient to a clinic or hospital. For instance, patients with manic depressive illness should be urged to obtain medical evaluation for possible lithium treatment. Nurses also have the opportunity to engage the patient in occupational therapy activities.

We will describe the psychiatric–mental health interventions under three categories: biologic or somatic, psychological–social, and behavioral. It is recognized that it may be arbitrary to refer to a particular treatment as social rather than behavioral or as psychological rather than social and thus have combined the psycho–social category.

SOMATIC INTERVENTIONS

The use of somatic intervention is an important aspect of the nurse's work with the patient. These interventions are generally classified as dependent nursing functions, for the nurse works in collaboration with the physician or psychiatrist. Standard VI defines this function.[1]

Psychopharmacological agents

The impact of drug therapy as a treatment for mental disorders has been truly revolutionary. With the development of new drugs since the 1950's, greater numbers of people have been able to return to their communities after hospitalization and more patients can be treated without hospitalization.

[1]Congress for Nursing Practice, *Standards of Psychiatric-Mental Health Nursing* (Kansas City Mo.: American Nurses' Association, 1973), p. 4.

STANDARD VI

KNOWLEDGE OF SOMATIC THERAPIES AND RELATED CLINICAL SKILLS ARE UTILIZED IN WORKING WITH CLIENTS

RATIONALE: Various treatment modalities may be needed by clients during the course of illness. Pertinent clinical observations and judgments are made concerning the effect of drugs and other treatments used in the therapeutic program.

Assessment Factors:

1. Pertinent reactions to somatic therapies are observed and interpreted in terms of the underlying principles of each therapy.

2. A patient's responses are observed and reported.

3. The effectiveness of somatic therapies is judged and subsequent recommendations for changes in the treatment plan are made.

4. The safety and emotional support of clients receiving therapies are provided.

5. Opportunities are provided for clients and families to discuss, question and explore their feelings and concerns about past, current or projected use of somatic therapies.

These drugs are classified as antipsychotic (major tranquilizers), mood regulating agents, minor tranquilizers, and sedatives and hypnotics.

Major tranquilizers Four groups comprise the antipsychotic or major tranquilizers: the rauwolfia alkaloids such as reserpine, the phenothiazines such as Thorazine, the thioxanthenes such as Taractan, and the butyrophenones such as Haldol.

The major tranquilizers are all effective in treating symptoms of the functional psychoses; they all may produce extrapyramidal symptoms as side effects; they lower the seizure threshold; they produce little or no physical tolerance or craving.

Reserpine. This tranquilizer is a natural complex chemical found in the juices of an Indian shrub called snakeroot (*Rauwolfia serpentina*). It is rarely used as an antipsychotic since the phenothiazine and butyrophenones are all more effective. Side effects from the drug are depression, hypotension, and upper gastrointestinal distress in addition to the general side effects of the major tranquilizers.

Phenothiazines. The phenothiazines are most effectively used in the treatment of schizophrenia, although they may also be beneficial in treatment of other functional psychoses, mania, agitated depressions, and behavioral disorders resulting from organic brain disease. The antipsychotic effects of the various phenothiazines are similar. The specific drug is chosen for maximizing or minimizing a particular side effect.

177

Commonly used phenothiazines are:

Generic	Brand	Daily Dosage Range
Chlorpromazine	Thorazine	50–1500 mg
Fluphenazine	Prolixin, Permital	1–45 mg
Perphenazine	Trilafon	8–64 mg
Prochlorperazine	Compazine	5–150 mg
Thioridazine	Mellaril	50–800 mg
Trifluoperazine	Stelazine	4–40 mg

Side effects of phenothiazines and management of this medication are as follows:

1. *Subjective discomfort:* Patients may complain of dry mouth, stuffy nose, blurred vision, drowsiness, and dizziness when getting up from a sitting position (associated with orthostatic hypotension).

2. *Dermatological complications:* Photosensitivity is common with discoloration of the skin with itching and burning. Patients should be advised to avoid exposure to sunlight. Allergic skin rashes also may occur.

3. *Blood dyscrasias:* Leukopenia and agranulocytosis have been reported on patients using chlorpromazine. Patients should be advised to report fevers and infections (e.g., sore throat) promptly. Blood counts are then taken, and if a dyscrasia is present, the phenothiazine is discontinued and antibiotics started.

4. *Jaundice:* Most cases of jaundice occur within the first few weeks. If this occurs, the phenothiazine is discontinued.

5. *Convulsions:* Phenothiazines reduce the convulsive threshold and in susceptible patients spontaneous convulsions may occur. Convulsions may also occur if there is withdrawal of an anticonvulsant medication (e.g., a barbiturate; meprobromate) followed by administration of a phenothiazine.

6. *Failure of autonomic reflexes:* Phenothiazines interfere with the autonomic response to stress necessary to raise blood pressure and increase cardiac output. This may endanger the patient who is exposed to unexpected stress.

7. *Accident risk:* There may be a decrease in normal visual, auditory, and kinesthetic perceptions, and in motor skills and coordination. Although people who use phenothiazines are permitted to drive cars or operate machinery, they are advised, for their own safety and the safety of others, to use extra caution and judgment in performing these tasks.

8. *Extrapyramidal symptoms:* Large doses of phenothiazines usually lead to the appearance of Parkinsonian symptoms. These symptoms are tremors, muscular weakness, dyskinesias (defect in voluntary movement), akathisia (jittery movements), dystonias (do not mistake for conversion reaction). Most of these symptoms respond to anti-Parkinson agents such as cogentin or artane.

Thioxanthenes. The thioxanthenes are chemically related to the phenothiazines and have similar therapeutic effects. The brand drugs from this group include Taractan and Navane.

Butyrophenones. Butyrophenones have therapeutic qualities similar to the phenothiazines. However, they are less prone to stimulate the appetite and are less likely to produce orthostatic hypotension. Innovar, Haldol, and Serenace are brand names for this group.

Mood regulating
agents

Tricyclics. The tricyclics, generally the most effective antidepressant medication, are chemically related to the phenothiazines. The commonly used drugs in the treatment of depression are as follows:

Generic Name	Brand Name	Average Daily Dose
Imipramine	Tofranil	150 mg
Amitriptyline	Elavil	150 mg
Desipramine	Norpramin	150 mg
Nortriptyline	Aventyl	50 mg
Doxepin	Sinequan	150 mg

Patients should be told that it will take a period of from 1–3 weeks before the drug will have a favorable effect.

Amine oxidase inhibitors. The inhibitors of momoamine oxidase (MAO) are of lesser clinical importance than the tricyclics. The more popular drugs of this group are Marplan, Niamid, and Nardil.

MAO inhibitors stimulate the central nervous system. The series of changes are similar to those described for amphetamine: wakefulness, euphoria, respiratory stimulation, excitement, and after large doses, a toxic psychosis.

A second effect is sympathoplegic in that postural hypotension occurs and cardiac output is reduced.

Central nervous system stimulants. All of the compounds in this group have a chemical and biologic similarity to ephedrine and amphetamine. The sympathominetic effect is constricted blood vessels, elevated blood pressure and pulse, and dilated pupils. Central nervous system stimulation symptoms are wakefulness, decrease in fatigue, and induced euphoria.

Common drugs of this category are as follows:

Generic Name	Trade Name	Daily Dosage
Amphetamine	Benzedrine	5–15 mg
Dextroamphetamine	Dexedrine	5–15 mg
Methamphetamine	Methedrine	5–15 mg
Phenmetrazine	Preludin	25–75 mg
Methylphenidate	Ritalin	10–30 mg

The clinical uses of these drugs are the control of obesity, as euphoriants and antidepressants, to improve psychomotor performance, to decrease hyperkinetic states in children, and to treat narcolepsy (involuntary lapses into normal sleep).

Because of drug abuse, many hospitals are now restricting the use of these stimulants to the treatment of hyperkinetic states and narcolepsy.

Lithium salts. Lithium salts are being used in the treatment of patients with manic-depressive illness. Maintaining the patient on the medication appears to have a preventive value for future episodes of both manic and depressive episodes.

The medication is given as lithium carbonate. The medication is preferably given after meals to avoid gastrointestinal disturbances. Serum lithium levels are monitored at frequent intervals.

Minor Tranquilizers

The minor tranquilizers or anti-anxiety agents are widely used for the symptomatic treatment of anxiety and tension in nonpsychotic patients. These medications have limited effectiveness; the placebo effect is great; they seem to act as sedatives; they have little specific action. Habituation, sensitivity, and withdrawal reactions may occur with almost all these medications. Although barbiturates also reduce anxieties, the anti-anxiety agents are more effective, less addicting, produce less excitement, and are safer in case of overdoses.

Commonly used minor tranquilizers are as follows:

Medication	Dose	Side Effects and Contra-indications	Comments
Meprobamate Miltown Equanil	400 mg t.i.d. or q.i.d.	Habituation; Sensitivity; Drowsiness; Withdrawal	A mild sedative with a wide margin of safety
Chlordia- zepoxide-HCl Librium	10–20 mg t.i.d. or q.i.d.	Habituation; Paradoxical reactions with ataxia or excitement	Probably more potent than meprobamate
Diazepam Valium	5–10 mg t.i.d. or q.i.d.	Fatigue; Drowsiness; Ataxia	Comparable to Librium
Oxazepam Serax	10–15 mg t.i.d. or q.i.d.	Drowsiness; Dizziness; Excitement	Comparable to Librium
Hydroxyzine Vistaril Atarax	25 mg t.i.d. or q.i.d.	Drowsiness	Safe, nonspecific, probably less likely to be habituating

Sedatives and hypnotics

Hypnotic–sedative drugs have two purposes: to induce sleep and to relieve anxiety. If given in progressively larger doses, sedatives will decrease anxiety and produce sedation, ataxia, general anesthesia, and ultimately medullary depression and death. Repeated and continuous administration causes habituating physical dependence and a withdrawal state.

There is increasing concern that many of the hypnotics lose their potency in a short period of time and that they ultimately interfere with normal patterns of sleeping.

Commonly used hypnotics are as follows:

Medication	Dose	Side Effects and Contra-indications	Comments
Pentobarbital Secobarbital	100 mg HS 100 HS	Habituation Sensitivity Overdose Suicide	Usually preferred for most patients, but not for the elderly or others who have to get up at night. To increase effectiveness, add 50 mg diphenhydramine (Benadryl) or 50 mg chlorpromazine (Thorazine)
Diphenhydramine (Benadryl)	50 mg	Minor atropine-like action	Preferred medication for mild sedation, for the elderly, and for those who react to sedatives by having hangovers.
Chloral hydrate	0.5–1 mg	Long-term use inadvisable— some patients develop "intoxication"	Quite safe; particularly for 5–10 days or while the patient is in the hospital
Sodium amytal barbital combination	200 mg sodium amytal and 200 mg barbital can be given orally (in liquid form) at bedtime to a disturbed patient who needs 8–10 hours of sleep.		
Paraldehyde	10–15 ml	Respiratory insufficiency	Useful for treatment of acute alcoholism

Drug management

After concentrating on the dosage and side effects of the psycho-pharmacological agents, a word relevant to the art of drug management by the nurse needs to be said. Not all patients are eager for medication nor are they totally reliable in self-administration of medication in the home setting. One essential component of ensuring safety in drug management is to engage the cooperation of the patient in his drug treatment. Some patients do not like to take medication because they feel out of control of their lives because of the power of the drugs. If the dosage is ordered four times a day, they may feel that two or three times a day is enough. Some patients feel that any drug is potentially addicting and even the word medication makes them fearful. Teaching about medications and their usage is one of the nurse's functions.

The nurse, especially when working in the community setting, should make detailed inquiries about the patient's method and regularity of taking medication. The nurse may ask specifically how many pills, how many times a day, what does he do if he forgets a dose, does he ever cut down on his medication. Answers to these questions give the nurse a framework for working with the patient on the administration of medication.

Convulsive therapies

Electroconvulsive therapy Electroconvulsive therapy (often abbreviated to ECT) was first introduced by two Italian psychiatrists, Ugo Cerletti and Lucio Bini, in 1937. The treatment consists of inducing a generalized grand mal convulsion by applying an electrical current to the head.

The treatment originated from the mistaken observation that epilepsy and schizophrenia were not likely to occur in the same patient. It was concluded that convulsions might serve as a treatment for schizophrenia. It was then learned that ECT was even more effective in treating some of the depressions.

ECT is used for both inpatients and outpatients. Because the apparatus needed for the entire treatment consists of a portable ECT box that can easily be carried and only needs a 110 AC voltage, therapy can be administered in any setting if necessary.

The patient usually receives 3 treatments per week. A minimum of 6 treatments, an average of 9 treatments, and a maximum of 25 treatments are considered within a normal range for a single course of treatment.

ECT is primarily indicated in the treatment of the serious depression where drug therapy has failed, has produced untoward side effects, or where treatment cannot wait for the onset of action of drugs. ECT may also be used in the treatment of acute mania, catatonic excitement, or catatonic stupor.

Management of the patient The patient is always told of the treatment. The physician generally discusses this treatment with the patient. The term electric shock may upset some patients and a more technical word to use is convulsive therapy or treatments.

The patient is told that a transient period of memory loss will occur following the treatment and possibly longer for recent events. If the patient is told that he will be asleep, will receive a treatment, and will wake up before an hour has passed with no memory of what happened, it is likely he will cooperate. It is customary to have permission forms filled out prior to the first treatment.

The steps involved in the treatment are:

1. Thirty minutes prior to treatment the temperature, pulse, respiration, and blood pressure are taken and any unusual findings reported to the physician. At this time the patient is reminded of the treatment and should be toileted to prevent incontinence during the treatment. Dentures and eyeglasses or contact lenses should be removed and food withheld or instructions given that nothing should be taken by mouth for at least four hours previous. This will prevent any complications arising from aspiration during the treatment.

2. 0.8 mg of atropine sulphate subcutaneously is administered 30 minutes prior to treatment to decrease bronchial and tracheal secretions. This reduces the chance of respiratory embarrassment due to excessive secretions.

3. At the treatment table the anesthetist administers a quick-acting anesthetic such as intravenous sodium pentathol. The administration of an intravenous muscle relaxant such as succinycholine chloride (Anectine 10–30 mg IV at 0.5–5 mg/min.) is combined with the anesthetic. Positive pressure oxygen is administered for 2–3 minutes until the muscular paralysis caused by the succinylcholine disappears and the patient breathes spontaneously.

4. Nursing care during the convulsion is aimed at controlling the patient's body by holding the patient firmly in order to reduce the chance of dislocation and fractures. The convulsion itself starts with a tonic spasm of the entire body, followed by a series of clonic, jerking motions, markedly in the extremities. An airway is inserted after the anesthesia is administered in order to prevent the patient from biting his tongue or lips during the treatment. The patient usually sleeps for 20–30 minutes after the treatment and remains confused for 30 minutes more.

5. During the recovery stage the respirations and blood pressure are taken. The nurse stays with the patient until he is awake and able to answer simple questions and can care for himself. Since the patient will be in a confused, hazy state after the treatment, it will be necessary to have someone accompany him back to the ward, if he's an inpatient, or to have someone drive him home, if he's an outpatient. Emotional support is needed to help the patient feel more secure and relaxed as the confusion and anxiety decrease.

Modifications of ECT produce effects other than the classic convulsions. The electrical current can be regulated so that it merely stimulates the brain (this can be useful in the treatment of severe drug intoxications). The current can be regulated to produce a loss of consciousness and sustain a minimum of quivering muscles. This kind of treatment is called *electro-narcosis* and usually lasts from 3–5 minutes.

Another technique of convulsive therapy is the use of a drug such as

Indoklon to induce the convulsion. In this method the patient is given the medication intravenously or by inhalation.

Insulin treatment

In 1933 in Austria Manfred Sakel (1900–1957) developed the method of insulin shock in treating psychosis. The purpose of insulin coma therapy is to induce a coma by the administration of increasing doses of regular insulin to a fasting patient. Hypoglycemic shock is effected this way.

The procedure involves the patient's receiving an initial dose of 15 units of insulin with daily increases until the coma is reached, about 2–3 hours after injection. Insulin doses needed to reach the coma vary from about 60 units to several hundred units. Coma usually occurs in 7–10 days. The dangerous stage of insulin coma therapy is during the early coma stage. The coma periods are gradually extended to an hour. The coma is terminated by awakening the patient through tube feedings of sugar solution. High carbohydrate feedings are given as soon as the patient is awake. Patients generally receive 30–50 comas averaging 5–6 per week.

This method of treatment requires a well-trained physician and nurse team. The treatment team is necessary because of the precarious and time-consuming aspects of each stage of coma. The shortage of professionals and expense during World War II made this method less practical. After the 1950's the increased knowledge and use of psychotherapy, psycho-pharmacology, and convulsive therapies have caused insulin therapy to lose much of its practical importance. The complications of this method, for example, the patient's failing to awake from coma or the development of acute and lasting symptoms of cerebral and cardiovascular damage, are not found in the more contemporary somatic therapies.

Other somatic treatments

Psychosurgery   The modern method of psychosurgery was described by a Portuguese physician, Ega Moniz, in the 1930's. For this he earned a Nobel prize.

Neurosurgeons have since attempted several variations of various surgical techniques from the original method. The objective of almost all lobotomies is the cutting of tracts between cortex, subcortex, and basal ganglia. If cortical tissue is removed, the procedure is called a *lobotomy*. If only white fibers are severed, the procedure is called a *leucotomy*.

Although lobotomy has lost its clinical importance, there is some resurgence in interest in psychosurgery by using surgical techniques producing less brain damage.

Hydrotherapy   The use of water as a relaxant has long been documented. Spas and baths are still popular in Europe and other cultures and resorts advertise regimens of exercise, swimming, and massage. Water is equated with pleasure and relaxation.

The water bath as a somatic therapy for disturbed behavior was popular prior to the 1950s and the advent of drug therapies. The patient was placed in a large tub filled with carefully maintained warm water. Then he was covered with a sheet of canvas so that only his head protruded. Close supervision of patients by the nursing staff was essential to maintain their safety. The interpersonal aspect of this type of supervision undoubtedly was as effective as the soothing water bath.

PSYCHO–SOCIAL INTERVENTIONS

Standard X includes the practice of individual as well as group psychotherapy in defining rationale and assessment factors.[2]

We will define psychotherapy for this section as a professional interpersonal situation between a socially acknowledged healer and a suffering person. The individual psychotherapy may be divided into the analytic technique and the directive and nondirective technique. All therapies involve support, direction, and goal setting. All therapies involve learning.

STANDARD X

THE PRACTICE OF INDIVIDUAL, GROUP, OR FAMILY PSYCHOTHERAPY REQUIRES APPROPRIATE PREPARATION AND RECOGNITION OF ACCOUNTABILITY FOR THE PRACTICE.

RATIONALE: Acceptance of the role of therapist entails primary responsibility for the treatment of clients and entrance into a contractual agreement. This contract includes a commitment to see a client through the problem he presents or, if this becomes impossible, to assist him in finding other appropriate assistance. It also includes an explicit definition of the relationship, the respective roles of each person in the relationship, and what can realistically be expected of each person.

Assessment Factors:

  1. The potential of the nurse to function as a primary therapist is evaluated.

  2. The accountability for practicing psychotherapy is recognized and accepted.

  3. Knowledge of growth and development, psychopathology, psycho–social systems and small group and family dynamics is utilized in the therapeutic process.

  4. The terms of the contract between the nurse and the client, including the structure of time, place, fees, etc. that may be involved, are made explicitly clear.

  5. Supervision or consultation is sought whenever indicated and other learning opportunities are used to further develop knowledge and skills.

  6. The effectiveness of the work with an individual, family, or group is routinely assessed.

[2]Congress for Nursing Practice, *Standards of Psychiatric-Mental Health Nursing* (Kansas City, Mo.: American Nurses' Association, 1973), p. 6.

Individual therapies

Classical psychoanalysis

Psychoanalytic treatment is an intense and lengthy procedure. Sessions are usually 50 minutes in duration four or five times a week. It is not unusual for analysis to last from 3 to 5 years (300–2000 sessions). Using the techniques introduced by Sigmund Freud, the analyst connects the patient's inner life and private and unconscious wishes and conflicts with his behavior and his goals. One goal is to gradually integrate the previously repressed material into the structure of the personality. The technique of free association means full and unedited reporting of psychic events. The analyst listens, clarifies, and interprets. Psychoanalysis requires self-control and a capacity for self-reflection. The patient usually lies on a couch and the analyst sits behind him.

Psychoanalytic psychotherapy

This technique is also referred to as *dynamic psychotherapy*. Patients are seen in a 50-minute hour usually once to three times per week. Patient and therapist usually sit opposite each other. Topics are introduced by the patient's telling his thoughts and experiences. The emotions are focused upon. The therapist helps by listening, clarifying conscious problems, and interpreting preconscious conflicts.

The therapist thereby teaches the patient to make correct observations and formulations by increasing his awareness. He helps him to differentiate the real from the unreal and what can be changed from that which cannot. The relationship is permissive in that the patient may say anything he feels.

Directive and supportive psychotherapy

Systematic approaches are made to help change the patient's attitude and behavior by encouraging him to accept the values and way of thinking of the therapist. In the therapeutic setting the patient must have confidence in the therapist in order to do what is suggested or advised. The techniques are direct suggestion, advice, faith in authority, praise, sustained verbal encouragement, and manipulation of the environment. This latter technique involves the therapist's suggestions on going to school, obtaining employment, recommending a vacation, or advising foster care.

Client-centered therapy

Carl Rogers introduced this structured, permissive relationship in which the "client" aims to gain an understanding of himself. The therapist reflects the client's feelings via nondirective techniques. Diagnosis is felt to be unimportant. The client gains a positive regard for himself through his relationship with the therapist.

Reality therapy

The main technique of reality therapy is confrontation. The therapist confronts the patient with the reality of the situation. Defenses are hammered at and diagnosis is felt to be unimportant. Illness and pathology are seen as a defense and are therefore pushed aside. For example, if the patient talks of hearing voices, the therapist would essentially tell him that this was unreal and crazy talk. The point of view is that confrontation affords a minimum of distortion in interpersonal situations.

Group therapies

Joseph Pratt, a Boston physician, first introduced therapy with a group in a medical setting in 1905. He gathered together and talked with patients all of whom had tuberculosis. The positive therapeutic results were transferred to other groups of patients.

The concept of group therapy has greatly expanded in the past decade. Carl Rogers has called the intensive group experience movement "one of the most rapidly growing social phenomena in the U.S. . . . perhaps the most significant social invention of this century."[3]

A recent survey reported by Irvin Yalom discloses a bewildering array of group approaches: psychoanalytic groups, crisis groups, psychodrama groups, Synanon, Recovery, Inc., Alcoholics Anonymous, marathon encounter groups, marital couples groups, family therapy groups, traditional T-groups, multimedia groups, and Gestalt therapy groups. Yalom emphasizes that many of the groups are designated as therapy groups; others straddle the blurred boundary between personal growth and therapy.[4]

If we review the groups according to their curative factors instead of on the basis of what the titles of the groups imply, we see that the array of group therapies seems a bit more organized. Yalom categorizes groups with similar goals[5] as groups which aim for providing support, suppression, and inspiration (Recovery, Inc., Alcoholics Anonymous); groups which aim for the restoration of functioning and the re-institution of old defenses (groups on acute, rapid turnover psychiatric wards); groups which aim for the maintenance of reality testing and prevention of ward friction (groups on long-term psychiatric wards); groups which aim for the building of new defenses and change in coping style and characterological structure (groups of patients with neurotic and characterological problems).

Therapists, depending on professional training and personality style, will master a system of therapy that fosters the growth of the curative process in clients. Of extreme importance is that in addition to the presenting method of operation and appeal, there is a basic framework to the therapy and an organized method to promoting growth in clients. Yalom identifies the curative factors of group therapy, that is, how group therapy helps clients in the following categories. These categories, in rank order of preference of group therapy patients, resulted from a study conducted by Yalom.[6]

1. *Interpersonal learning (Input).* The group's teaching me about the type of impression I make on others; learning how I come across to others; other members honestly telling me what they think of me; group members pointing out some of my habits or mannerisms that annoy other people; learning that I sometimes confuse people by not saying what I really think.

[3]Carl Rogers, "Interpersonal Relationships: Year 2000," *Journal of Applied Behavioral Science,* **4** (1968), 265–80.

[4]Irvin D. Yalom, *The Theory and Practice of Group Psychotherapy* (New York: Basic Books, Inc., 1970), p. vii.

[5]Ibid., p. viii.

[6]Ibid., pp. 60–81.

2. *Catharsis*. Getting things off my chest; expressing positive and negative feelings toward another person or toward the leader; being able to say what was bothering me instead of holding it in.

3. *Group cohesiveness*. Belonging to and being accepted by a group; continued close contact with other people; revealing embarrassing things about myself and still being accepted by the group; feeling alone no longer; belonging to a group of people who understand and accept me.

4. *Insight*. Learning that I have likes or dislikes for a person and reasons which may have little to do with the person and more to do with my hangups or past experiences with people; learning why I think and feel the way I do; discovering and accepting previously unknown or unacceptable parts of myself; learning that I react to some people or situations unrealistically; learning there are reasons I am the way I am which has to do with my early life.

5. *Interpersonal learning (Output)*. Improving my skills in getting along with people; feeling more trustful of groups and other people; learning about the way I related to the other group members; the groups's giving me an opportunity to learn to approach others; working out my difficulties with one particular member in the group.

6. *Existential factors*. Recognizing that life is at times unfair and unjust; recognizing that ultimately there is no escape from some of life's pain and from death; realizing I still face life alone; facing the basic issues of my life and death and thus living my life more honestly and being less caught up in trivialities; learning I must take ultimate responsibility for the way I live my life.

7. *Universality*. Learning I'm not the only one with the same problem; seeing that I was just as well off as others; learning that some others have some of the same bad thoughts and feelings I do; learning that others had parents and backgrounds as unhappy or mixed up as mine; learning that I'm not very different from other people gave me a "welcome to the human race" feeling.

8. *Instillation of hope*. Seeing others getting better was inspiring to me; knowing others had solved problems similar to mine.

9. *Altruism*. Helping others gives me more self-respect; putting other's needs ahead of my own; forgetting myself and thinking of helping others, giving part of myself to others; helping others and being important in their lives.

10. *Family reenactment*. Being in the group was like reliving and understanding the family in which I grew up; helped me to understand family hangups; group was like my family and helped me understand past relationships.

11. *Guidance*. The leader suggesting or advising me to do something; group members suggesting or advising me to do something; someone in the group giving me a definite suggestion about a life problem; group members advising me to behave differently with an important person in my life.

12. *Identification*. Trying to be like someone in the group; seeing that others could take risks; adopting mannerisms or the style of another group member or the group leader.

Role of the therapist

The initial task of the group leader is to create and convene the group. Once the group begins, the leader attends to fostering group maintenance and culture building by recognizing and negotiating factors that threaten group cohesiveness: tardiness, absences, scapegoating, subgrouping, disruptive extragroup socializing. The leader helps the group build norms conducive to therapy such as nonjudgmental acceptance, involvement, self-disclosure, expression of conflicts and affections. To accomplish tasks, group leader has two basic roles in the group: she is a technical expert or social engineer and she is a model-setting participant.

In summary, a full exploration of the theory and practice of group psychotherapy involves discussion of the techniques of the leaders, the selection of clients, the composition of therapy groups, stages of group process, and training and research in group therapy.

Family therapy

Family therapy, as a well-conceptualized treatment model, started in the late 1950s in several geographic areas of the United States. It developed as psychotherapists found that their traditional individual or one-to-one approach led to two kinds of stalls:[7]

1. A person who made progress would slip back, and the slips seemed to relate to something happening in the family.
2. Sometimes, when a person improved, other family members improved, other family members would get worse. It seemed as though the problem was just moving around the family.

From such observations, it became clear that therapists who were seeing couples and whole families together soon found that family groups have certain factors that are not operating visibly when only one member of the family is seen. Psychotherapists began studying family systems and learning that the systems were more powerful than the sum of their individual parts. From this, therapists began to deal with the synergistic—the feedback circle has more power than the sum of the powers of its parts—qualities of the systems.

As family therapy has continued to develop, new techniques and methods have emerged. Family therapy usually takes a more active form than the classical models of individual psychotherapy. Family therapy is practiced by a wide variety of professionals, for example, psychiatric nurses, social workers, psychologists, psychiatrists, and family physicians.

The majority of people have lived their lives either as children or parents. Thus, the experience of family therapy—involving family members—is not an unusual concept to present to a client. The family is a subsystem of society and the individual is a subsystem of the family. In most societies the family is the unit for child-raising. It is a significant variable in the emotional life of the individual and society.

[7]James J. Bulger, D. Donald Dettore, George A. Donnally, David C. Eilaud, Jr., Sidney Gerhardt, Charles H. Kramer, Margaret D. Sheely, and Barbara L. Thompson, "Roundtable/Family Therapy," *Patient Care,* **8,** No. 17 (1974), 180.

Family therapy pays attention to psychological or intrapsychic events as well as to extrapsychic events in the family and community environment of the individual. Various definitions of *family* may be given to identify its structure. In general, the term *nuclear family* is given to the immediate members of a group living together. The term *extended family* usually refers to significant people outside the nuclear family such as aunts, uncles, cousins, grandparents. Various family functions have been identified within the family, for example, dealing with affectional and biological needs of family members, child-raising, material maintenance, replacement of members for society, and social control.

Systems theory is often used as a theoretical framework in family therapy. A therapist quickly realizes the impact of the relationship system in a family when he gives advice and soon observes that no change is occurring. Relationship systems within a family mean that when there is a change in one person, it affects all persons in the system. Also, all those reactions have an effect on the original person and this closes the circle. Once the circle is closed (with this feedback going on), the system takes on properties of its own and an idea or an attitude can go around and around and escalate. The positive power in such a system is that when it is synchronized, it works very well. When it is not, the family structure is threatened and weakened and is vulnerable to divorce, alcoholism, drug abuse, and all kinds of lesser problems.

Intervention at an early point in a family crisis often aids the family in getting back to a normal style of functioning fast. It is a longstanding problem that takes considerable professional investment of time.

Assessment of the family

In making a family evaluation, Henry Grunebaum identifies the following parameters as essential to assess in making a family diagnosis:[8]

1. The family issue and the affects. An increasing amount of research is being done in delineating the stages of family life issues and the tasks that are involved in each stage. For example, the first stage of family life requires that provisions be made for housing, food, finances, and health. A second stage is the entry of a third person to the family, as for example, through adoption or birth of a child or addition of an adult member. The task for this stage is the dyad adapting to a triad relationship which in turn may affect the woman's career and the couple's recreational patterns.

Other family issues include children's schooling and exit from the household, onset of grandparenthood, illness, and crisis situations. The impact of the couple's career patterns often becomes significant in influencing family structure.

Families generally seek help with a family issue when they are unable

[8]Henry U. Grunebaum, *The Practice of Community Mental Health* (Boston: Little, Brown & Company, 1970), pp. 57–78.

to cope with the situation. During the evaluation, we suggest assessment of the following questions:

1. What is the target issue of conflict?
2. How does the family deal with emotions?
3. How have parents taught their children to cope with their feelings?
4. In what way do the parents present themselves as sex-role models?
5. How are limits set in the family?
6. What is the relationship between the husband and wife? Do they form a parental coalition in terms of giving unity of direction and each providing emotional support in carrying out parental functions?
7. What is the nature of the siblings' relationship to one another?
8. What family issues are identified explicitly and implicitly?

2. The defenses, cognitive capacities, and communicative abilities of the significant members. This area identifies the peoples' assets and liabilities available to resolve the issue. A second important area to assess is the capacity of the family to cope with the issue and its subsequent affects (emotions). It is important to identify the nature and effectiveness of family defense mechanisms. These are assessed by observing how family members handle emotions. For example, if one person uses such narcissistic defenses as denial, projection, and distortion, it will be difficult for him to assume responsibility for his own feelings.

Cognitive and communication abilities are important in order to resolve an issue because the person must be able to focus his attention and think clearly about the issue of concern. Family members often do not perceive the ways in which they contribute to family problems. In such cases, sometimes when individual behavior is brought to their attention they are able to correct the situation. In other cases, the person is unable to see the effect.

3. The willingness of family members to undertake therapeutic tasks that lead to changes. This point is critical in evaluation. All too often professionals overestimate the family's resistance to participation. The clinician is an outsider and families have a set way of dealing with outsiders.

This question is especially important when one member of the family seeks treatment without the others. The therapist must evaluate whether or not the individual's situation allows him an opportunity to progress independently. However, the labeling of one family member as "patient" often relieves the anxiety and obligation of other members to deal with the issue and change their behavior.

There are three variables to consider in the situation in which one member presents for treatment. First, is the family willing to participate in resolving the issue? Second, if the family is unwilling or unable to change, can they accept support and guidance? And third, is the family totally unable and unwilling to accept any help?

In summary, the clinician can evaluate three areas during an initial family interview: the issue that is triggering the family difficulties and the underlying affects that prevent the family from coping with it; the problem-solving skills of the family; and whether or not the family is willing to change in the overall goal of family growth.

Couples therapy

Couples therapy is a variation of family therapy in that only the couple is treated. Within couples therapy there are several treatment models:

1. *Individual psychotherapy for each partner by two therapists.* The two therapists may or may not confer with each other on the progress of their clients.
2. *Individual psychotherapy for each partner by a single therapist.* There may or may not be occasional conjoint meetings.
3. *Conjoint therapy with a single therapist or with two therapists.* The couple is seen together with one or two therapists.
4. *Couples group psychotherapy.* Several couples meet with a single therapist or co-therapists.

The selection of the treatment model generally depends on the careful assessment and evaluation of the following questions:

1. Are the couples' difficulties specific to their relationship?
2. Are the couples committed to and able to work on their problems?
3. Are the problems acute and ego-alien or are the problems chronic and ego-syntonic to both partners?

The selection of the treatment model often is as follows:

1. The separate treatment of couples is usually indicated (1) when their relationship does not appear to be the problem of greatest priority and when either developmental issues or severe psychopathology in one partner is very evident; (2) the couple is not emotionally committed to the relationship or committed to working out their difficulties.

2. Conjoint therapy is usually indicated when the couples are emotionally committed to the relationship. They are able to communicate with each other, and problems are experienced both within and outside the marriage. If the problems are acute and ego-alien, conjoint treatment is indicated.

3. Couples group psychotherapy is indicated when problems are long standing and ego-syntonic, that is, their problem marriage is a way of life. The couple often can gain some objective evaluations of their problem from other couples. For example, the group may support the wife that her husband should not yell and beat her. However, they may also point out that the long-suffering wife may be provoking the husband's behavior.

Groups tend to be most satisfactory when member couples share a similar life issue. For example, a couple with several children currently in school may deal with the issue of the wife's seriously pursuing a career and the subsequent changes in the family structure.

Social network therapy

An extended kind of group therapy is social network therapy. A *social network* may be defined as a group of individuals who have some kind of relationship in each other's lives. A typical social network of a family includes all members of the kinship system, friends of the family, friends of kin of the family, and neighbors.

The goal of bringing as many people of the social network together is to increase communication, particularly between the clients and their kin, friends, and neighbors. The therapeutic potential of gathering networks together in one place at one time with the purpose of strengthening the organization of relationships is documented in crisis situations such as grief or disasters. Also, tribal meetings for healing purposes are well described in varying cultures. The overall goal is to make the entire group involved in the issue at hand and to supply a strong sense of group support, reassurance, and solidarity.

Occupational therapy[9]

The goal of occupational therapy is the socializing of patients by countering the regressive aspects of the psychiatric illness. The aim is to increase self-esteem and to teach new occupational skills. A basic principle of occupational therapy is that people learn through activities.

Occupational therapy is an essential part of the total treatment program for a patient. Similar issues may be explored as in talking (psycho) therapy but in different ways. For example, the patient may say, "I want to gain more confidence." The occupational therapist then engages the patient in an activity and continues to talk about the issue of gaining confidence, but the patient is learning through his actions. This is in contrast with psychotherapy in which the patient has to verbally recall previous situations of success or failure in confidence.

Entry process in the occupational therapy setting Assessment of the patient begins the moment he walks toward the occupational therapy room. Is the patient hesitant about coming into the room? How does he walk in? Does he seem fearful to be in the room? Once the patient is in the room, his reaction to the room as well as to the therapy should be observed. Occupational therapy rooms tend to be very colorful and perceptually stimulating with art work and materials displayed in the room.

If this is the first time that the patient goes to the occupational therapy department, the therapist orients him to the room and explains the purpose of the therapy. Then the patient is asked to select an activity. Some patients say, "I don't know what I want to do. You pick one." Other patients may say that they do not like activities or that the activities are too hard. These

[9]This section was prepared in consultation with Dawn Huber Warrington, O.T.R.

responses are very meaningful. Is the person trying to say that he has trouble making decisions or that he is dependent or that perhaps he has had so many failures in his life that he does not even want to take a chance on making an occupational therapy item? The therapist then collects more data to confirm or reject possible interpretations.

If the therapist decides that a patient needs help with decision making, she might take two items and ask the person to pick one. This action narrows the choice and most people can select one item. The patient is also asked if there is someone he would like to make an activity for. This question provides data on who is important to the person at that particular point in time.

The occupational therapist might ask the person to look around the room and select an item to try. After selecting one, the person is asked to talk about why he selected it. Some people say they have never tried such an item or maybe they like the looks of the activity.

Setting goals   Ideally, the patient sets his own goal. The therapist may have to negotiate the goal. The therapist asks if the activity is realistic, and, if necessary, the person may have to change his goal. For example, one patient wanted to build an electric organ. This turned out to be unrealistic because of the size of the occupational therapy room facilities. The patient was helped to select a smaller project that could be finished within a certain time period and within the room space. The important part of the goal was that the person chose to do something he had always wanted to do and the therapist helped negotiate the goal so that the person was successful in some aspect of the overall request.

Different patients have different goals. For example, the adolescent with impulse control difficulties may want a project that he can finish fast in one day. After the patient completes the project, the therapist may try to negotiate an activity that would take longer in order to increase the patient's attention span. A good project for this goal would be an item that required cutting, staining, and then glazing, for example, a multi-phase project. The adolescent is supported as he tolerates the time delay in finishing the project.

Some patients select projects that are not therapeutic to their problems. For example, a depressed patient who selects knitting becomes involved in a project that is repetitious and has no interactional stimulus. Knitting is better for someone with impulse control problems because it helps set internal limits on the patient. The depressed person needs interpersonal stimulus and an activity that requires that the therapist come back frequently for reinforcement or a project that requires that the person ask many questions.

Projects   There are many occupational therapy projects which are goal-directed in terms of the patient's therapeutic progress with life problems. Some of these projects follow.

Decision-making
situations   The therapist asks the patient which color or which material she wishes to use. These data help to evaluate the patient's ability to make a decision.

Ranking of projects	Projects are ranked from easy to complex. A project such as painting-by-number is usually considered a no-fail project unless the person cannot concentrate well enough to stay within the lines. A complex project would include multiphases.

Establishing interpersonal relationships

Activities aid in strengthening object relationships and reality testing. If a project is a success (for example, growing a plant), the success helps to build self-esteem and others will comment on it. The socialization aspect in the occupational therapy room is important. In one case, a patient had a difficult time sitting in a group and sat outside the circle which had gathered around the table used for working on projects. The therapist talked with the patient and found out that she was fearful of sitting in the group. The therapist suggested to the patient that when she felt comfortable, she should try to sit at the end of the table instead of outside the circle and that she should try to work her way gradually into the circle. Since the activity the patient was working on helped to provide the entry into the circle, this was an important step for her. Also, sitting around a table encourages patients to ask each other for input to their activities. It helps patients reach out to others and to find out that others, and not just the staff, care and can be helpful. Usually, the therapist does not know how to do all the activities that are available. When there is one that the therapist does not know, she and the patient get the instructions and learn together. This encourages the cooperative effort and decreases the omnipotence of the therapist. Other patients may know better how to do an activity and their expertise is very much encouraged.

Expressing feelings

An important therapy is encouraging patients to express their feelings. In one case, an angry patient was not talking in psychotherapy. She came into occupational therapy and took a hammer and piece of wood and pounded away on the wood. During the second week of her hospitalization, the occupational therapist asked her to label each indented area in the wood. She did and identified anger at having to be in the hospital, anger at her husband, anger at her doctor, anger at her child. Identifying the anger was the first step in beginning to express and talk about the feelings. As in this case, many patients find it helpful and therapeutic to pound away at something, such as leather or an ashtray, in a constructive way.

Freeing people

Working on projects is one way to free people emotionally. Occupational therapy tries to bring into the therapy what is occurring in their outside environment. For example, one man had a history of losing four jobs in one year, recently divorcing his wife, and leaving his family. These data imply that this man starts something and then stops. Where during occupational therapy the therapist observes that he starts a project and then leaves it before it is finished, she might say, "I see you have started three different projects here and are having difficulty finishing them. Does this happen in your personal life?" In another example, a patient has an impulse control problem and the therapist observes that he starts many different projects. This lack of following through can be confronted as he works on the project. If the patient is a

195

dependent person, he may be encouraged to move into more independence. The therapist can encourage him to help another person with a project that he himself has already completed.

There are particular kinds of material that help people relax. These materials are crayons, watercolors, charcoal, and oil paints. In matching the dynamic issue of a person, if the dynamic issue is to be successful, he should be given something that is difficult, such as working with crayons. For the person whose dynamic issue is control, he may do best working with watercolors.

Evaluation of activities   In evaluating a patient's progress it is necessary to look at the whole process from beginning to end in all areas. What feelings is the person struggling with—depression, anxiety, lack of confidence—and how does he move from that position? How does he deal with feelings and with other people? What can occupational therapy teach him?

When the therapist evaluates the activity, she must find out the goal of the person. Were the goals too low or too high? For example, evaluate two different people who worked on making ashtrays. One ashtray has good color, and is neatly done and structured. The other ashtray is bizarre with contrasting colors and strange arrangements. The first ashtray may be considered good, but it may mean that the person is too controlled and rigid. The second ashtray may be good because the person was depressed and restricted and was able to loosen up and do something very abstract. The kind of activity and what it means in terms of the goal of the patient must be carefully evaluated.

In evaluating the progress of the person, the therapist may test the thought process. When she instructs a patient on an activity, she may omit one step in order to see if the patient is able to figure out the missing step. At the end of the project, the therapist evaluates how the person compensated for the missing step. If he managed well, that is a success and he is told this in the evaluation process.

Art therapy

Art therapy may be part of the occupational therapy department or activities therapy department or it may be a technique the nurse wishes to use in working with a patient. People who cannot express themselves verbally can often put their thoughts on paper. The use of art therapy encourages a person to reach a part of his potential not realized before. Art therapy helps people express what they feel in terms of color and design. For example, in one case, a patient drew a picture of a house, but she did not sign the picture. When asked about this, she expressed ambivalence about going home for the weekend. This information was helpful in the planning session for her visit home in terms of what she anticipated and how she might cope with certain situations.

After the patient has completed a painting or picture, the therapist asks the patient to explain the picture. The therapist may ask what the colors mean or what a certain shape or object is. It is very important to let the patient explain. The therapist cannot interpret what it means, but she can help clarify what the patient is trying to say. For example, one patient drew a multicolored picture in which there was a tree. The patient's interpretation of this was that she felt like the tree—lonely with the sun all around but she could not feel the sun.

In another case, the patient drew a picture of her previous weekend at home during which she had had anxieties and fears. Many conflicts had developed and she became angry at her husband and returned to the hospital feeling very depressed. She drew a picture of a rainbow with many colors and talked about each color in relation to her weekend. She said that whenever she is pushed, she gets angry and depressed and nothing comes out. The rainbow showed this change.

Another therapeutic technique is to take pictures drawn previously by the person and show them to him to see whether or not progress is being made. Pictures may be compared as to how the choice of colors changed and what objects mean within the picture. Color usually means feelings. Often, as anger and hostility decrease, there is an increase of feelings, typified by yellow or bright colors.

Art therapists can see change over time. For example, instead of many colors being run together, subsequent pictures will show definite boundaries. In exploring this with the patient, it may be learned that issues were clearing in her life and that the patient was able to talk about this in art therapy. In one case, a patient said that the brown color used in the painting were the pills she took and they helped her not to lose control. In every picture she used the color brown. This patient used to lose control and throw plates and furniture, a behavior that frightened her. Her goal was to have control and one way to have control was to take pills or to put the color brown in her paintings. Through talking about her paintings in art therapy, it came out that her father had deserted the family when she was in the second grade. As an adult, she sees her children starting grammar school and she fears that her husband will divorce her and desert her. The color showed this in her work. Her talking about these issues and her painting showed definite evidence of her gaining control over this fear.

Occupational therapy departments may offer additional activities for patients. Music therapy may strengthen the artistic and creative potentials in patients. Poetry or play reading are activities that may be regularly planned for small groups of patients.

BEHAVIORAL INTERVENTIONS   Behavior therapy is a method of treatment to alleviate specific behavioral problems as quickly as possible by controlling the learning behavior of the patient. Three principal ways of controlling or modifying human behavior exist:

1. Behavior can be modified by changing the stress factors that produce the maladaptive behavior. For example, the student doing poorly in one class may do effective work under the guidance of another instructor.

2. The type of behavior occurring in a particular situation can be changed or modified. For example, the obese person can be taught to substitute low-calorie foods for high-calorie foods.

3. Some behaviors are learned because the outcomes are satisfying. For instance, if a person becomes anxious when he has to talk in a group situation, his anxiety may be modified by exposing him to repeated satisfying and nonfrightening group experiences.

In contrast to the psychotherapies that focus on thoughts, feelings, and behavior of patients, the behavioral approach addresses itself to the patient's overt behavior that is presenting the problem.

Desensitization therapy

Desensitization therapy was introduced by J. Wolpe in the early 1960s. This therapy marked an important milestone in the treatment of phobic disorders. In this therapy the patient is taught to relax and then a series of the fear situations is suggested gradually through progressive steps. The patient is flooded with fear from these described, imagined, and audiovisually induced situations. The forced exposure to the feared stimulus while the response is prevented facilitates extinction of the fear.

Implosive therapy

The behavior therapy similar to desensitization therapy (or response prevention) is called *implosive therapy* (or *flooding therapy*). M. Z. Hussain reported gradual symptom improvement in a study group of 40 patients with social phobias. These people complained of going out alone into open spaces or into shops, crowds and streets; traveling in cars, buses or trains; remaining alone; and participating in other social situations. This method of treatment included six 45-minute sessions, which were held twice weekly, of flooding or desensitization assisted by 20 cc. of intravenous saline infusions or thiopental solution. This therapy enabled patients to suppress their avoidance behavior adequately. The results obtained and the speed of relief are significant findings in the treatment of phobias to date.

SUMMARY

This chapter described the various psychiatric treatments under three categories: (1) somatic (psychopharmacological agents, convulsive therapies of electroconvulsive therapy and insulin coma, psychosurgery, hydrotherapy); (2) psychological (individual therapies) and social (group therapies and occupational therapies); (3) behavioral (desensitization and implosive therapy).

REFERENCES AND SUGGESTED READINGS

Black, Barbara (1970). "Unit System—The Third Revolution," *American Journal of Nursing,* **70,** No. 3, 515–19.

Duran, Fernando, and Gerald D. Errion (1970). "Perpetuation of Chronicity in Mental Illness," *American Journal of Nursing,* **70,** No. 8, 1707–09.

Gardner, Kathryn (1971). "Patient Groups in a Therapeutic Community" *American Journal of Nursing,* **71,** No. 3, 528–31.

Haller, Linda Lacey (1974). "Family Systems Theory in Psychiatric Interventions," *American Journal of Nursing,* **74,** No. 3, 462–63.

Hussain, M. Z. (1971). "Desensitization and Flooding (Implosion) in Treatment of Phobias," *American Journal of Psychiatry,* **127,** No. 11, 85–90.

Kline, Nathan S., and John M. Davis (1973). "Psychotropic Drugs," *American Journal of Nursing,* **73,** No. 1, 54–62.

Lerner, Arthur (1973). "Poetry Therapy," *American Journal of Nursing,* **73,** No. 8, 1336–38.

Loomis, Maxine E., and Judith T. Dodenhoff (1970). "Working with Informal Patient Groups," *American Journal of Nursing,* **70,** No. 9, 1939–44.

Lyon, Glee G. (1971). "Stimulation through Remotivation," *American Journal of Nursing,* **71,** No. 5, 982–86.

Monea, Helen Pazdur (1974). "A Family in Trouble (A Case Study of a Family in Conjoint Family Therapy)," *Perspectives in Psychiatric Care,* **12,** No. 4, 165–70.

Morgan, Arthur James (1973). "Minor Tranquilizers, Hypnotics and Sedatives," *American Journal of Nursing,* **73,** No. 7, 1220–22.

Pesso, Albert (1969). *Movement in Psychotherapy: Psychomotor Techniques and Training.* New York: New York University Press.

Racy, John (1969). "How a Group Grows," *American Journal of Nursing,* **69,** No. 11, 2396–2402.

Speck, Ross V. (1967). "Psychotherapy of the Social Network of a Schizophrenic Family," *Family Process,* **6,** No. 2, 208–14.

Yalom, Irvin D. (1970). *The Theory and Practice of Group Psychotherapy.* New York: Basic Books, Inc.

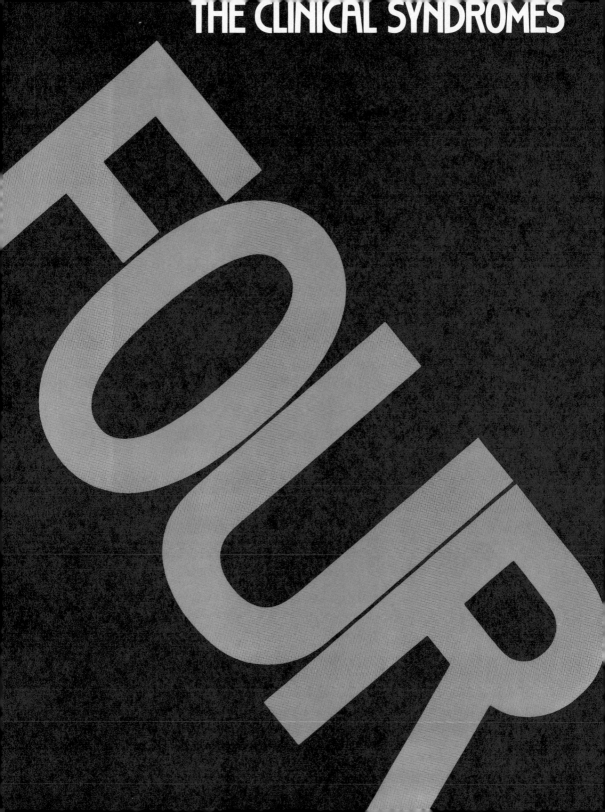

FOUR

The psychiatric diagnostic classification is constantly under debate. Some mental health professionals take the position that diagnosis leads to labeling and stereotyping patients. They feel that the patient's unique problem in living should be the primary and only concern of the helping staff. Therapeutic efforts are viewed as being geared to the patient and his problem in coping in this society. They do not see any relevance in trying to classify patient symptoms into diagnostic categories. Treatment plans, via this concept, tend to be on an intuitive basis with justification in the art of mental healing.

Some psychiatric nurses feel that the diagnostic categories are not relevant to the practice of psychiatric nursing and they advocate teaching by concept of behavior patterns and subsequent nursing care to these patterns.

The opposing position is taken by clinicians who feel there is a need for some logical ordering of patient difficulties and through this process, clinical judgment regarding treatment plans and goals are developed.

We agree with both positions. Paying attention to the immediate concerns of the individual as well as his particular behavioral style is essential. And the diagnostic categories of psychiatric disturbances are important because nurses continually deal with mental health professionals who do use the terminology. Nurses need to be able to discuss patient care within such a framework.

Every clinical symptom and category can be regarded as an expression of psychic distress. Part Four discusses the products of emotional distress as expressed through thoughts, feelings, and behavior. Chapters in Part Four are as follows:

FEELINGS, THOUGHTS, AND BEHAVIORS

12

The mind expresses its distress through feelings, thoughts, and behaviors. For instance, a troubled person may *feel* anxious or depressed, *think* in an obsessional or psychotic manner, and/or *behave* impulsively. Sometimes feelings, thoughts, and behavior are simultaneous manifestations of psychological distress. Often, however, only one or two of these three dimensions are apparent in a given patient.

Even if nurses are not aware of the diagnostic category or syndrome of a given patient, they can explore each troubled feeling, thought, or behavior as a meaningful subject of study and concern. For example, the understanding of a patient's sadness is important whether the diagnosis is neurosis or schizophrenia.

Psychiatric diagnostic categories will be discussed in this part of the text. These categories may be viewed as syndromes of specific patterns of pathological feelings, thoughts, and behaviors that tend to occur together in groups of people. For instance, a patient who feels elated, has pressured and tangential thinking, and behaves with poor judgment may be suffering from manic-depressive illness. These syndromes can be easily learned once the nurse understands how to observe the specific feelings, thoughts, and behaviors.

Mind–body similarities

There are several similarities between the mind's expression of psychological distress and the body's expression of medical distress. For example, a single manifestation of distress may result from a variety of clinical conditions. In medicine, diarrhea may be a manifestation of infection, ingestion of toxic materials, anxiety, obstruction, or other causes. In psychiatry, anxiety may be a manifestation of schizophrenia, various neurotic conditions, or situational reactions. As another similarity, both the mind and a particular organ can manifest their distress in a limited number of ways, regardless of etiology. For instance, pathology in the lower gastrointestinal tract, whether caused by an ulcer, a tumor, inflammation, or trauma, can manifest symptoms in limited ways: pain, bloating, diarrhea, constipation, or bleeding. Psychological distress, as we will show, is limited to expression by feelings, thoughts, and behavior.

Normal and abnormal symptoms

A symptom, depending on the associated conditions, may be a manifestation of a normal or a pathological state. For example, constipation would be normal if it resulted from a change in diet. It would be abnormal if it resulted from a tumor or an obstruction of the intestinal tract. Intense sadness would be normal following an important loss and abnormal when there is no good reason for the mood state. Certain symptoms are always abnormal regardless of the associated condition. In general medicine, vomiting blood or passing blood in the urine is always abnormal. In psychiatry, suicidal behavior and visual hallucinations are always abnormal.

Symptoms as a defense

Symptoms in medicine and psychiatry often perform defensive functions. For instance, a fever may be viewed as a defense against an infection in the body. It is also useful in following the progress of an illness. Vomiting following the consumption of contaminated food functions to expel or "defend against" the irritant. Following staphylococcal infection, an abscess functions to wall off the infection.

Similarly, a delusion may be an attempt by the mind to protect itself from something more painful. It may be easier to think unreal thoughts than to face an overwhelming situation. There may be less anxiety in fainting than in facing the fright of an aggressive encounter. It may be easier to develop an obsessional thought than to feel like hitting someone. Or it may be safer to forget to attend class than to tell the instructor the homework was not completed.

Based on the above observations and theories, we will show in this chapter how pathological thoughts, feelings, and actions are reactions to and defense against overwhelming but genuine human feelings. The nursing management of these conditions will become evident.

FEELINGS   Feelings are subjective mood states. They may be pleasant and enjoyable or they may be painful and uncomfortable. Human feelings are numerous; the differences among them may be subtle. To identify just a few:

Alienation	Exasperation	Indifference
Anger	Fear	Isolation
Anxiety	Frustration	Joy
Caution	Guilt	Loneliness
Contentment	Happiness	Love
Delight	Helplessness	Resentment
Disgust	Hope	Respect
Distrust	Hopelessness	Sadness
Embarrassment	Hostility	Suspicion
Envy	Inadequacy	

The state of mental health includes the capacity to bear and tolerate certain kinds of feelings, even when they are painful or unbearable.

When the feeling is unbearable, two situations may occur. First, another feeling may be substituted as an avoidance or defensive technique. For example, anger may be used to avoid feelings of closeness or love; depression may be used to avoid sadness; elation may be used to avoid anxiety or depression.

Second, abnormal states of action or thought function to avoid the genuine affective states. For instance, a patient suffering from overwhelming anxiety may break a window or begin to hallucinate.

Following are descriptions and examples of a few commonly seen feelings.

Anxiety

Anxiety is most often described as an uncomfortable feeling state. It is characterized by a subjective sense of impending disaster. The common physical or somatic alterations in the body systems associated with anxiety may be experienced as follows:

CIRCULATORY SYSTEM: perspiration, clammy hands, flushing, blushing, feeling hot or cold.

RESPIRATORY SYSTEM: heavy breathing, sighing respirations, hyperventilation, dizziness.

GASTROINTESTINAL SYSTEM: abdominal pain, anorexia, nausea, dry mouth, diarrhea, constipation, butterflies in the stomach.

GENITOURINARY SYSTEM: urinary frequency, various interferences with sexual function.

MENTAL FUNCTIONING: impaired attention, poor concentration, impairment of memory, changes in outlook and future planning.

EMOTIONAL REACTION: irritability, mood change, dream disturbances, changes in relationships with family and friends.

The above symptoms of anxiety are known to all of us. A useful way to view the normal feeling of anxiety is that it does not involve repression. One can consciously feel and acknowledge it and by so doing, keep it proportionate to the threat.

Neurotic anxiety, however, is a reaction disproportionate to the threat. This kind of anxiety and its results are discussed in Chapter 14.

Anxiety may be regarded as pathologic when it is severe and persistent or when it seems to be triggered by some minor cause. Sometimes the individual's previous experiences cause an automatic reaction. To one man the presence of a policeman may provoke an anxious anticipation; to another the same policeman elicits a feeling of protection and safety.

To some students the instructor, when returning an examination paper, incites a feeling of anticipation and curiosity. To other students the action produces fear and anxiety.

Within normal limits anxiety can be motivating and useful in a productive, affirmative way. Examples of this kind of anxiety which is viewed from three different responses follow:

> Students are scheduled for a final course examination. The grade for the test will be the final grade for the course because no other exams or papers were assigned.

> Student A is anxious and admits it. She spends the evening before the exam reviewing her notes and rereading chapter summaries for 4 hours. At midnight she decides to go to bed and sets the alarm for 6:00 A.M. so that she can have an hour of study before going to class.

> Student B is anxious and admits it also. She spends the evening before reading the supplementary readings assigned for each class, talks with three upperclassmen who have taken the course, skips supper and stays on black coffee and dexedrine through the night until she falls asleep at 3:00 A.M.

> Student C says that last-minute studying for an exam is useless. She feels that if you haven't read the chapters as you have gone along, you won't learn anything by cramming. She has been invited to a party and decides to go rather than to stay home to study. She comes home at 1:00 A.M. and goes to bed.

These three examples show typical ways that students may react to the same stimuli of an examination. Each anxiety level is different and for each student the anxiety served its own purpose. The results of the examination showed that Student A got a 90%, Student B a 70%, and Student C a 75%. Discussions with the students after the examination revealed that Students B and C could have understood and coped with their anxiety to better advantage. Student B became too anxious and thus exhausted herself and flooded herself with too much studying. Student C denied the anxiety and thereby did not show her full potential on testing because she was physically and mentally exhausted from activities unrelated to studying. When these two students were reexamined, Student B achieved an 80% and Student C an 88%. These scores were truer indicators of their real understanding of the course because the anxiety had been identified and resolved.

Love and other positive feelings

Love and human closeness may be difficult feelings for many people to bear. In current society people are frequently more comfortable discussing matters of aggression and sex than matters of love and fondness. Can you imagine a friend coming up to you and saying, "I am very fond of you. You are a very fine person." Almost everyone would become uneasy.

People may avoid being loved by expressing hostility or by withdrawing. In psychiatric nursing the patient commonly explains his fear of closeness as a protection against being rejected or as a protection against his fear of wanting too much.

Anger

Anger may be an appropriate response to a frustrating situation. Some people, however, use the feeling of anger to defend against human closeness.

It is paradoxical that those to whom we feel closest can provoke our anger and cause us to behave in unpleasant ways. The important people in our lives evoke both the greatest joy and the strongest anger. Instead of bearing this human feeling of love, people often use defensive techniques. For example, when someone slams a door or berates another person, his behavior may be a response to a critical remark just made by a close friend, an insensitive spouse, or an indifferent parent.

The anger may also be a defense against a real feeling of helplessness. That is, if a person feels weak, ineffective, and overwhelmed by this feeling, it may be easier for him to get angry to show that he is the big tough guy. For example, the grade-school bully who goes around pushing other children may really be overcompensating for feelings of helplessness.

Another example is the patient who comes into the hospital ward outraged at how dirty the ward looks or how inefficient the ward seems to be or wants to know why the staff cannot be therapeutic. That person may be defending against his own feelings of anxiety, helplessness, or insignificance by trying to be critical of the ward.

Nursing management of feeling states

The first task of the nurse in observing the patient and his feeling state is to assess the feeling. Identifying the feeling and the degree of anxiety accompanying it is important. The following questions may serve as a guide in this process:

1. What is causing the feeling? What is the precipitant?
2. Is it anxiety or a specific feeling?
3. Can the person talk about the feeling?
4. What is the current life situation for the person?
5. Is the person taking any drugs or medications?
6. Does talking with the person increase or decrease the feeling?

After observing and identifying the feeling state, the nurse may try to decide whether the feeling is genuine or a defense against another unexpressed or unbearble feeling. Nurses do not uncover or point out the feeling; instead, they make it possible by their support to help the patient talk about the feeling.

Nurses deal with the feelings of patients by helping them put the feelings into words. This may lead to the patient's discovering feelings of which he was not previously aware. This technique helps him to be in touch with his feeling. For example, the patient talks of his extreme anger with his wife. As the nurse sits and listens to him and his description of real situations, she helps him to bear the pain he has been avoiding. As he expresses his feelings to a therapeutic person, he may not have to be so angry with his wife and he may be able to look at other feelings he has, perhaps the positive feelings. The anger has prevented him from feeling close to her.

Sexual feelings are another area in which people are hesitant to express themselves. The therapeutic person helps the patient to bear these feelings—

to tolerate them and to talk about them. The goal is to help the person learn how to not push the feelings from consciousness or defend against them or act inappropriately on them.

Boredom and apathy are also subjective feelings common to many people. They are evoked by situations that one would rather not be in. For example, a person would like to prolong the weekend, but he must go to work on Monday. This presents the person with transitory feelings of apathy.

The nurse helps the person to bear feelings that are unbearable. Putting the feelings into perspective helps the person understand how the feelings originated and what brings them out. The more a person can gain control of the feeling with words and understanding, the easier it is to bear.

THOUGHTS   Thoughts are pathological when they interfere with productive activities and when they defend against normal feeling states.

One kind of pathological thought is a wish or a fantasy that interferes with a particular feeling, relationship, or goal. For instance, an adolescent may substitute a fantasied love affair with the "perfect girl" rather than risk the threat of rejection by a real girlfriend. Another kind of pathological thinking is psychosis in which the patient avoids reality by denying it. Psychotic thinking will be discussed further in Chapter 15.

Another way of viewing pathological thinking is to examine defense mechanisms that represent the mind's attempt to deal with anxiety.

Defense mechanisms

Defense mechanisms are used by people as a means of avoiding pain by thinking. These mechanisms, although universally used by people, are intellectual techniques to avoid pain. Some of those commonly used mechanisms are explained in Chapter 4.

The nurse needs to understand the defensive mental techniques for two reasons: first, to understand the defensive position of the patient in order to be therapeutic; and second, to describe it in order to help formulate the syndrome or diagnostic category.

Nursing management of thinking defensive techniques

In normal dialogue with a person who is not using grossly pathological defensive thinking techniques, the nurse can sit and listen to the person, she can feel involved, the patient can feel that the nurse understands, and she can have a sense of progression in the nature of the discussion. But when patients use neurotic or psychotic thinking, it is common for nurses to get a feeling that they really do not understand, that they felt bored, that their mind wandered, that they did not feel engaged, that the patient really did not say what was bothering him. They feel that something superifical happened. In fact, that is true because something superficial did happen. The patient was avoiding the real issues of concern to him. These are some of the clues that indicate a patient is using defensive thought techniques. By using these techniques the person avoids saying what counts, what is painful, and what is meaningful.

After being lectured to by a patient who has been intellectualizing for an hour, the nurse really does not learn anything. She feels that she has heard a lecture rather than a meaningful discussion. After sitting with a patient who is sad, but who in fact has been telling jokes for the whole hour, the nurse feels like saying, "I don't know where that person is or where I am." The patient has managed to put her off. The jokes are avoidance techniques to avoid dealing with her. The nurse knows it even though it is difficult for her to put her finger on this.

As soon as the nurse is able to notice the avoidance during the interview, then she may be able to say, "It sounds to me as though there are a lot of painful things you want to say that are difficult to talk about." Somehow she communicates to the patient that it is acceptable for him to tell her the feelings and that she is prepared to hear them. An alternative to helping the patient is knowing what the issues are and how the person must really feel. For example, if someone has lost a spouse prior to coming to the hospital, the nurse can assume that the person is experiencing sadness. And if the person shows no sadness at all, then she knows what to expect and can help the person with the feeling. We use this approach because clinical knowledge shows us the kind of feelings that usually occur with grief.

The goal of the nurse is to translate the patient's defensive thinking into nondefensive, direct thinking.

BEHAVIORS   A third way in which people express psychic distress is through their behavior. The normal discharge of actions is through motor activity or goal-directed, problem-solving behavior. For example, if your foot is hot, you take it off the radiator. If you feel you must kick the radiator, you would be overreacting to the situation.

People use gymnasiums to release tension. Husbands waiting for wives to give birth pace the floor. Waiting for a telephone call or a date inspires people to use motor activity. Some people knit or sew as a means of handling agitation. These are all normal ways of dealing with feelings through actions.

Sometimes the behavior is not productive and does not relieve tension, but instead it gets the person into more trouble. It can become pathological. When you are tense, it is not helpful to break a window or door because you generally have to pay penalties for these actions. If you are angry at the authorities and you damage property to get back at them, you generally must pay a penalty, but if you call someone and tell him what is on your mind, the behavior tends to be more adaptive.

The other extremes may be seen in the bizarre behavior of the schizophrenic person or the manic behavior of the affective disorders or the antisocial acts of robbery, rape, murder, and of alcoholism, suicide, and drug abuse.

Nursing management of behavior

Some people learn to deal with anxiety or overwhelming feelings by behavior rather than by thinking out the problem or by putting it into any emotional perspective. For example, the acting-up patient may become suicidal when hospitalized and prevented from acting on his feelings. The nurse is making the patient feel the feelings that he is trying to defend, deny, or avoid.

The nurse can help patients verbalize the feeling and understand it. The patient needs to be taught how to put time between the overwhelming feeling and his action. For example, if the patient were to say, "My brother said something rotten and I felt so angry I smashed him," the nurse would intervene by saying, "Your brother said something rotten; you felt angry. Tell me what that feeling was like."

Nurses try to teach the patient to put into words that which he normally acts on immediately. They try to teach him to delay the action by increasing his verbal skill and his understanding of the feeling. When he is about to act in a destructive manner, she sets limits on the behavior.

SUMMARY   Part of a mentally healthy state is being able to bear certain kinds of painful feelings. This implies not avoiding the genuine painful feeling by using other defensive feelings or not substituting behavior or a thought disorder for that feeling. That is not to say that all feelings are normal or that the expression of feelings is always healthy or appropriate; however, bearing certain genuinely painful feelings is often the healthiest way to deal with certain conditions.

DEPRESSIONS AND SUICIDAL BEHAVIOR

13

Depression is a common complaint, not only among psychiatric patients, but also among large numbers of people who are not psychiatrically ill and who may never seek psychiatric help. The apparent widespread phenomenon of depression is probably related more to the lack of specificity of the word than to the prevalence of psychopathology in society. In everyday use, depression may refer to almost any unpleasant feeling including sadness, boredom, apathy, even anger. As a result, when someone says he is depressed, we know very little about how he is feeling except that the person would rather feel differently.

In clinical psychiatry and nursing the meaning of "depression" is clearer, although ambiguity remains. The various meanings follow:

1. A normal mood state or an abnormal mood state which may accompany any psychiatric disorder.
2. A syndrome or symptom complex.
3. A disease process or diagnostic category.
4. A complex of psychodynamic mechanisms.

The nurse must understand the various meanings of depression in order to make decisions on the nursing management of the patient. This chapter describes the four meanings and the nursing management for each case.

DEPRESSION VIEWED AS A MOOD STATE

This mood state of depression may occur in a normal person, in a patient with a psychiatric syndrome, or in a medical patient. Anyone can experience depression.

The mood of depression may be described as one of despair, gloom, a sense of foreboding, a feeling of emptiness, or a feeling of numbness. This mood state may be qualitatively and quantitatively different from other mood states. Whether or not the mood of depression in normal people differs from the mood of depression in people who have clinical depression is a matter that has not yet been decided. The same word is used, but it is not clear whether or not there is a clinical differentiation between the two.

213

When patients who have recovered from a severe, retarded depression are asked to compare the everyday kind of depression with this kind of clinical depression, they reply that the two kinds of depression are very different. Patients say that the severe depression comes over them like a very dark cloud but the depression of everyday life is more transitory.

It is clinically important to distinguish between the mood of depression and the mood of sadness.[1] The emotion of sadness may so resemble pathological depression that mental health professionals sometimes fail to note the distinction between the two. Consequently, the normal emotion of sadness may be improperly treated by antidepressant medications or by a referral for psychotherapy. This distinction between sadness and depression may be as relevant to the management of the depressed patient as the distinction between the murmur of mitral insufficiency and the functional heart murmur is to the medical management of the cardiac patient. In the cardiac situation the heart murmur sounds the same, but the conditions are very different from the medical treatment aspect. Similarly, two people can look sad and depressed, but etiology and psychiatric treatment for each one may be very different.

Sadness is experienced as a normal feeling in a variety of situations: the loss of a loved one through death; the loss of one's children through their maturation and leaving home; graduation from school; observing the aging in one's parents; the loss of friends and a familiar neighborhood through moving; observing the aging process in oneself; failing an exam; changing jobs; ending a marriage; finishing a good book; experiencing a change in body image, for example, the loss of hair or teeth; the loss of an organ through surgery; giving up a life's dream; the knowledge of one's impending death.

In many of these situations and circumstances groups of people gather together to assist one another in bearing the sadness, for example, at farewell parties, marriages, birthdays, graduations, the bedside, and the graveside. Granted, many of these losses may and often do lead to a depression.

A patient who is unable to experience sadness often presents himself for psychiatric care with this depressive mood state as an important clinical feature. He may be reacting with functional complaints to some loss in his personal life or he may be reacting to a loss resulting from a medical diagnosis or procedure. This patient then presents himself with symptoms of gloom, despair, and feelings of emptiness.

Depression may occur because this person is unable to bear his sadness. Instead of acknowledging and facing the loss, he feels numb or detached. He denies the loss by saying, "It couldn't have happened. It is beyond belief." The denial may even take the form of a psychosis. If the patient is depressed over something he has done, he may project the blame onto someone else or criticize himself in a totally unreal or highly exaggerated way. His agitation relieves his tension. His motor retardation keeps his

[1]Aaron Lazare, "The Difference between Sadness and Depression," *Medical Insight*, **2**, No. 23 (1970), 23–26.

mind from active thinking. In other words, the patient avoids his sadness by depressive symptoms: he feels nothing, denies the loss, avoids responsibility by projecting the blame, and uses motor activity. Depression, then may be viewed as a defense against sadness and grief.

There are a number of "acting out" behaviors that a patient may use to avoid feelings of sadness or grief. He may drink, eat, or sleep excessively, or behave impulsively. Patients may also use pain as a depressive equivalent to avoid sadness and other painful affects.

DEPRESSION VIEWED AS A SYMPTOM COMPLEX

The multitude of differences evident in people who are depressed is impressive. Although 100 depressed people may have certain similarities, they will have more differences than they will similarities. The problem is how to classify and how to deal with the differences.

One way clinicians differentiate between the depressive syndromes is by designating the depression as being either retarded or agitated. These terms describe the motor activity of the patient. A second way of differentiating is by calling the dichotomies either neurotic or psychotic depressions. These terms describe the patient's ability to cope with reality and everyday situations.

A dichotomy that is felt to have considerable clinical value is the *reactive* and *endogenous* distinction. These terms describe various symptomatic characteristics of a depression.

The first distinguishing concept between these two depressions is based on the precipitating event. The precipitating event in the reactive depression is much clearer to identify, whereas in the endogenous depression the precipitant is not evident. For example, the precipitant in the reactive depression might be the death of a family member or the loss of employment. The psychiatric history of the person having an endogenous depression shows no clear-cut event that precipitated the depression.

The symptom clusters differ in each depression. The reactive depression includes the presence of a precipitating event, difficulty getting to sleep at night, feeling worse as the day progresses, and weight loss of less than 10 pounds.

The symptom cluster in the endogenous depression often has retardation of thought and action, substantial weight loss (greater than 10 pounds), feeling that the depression came on gradually and out of the blue (no clear-cut precipitate event), feeling worse in the morning but becoming better as the day progresses (diurnal variation), and feelings of worthlessness.

The concept of reactivity is also a distinguishing factor. That is, the reactive depression has the characteristic of the stimulus of the environment producing a positive effect on the patient. The patient responds to environmental stimuli. When people are around or the nurse smiles and is cheerful, these people are able to respond positively and do state that they feel better.

The person with an endogenous depression does not react to environmental stimuli. The nurse sitting with this patient often feels the contagious effect of the depression. Nothing that is said or done by the nurse seems to have any effect on the patient. He remains engulfed in the depression.

The endogenous depression tends to be time limited, that is, the depression tends to run its course. There is likely to be a family history of depression with the endogenous group. There is presumed to be a possible biochemical aspect to the endogenous depression; perhaps because of the family histories and because it also responds well to somatic therapies. Another characteristic of the endogenous group is that these people tend to have obsessional personalities. These people have accomplished a great deal in their lives and are often successful people who seem to become depressed at certain periods in their lives, for example, the middle-age period. Because of their productivity, it is important to treat them as quickly as possible so that they can return to their work. The use of somatic therapy, and especially electroconvulsive therapy, facilitates this process.

Case history of reactive depression

The following is a case example of a reactive depression:

> A 68-year-old widow presents at a psychiatric hospital admission conference as a highly anxious, trembling, teary woman with alternate statements of complaints and sentimentalism regarding her family. She states her depression began one year previously when she was hospitalized for a cholecystectomy and bowel resection.
>
> Following a 3 month period in the hospital she went to live with her eldest son in a relatively small house where she had to sleep in the living room. The son was from her first marriage. She had had little contact with either him or his brother since they left home for the service 25 years earlier. The sons felt they had been on their own since adolescence when the mother had remarried after her first husband died.
>
> The sons felt that "mother didn't bother them too much until she found herself a widow again." The second husband died from a heart attack 2 years prior to her psychiatric admission. Since this loss, the mother had been trying to make arrangements to live with the eldest son in spite of the fact she had her own apartment in an apartment building for people over 50. She felt she was quite isolated there and did not join in the activities of the project. The sons said they were willing to do their share but felt she was capable of helping herself.
>
> The sons described the mother as being a difficult person to get along with and one who pushed people away from her by being too demanding.
>
> The patient did well until a year ago when she began to have physical complaints. She said that she had felt "depressed" since her second husband died. Since the surgery she has been extremely depressed, feeling that life was not worth living and was also unable to drive her car because she "felt so badly." Her previously neat obsessive personality changed and she did not pay attention to her dress or keep her apartment clean. There was a 4-pound weight loss and difficulty falling asleep. In the hospital she eagerly took her medications and was continually asking for more medicine. She created conflict between herself and patients by passing along gossip that the other patients resented. She was very reactive to the interpersonal stimuli on the ward. The diagnostic impression was reactive depression following surgery; the loss of her husband

who was the important person in her life; isolation in an apartment building where little contact was made with others and in which others were relatively intolerant of depressive behavior; and the sons' lack of involvement in her life.

Hospital course

During the hospitalization the patient was constantly pleading to have staff intercede with her sons to have her live with them. She became physically shaky whenever she was with staff and patients on the ward.

She was quite hopeful that after the wedding of her grandchild that the grandchild's room would become available to her to live in. When she realized that her son was not going to invite her to live with his family, she began to regress for about a 4-week period. This behavior took the form of her not getting out of bed in the morning, constantly demanding extra time by staff, demanding her meals on the unit, refusing to do her ward work or to become involved in ward activities, ward meetings, or group therapy. The therapeutic task for staff was to help her verbalize and resolve her disappointment over not being able to have what she wanted (to live with the son) and to help her reinvest in new activities such as interacting with patients, staff, and the ward activities.

Within the 4-week period she was able to deal with the feelings of loss and disappointment and did become sociable with staff and patients. She then decided not to live in a nursing home as she had previously thought was her only alternative, but was able to make plans to return to her own apartment. She went from full hospitalization to weekends in her apartment until she had made a few friends in the apartment building and now that she had this new interest she was discharged from the hospital. This step was accomplished 7 weeks following admission.

The nursing management focused on helping her to bear the feelings of her sadness and to deal realistically with the alternative of living in her own apartment, making new friends, and accepting the relationship her sons could offer her at this time.

DEPRESSION VIEWED AS A DISEASE PROCESS OR DIAGNOSTIC CATEGORY

Depressive illness, viewed as a disease process, would include such diagnostic categories as psychotic depressions, manic–depressive disorders, neurotic depression, and the involutional depressions.

Manic–depressive illness

Recurrent endogenous depressions are categorized under this diagnosis even though a manic phase may never have occurred. Often, however, a careful history may disclose that a few days prior to a depression the person showed some manic kind of behavior such as spending a large amount of money or impulsively taking a trip or behaving in an unusual way.

Manic behavior is viewed as the mirror of depression. The basic affect of the patient is one of euphoria. A cursory observation of the patient reveals that he looks happy, is totally unconcerned, and is free of worry. Manic or hypomanic people tend to have quick wits and possess good senses of humor. In the manic state the verbal and physical exertion of the person is greatly increased and he truly can exhaust himself to the point where he does not eat or take care of himself. Just as the depressed patient neglects himself in a self-destructive way, the manic person neglects himself by overactivity in that he does not have time for the reality details of eating, dressing, organizing his time. Similarly, the depressed person does not have the energy or interest to do these things.

The person with a depression may go into a manic phase from the depressed phase; this then accounts for a cyclic diagnosis such as manic–depressive, manic type or manic–depressive, depressed type. The cycle may be gradual or be of sudden onset. Recurrent depressions with no manic attacks are referred to as *unipolar depressions*. Recurrent manic attacks with or without depressive episodes are referred to as *bipolar depressions*. The following case illustrates the cyclic aspect of manic–depressive illness.

> Mr. Land stated that his problem was "recurring depression." He first began having "emotional problems" at 11 years of age. He described becoming dizzy in the library and running home to his grandmother (who lived with the family) in a "panic," His family physician referred him to a psychiatrist at that time. He described himself as a shy and introverted child but extremely overactive. He always felt "5 years ahead" of his peers both in maturity and physical skills. He felt that he was better than his friends except in the really important things like work. He has always felt inferior because his friends never had "depressive attacks."

> Mr. Land said that his attacks come every year and usually last about 3 months. They used to come in the winter but more recently have been coming in the spring or early summer. He describes himself as a "night owl" who constantly goes out with his friends (when not depressed) and is always the life of the party. He says that he goes from one extreme to another and that there is no in between. When "up" he is always rushed, has a very poor appetite, constantly going, doing things on impulse without thinking them through. When he is down and depressed, he constantly thinks about all the catastrophic things that could happen to him or his family. He wakes up "shaky" at night in "anxiety attacks" and cannot carry out the activities of normal living such as attending to his appearance. He withdraws from people, cannot concentrate, and everything "appears as if he were looking out from a walled-off vacuum." He becomes afraid to travel and usually has to leave his job.

> He knows he does not rest when he should and is like a "machine driving himself even when the fuel is low." He said that his depressive states usually follow some precipitating event such as being transferred to a new position in his work.

> He said that no doctor has given him an answer to "why it happens." Each time the depressions occur they "have to run their course." Once they are started, he cannot prevent himself from going into them and that they "engulf" him totally. He can usually see the symptoms coming on. He stated that the state is like "being dead; that everyone seems far away and although he usually loved people, he did not care about anyone at all." He has not felt suicidal during these periods.

> Mr. Land describes his father as a "great guy" but someone he cannot talk with. He has an older (middle-aged) cousin whom he greatly respects. He

frequently goes to him for talks in which the cousin "sets him straight" and gives him support and encouragement. He describes his mother as an "over-protective Italian" woman who spoiled him when he was a child; she gave him everything materially. She has always compared him to his older brother (who is 30) who is the "golden son" who can do no wrong. His mother still brings Mr. Land clothing and food whenever she goes shopping. His wife does not get along with his mother because she tries to interfere with the raising of the two children. Mr. Land said that his mother has always given money to "smooth things over."

Mr. Land was married 5 years ago and experienced a depression 2 months after the marriage. He said his relationship with his wife is presently "going very well." His wife does become upset when he is depressed and tells him to "try and fight it." He describes his wife as a sensitive woman. He said he does not want any sympathy from his family when he has these depressive periods because it only makes him feel worse.

The choice of biologic treatment in bipolar depressions is lithium carbonate.

Involutional depression

The classic involutional psychotic depression is felt to occur for the first time in the involutional ages (40–55 for women and 50–65 for men). These people have had no prior history of manic–depressive illness.

The personality of the patient prior to the illness is often stated to be rigid, overconscientious, and emotionally constricted. The illness may be viewed as a decompensation of the obsessive defensive life-style of the individual.

The onset of the illness is slow with an increase of hypochondriasis, pessimism, and irritability. The main symptoms are motor agitation and restlessness, a pervading anxiety and apprehension, and occasionally delusions associated with an exaggerated hypochondriasis and paranoid ideation.

The prognosis for untreated patients is poor. Treatment with psychotropic agents or electroconvulsive therapy is usually effective.

Questions are currently being raised about whether or not involutional depression is indeed a specific entity with its own etiology, natural history, and clinical picture.

The following is a case example in which the diagnosis between the reactive depression and involutional melancholia was not clear:

A 53-year-old married mother of a 32-year-old unmarried daughter presents with the feelings that people were laughing and talking about her lack of eyebrows. The woman had been depressed 2 years previously over excessive facial hair. This problem developed after her medical physician had prescribed hormonal supplements for menopausal symptoms.

The patient was an attractive woman who had formerly been a model. She had always been concerned about her looks and was fastidious in her dress. In helping the patient to unpack after the admission process, the nurse was impressed by the compulsive nature in which she removed her clothes from her suitcase and placed them in the bureau. The patient kept requesting assurance about her looks and kept repeating, "What will people think about my losing my hair and having no eyebrows?" In further discussions with the patient, she began to relate her many fears about getting older. She stated how she dreaded it and any slight physical change that she noted in her body was a reminder of her fears.

The nursing management of this patient focused on implementing the medical regulation and reduction of the amount of hormonal treatment she was receiving that had been aggravating her condition and causing the loss of hair. The ideas of reference (that everyone was laughing and talking about her) subsided and through talking with the staff, she was able to talk about her fears and gain some control over these feelings. She had reacted to the loss of control she felt within herself. Working on this issue and introducing structured new ways for her to be attractive through the use of cosmetics as well as the development of new interests helped her deal realistically with the issue of growing older.

DEPRESSION VIEWED AS A COMPLEX OF DYNAMIC MECHANISMS

A fourth way to view depression is to understand some of the psycho-dynamic theories that have been developed to explain the phenomenon of depression. These include a complex of dynamic mechanisms such as oral dependency, identification with the lost object, inhibition, anger turned inward, and specific dynamic issues.

The psychoanalytic theories regarding the dynamic structure of the depressions had their beginnings in Freud's paper, "Mourning and Melancholia."

Recent developments in psychoanalytic theory define depression as an ego state in which the individual's emotional expression of helplessness and powerlessness occurs. The depression, as an ego state, is characterized by loss of self-esteem in reaction to three dynamic issues: (1) the wish to be worthy, loved, and appreciated; (2) the wish to be good, loving, and unaggressive; and (3) the wish to be strong, superior, and secure. When these three aspirations are threatened, they lower the person's self-esteem and bring on a depression.[2]

1. The wish to be worthy, to be loved, to be appreciated and not to be inferior or unworthy. People who have these aspirations struggle with strong needs to be loved and cared for. These aspirations are viewed as oral issues which means these people have the potential to become depressed when the fear of not being loved or cared for occurs. They receive their "ego supplies" of being given to and cared for from people who are important to them. The depression may occur when someone who has cared about them leaves or dies.

2. The wish to be good, to be loving and not to be aggressive, hateful, or destructive. These people struggle with issues relevant to being in control and being good vs. not being in control or being bad. When these people feel that they are bad or out of control, they may be prone to depression. Sometimes when aggressive or angry feelings within the self become too painful to acknowledge, depression may occur. For example, when someone important to the patient dies, the patient may feel that he might have done something to prevent the death or that he might have contributed to the death. These feelings could precipitate a depression.

[2]Based on Edward Bibring. "The Mechanism of Depression" in P. Greenacre (ed.), *Affective Disorders* (New York: International Universities Press, 1953), pp. 13–48.

3. The wish to be strong, superior, great, secure and not to be weak and insecure. Some people, often men, become depressed when they lose in competition. They are concerned about being strong and winning and not losing. For example, a business failure or poor choice in the stock market may depress this kind of person. The person does not talk about not being loved or about whether he is good or bad in the moral sense, but he feels defeated and this is the issue with which he struggles.

In summary, that there is no right or wrong way to view depression shows the complexity in the field. We have presented four ways of viewing depression which nurses need to be familiar with as they collaborate with different mental health workers. Clinicians tend to find the point of view that provides the greatest therapeutic leverage for their treatment of the depressed person.

NURSING MANAGEMENT OF DEPRESSIONS

There can be no single way to treat depressions because, as we have attempted to show, there are many views of depressions and many kinds of depressions. We should expect, therefore, that a variety of treatment skills would be necessary. The nurse should view any single approach for all depressed patients skeptically. The treatment of edema is an analogous situation in medicine. There are several clinical entities that may produce edema (heart, kidney, and liver disease). The treatment for each variation differs in many respects.

The following nursing approaches are most frequently implemented by nurses in caring for patients with depressive behavior.

Bearing painful feelings

It may be very difficult and painful to sit with a depressed patient, but the situation and the patient require it. Being able to bear sadness and grief is made possible for many people by the presence of a caring person, who listens, who talks, and who shares the discomfort. A lonely person, whether because of circumstances or his own personality difficulties, may not be able to deal with the sadness in his life. The nurse helps the person to bear the feelings he does not want to bear alone. What is said to the patient is not as important as the fact that the nurse is present. The depressed patient is often desperately lonely and unable to cope effectively.

It is helpful to remember that depression is usually a time limited condition. Eventually the depression will lift, but much patience will be needed before it does. If it is difficult to allocate an extra amount of time listening to the sadness of the patient, the nurse might try to allot a specific amount of time she knows she can remain with the patient. Sitting and bearing the feelings are therapeutic for the patient even though the results of this approach are not immediately evident.

Resolving the feeling

Bearing the feeling of sadness is the first step in the total process of resolution and mastery of the feeling, but not everyone knows how to do this. In the course of their personality development, some people have never learned to cope directly with the experience and to discriminate between various feelings. Instead, they handle internal discomfort and distress by impulsive actions. Some people have never allowed themselves to experience feelings, because they have been taught that demonstrating sadness or any similar emotion is a sign of weakness.

To successfully deal with one's feelings means that a resolution of the feeling has occurred. That is, the person must make peace with the situation and its ensuing conflicts, feelings, and problems. In the situation in which the feeling of sadness caused by a loss must be resolved and peace made, the nurse can be of significant support to the patient during the process.

To resolve one's sadness, the feeling must be acknowledged cognitively and viscerally, that is, in the head and the heart.[3] The meaning of the loss must be thought about and talked about. The feeling, which may be accompanied by tears and by physical distress in the head, chest, stomach, and other portions of the anatomy, must be experienced. Only then can one give up and part with that which has been lost.

The nurse helps the patient express his feeling and she can specifically go over the reality details of his physical symptoms as he works to resolve his sadness. She listens, understands, and helps to bear the painful feelings of sadness so that the patient's pain is lessened by knowing that he is making peace within himself, that he is making therapeutic progress, that someone does care about him and his distress, that he is not alone in his sadness, that he is sharing it in a human way with another person.

When the resolution of sadness is optimal, people can move on to new obligations and opportunities.[4] For example, they can say: "I have lost someone whom I love, but I am able to love again." "I have not lost a son; I have gained a daughter." "I may have lost my uterus, but I am still a woman." "I may be older, but I am wiser and more free." "My dream has collapsed, but I am free of its tyranny." "My children no longer need me in the old ways, but I have something different and vital to offer them." Even the patient with a terminal illness must come to terms with his sadness if the remaining hours, days, or weeks are to have any human meaning.

Dealing with anger

There are some patients for whom anger turned upon the self in the classical Freudian way seems to cause depression. This phenomenon, however, is not a universal cause for depression as was previously supposed. There is a large group of depressed patients who seem to be angry and who seem willing to express their anger. The anger is not a primary cause of their depression. Anger turned upon the self is an overused and misunderstood concept in contemporary psychiatry and psychiatric practice, and nurses need to be aware of this.

[3]Lazare, "The Difference between Sadness and Depression," p. 27.
[4]Ibid., p. 30.

Because of this belief in the dynamics of anger in depression, some mental health workers feel that encouraging the patient to express the negative feelings and helping him be aware of them is a therapeutic approach. This technique will be effective for some but not for all depressed patients for the following reasons:

1. Anger turned on the self is not the cause of all depressions. To the contrary, many depressed patients have no difficulty in expressing anger.
2. Even when the patient has turned the anger on himself, helping him express his anger too quickly and without proper support may communicate to the patient that he is an angry person, a concept which may further depress the patient.

The formulation of issues over which people get depressed seems to indicate that many people in this present-day society have difficulty in getting close to other people. They become somewhat socially isolated. When a person becomes very isolated from caring people, he will invariably become depressed. This position may make him angry because he is isolated and miserable. The anger is really secondary to the condition he is in.

As we have said before, encouraging the person to express his anger may be antitherapeutic. The few people who care for him usually receive the full force of the anger and turn away in a natural withdrawal. The patient then says, "See, what happens. No one cares about me."

It is a far more helpful approach to explore with the person what it is that prompts him to socially isolate himself, why his anger affects others, and just what it is that gets him into the miserable and trying situations in the first place. It is therapeutic to help the patient find out what the psychological issue really is. The inability to express anger and anger turned on the self is one of many such issues.

Responding to the dynamic issue

An understanding of the concept of the intrapsychic issue is the basis for the therapeutic skill of determining and responding to the issue. If the assumption is that depression may be viewed as patients struggling with different dynamic issues specific to them, then each patient must be looked at separately.

For example, there are some patients who are demanding and clinging and want everything possible done for them. The nurse feels compelled to give the patient something. Other patients feel they are so without merit and worthless that they are not entitled to anything. Some patients say they hate themselves, but when the nurse contradicts them and says that they are fine people, they will become angry with the nurse.

To be cared for There are several things the nurse can do when a patient is depressed because he feels unloved and uncared for. The patient can be taught how to get those ego supplies he wants. He can be taught some of the social skills of how people develop important relationships. The nurse can help the patient look at situations in which he emotionally pushes away people with whom he could become close. For example, when a wife tells of how critical she is of her husband and says that nothing he does seems to please her, the nurse might say, "What I hear you saying is that your inclination is to push your husband away. It might be more helpful to listen to him more instead of constantly criticizing him." Helping the person who has a strict and hypercritical attitude to soften his approach is often a useful way to help teach more fruitful ways of interacting with people.

If the person is depressed because someone who cared about him is gone, the nurse can help the person grieve. By this process the patient can be helped to give up unrealistic aspirations. For example, if the patient says, "I wish I had my mother back even though she has died," the nurse can say, "You may not be able to have her back, but I can help you grieve so that your wishes will be more realistic." The nurse is often the replacement for the lost person during the grieving process.

When there is a longing for the external supplies that are now gone or have been cut off, the nurse can diminish the need for those supplies or the nurse can teach the patient new ways to get these supplies by helping the person to resocialize and not to be so demanding of others.

Control The nurse can help the patient to get his life back under control by helping him to reorganize his life. This involves the nurse's listening to the person describe in detail his usual style of life and then working with the person to restructure the disorganized parts of his life. Or the nurse can help to ease the patient's superego that demanded that everything be so orderly that the person's life became disorganized. The nurse can work at the control issue from both viewpoints.

Achievement When some people feel that they have failed and have not accomplished their goals, they may become depressed. The nurse can help these patients to reevaluate what they really want to accomplish and help them to readjust their goals. This might involve helping a patient to grieve a lost goal or a goal he had to give up. This may be seen in medical situations, for example, among paraplegics. The athletic person whose dynamic issue is to achieve really has a great deal of difficulty in this medical situation, because he has to give up his goals for athletic achievement.

The paraplegic who has the dynamic issue of being cared for may not become depressed in this situation because he may well thrive on the nurses' caring for him.

Determining the dynamic issue is very important in the nursing approach to the patient who is depressed.

Implementing the biologic model

In the hospital setting, somatic treatments are often prescribed by the psychiatrist in the medical treatment of a depression. Antidepressant medicines frequently are first tried before electroconvulsive therapy is used. In the administration of the medicine the nurse should carefully observe the symptom picture of the patient over the 24-hour period. The nurse can then confer with the physician about the patient's sleeping pattern, his degree of activity and involvement on the ward (which will indicate physical energy, ability to make decisions on the reality details of waking, rising, and dressing), eating, ward activities, and work. It is important for the nurse to record the patient's somatic complaints (frequency of distress, type and intensity of the disturbing complaint). The side effects of medication should be distinguished from the somatic aspects of the depression.

Electroconvulsive therapy is a second somatic treatment used in the medical treatment of depression. In addition to paying attention to the procedural details, as outlined in Chapter 11, the nurse also listens to and encourages the patient to express his feelings about the treatment. Following treatments, the nurse can be especially supportive through the period during which there is some memory loss and can help the patient to focus on the reality details and structure of the ward milieu and his mastering these activities. Feeling in control of these factors will help prepare the patient to reorganize his thinking and feeling about his own life.

Providing controls for the patient

Often the patient with a depression feels so low and has such little self-esteem and hope regarding his situation that he may lose control of his impulses. Loss of control may result in the patient's attempting to hurt himself through a self-destructive act.

When the patient cannot control his own impulses, the nurse assumes responsibility for the safety of the patient. Often this is one of the reasons for the patient's hospitalization. The nursing process for providing controls for the patient in the hospital setting is implemented by the one-to-one relationship, restricting the patient to observable areas on the ward, determining when the patient may leave the unit with staff or visitors or alone. The removal of potentially injurious items such as razor blades and scissors is usually part of the routine admission procedure for patients who have self-destructive impulses.

Although it is documented that the removal of all potentially injurious items will not necessarily ensure that a person will not hurt himself, removal of the items does help to decrease the impulsive gestures of the patient, for example, wrist slashing and swallowing of pills from hidden medications.

Providing controls is also essential for the person with manic episodes who can exhaust himself because of his excessive motor activity. The reduction of environmental stimuli that may be increasing the hyperactivity is an important consideration. The patient needs one-to-one contact until he can handle more complicated interaction or environmental stimuli.

The eating habits of depressed or hyperactive patients must also be observed carefully. The patient may either feel too unworthy to eat or may be too active to take the time to sit to eat. The nurse takes the time to ensure that time is set aside for eating and, if necessary, she stays with the patient until he is able to resume this reality detail by himself or in the dining room with the other patients.

The nurse should also assess the patient's sleeping habits and behavior. The depressed person may be unable to fall asleep or may be waking several hours after falling asleep. The patient in a manic episode may be too agitated to even try to fall asleep. Corrective measures by the nurse to reestablish positive sleeping behavior is indicated.

Evaluating the symptom cluster

The nurse in the community setting (in home visiting, in industry, in schools) needs to know what symptoms to evaluate in the depressed person. Because somatic therapies are so helpful, especially in the endogenous depressions and the manic episodes, the nurse, by evaluating the symptom cluster, may refer the patient for somatic treatment or medication.

One of the ways to determine the severity of the depression is to evaluate the symptom cluster. Inquire about specific symptoms such as weight loss, sleeping patterns, feelings of hopelessness and worthlessness. Look for symptoms of withdrawal from activities and previous interests, interactions with family and friends, work productivity and relationships with fellow workers.

The assessment of the symptom cluster enables the nurse to determine if the patient is suffering from a depression of the endogenous type or the reactive type. When the nurse discovers an endogenous cluster of symptoms, she should give serious thought to referral for medical treatment. The symptoms of severe weight loss, psychomotor retardation, diurnal variation, hopelessness, worthlessness, and inhibition of feelings are all of the endogenous type of depression. These people usually respond well to antidepressants and/or electroconvulsive therapy.

In the endogenous depressed patient the premorbid personality is quite good and the person tends to describe the depression as "coming out of the blue." He feels enveloped in the depression but then it may suddenly lift. The medicines work well as a biochemical factor in reversing the symptomatology. When the nurse assesses this kind of depression, she might immediately think to herself, "Here is a penicillin type of depression and the patient should see a physician." The medical model of treatment is indicated.

When the nurse assesses a reactive cluster of symptoms in a person in the community, and if the depressive symptoms are not too severe and are related to an environmental stress, it is more likely that the patient can be treated by interpersonal intervention. The community mental health nurse may decide to treat the depression with a social or intrapsychic model or she may refer the person to a local mental health center.

When the nurse sees a patient who is suffering from a manic episode, she should consider immediate referral to a physician so that medication with lithium carbonate may be prescribed.

Handling subjective feelings

Subjective feelings indicate the many different reactions that nurses may have to the depressed patients. As previously stated, it is difficult for many people to know how to talk to and be therapeutic with a depressed person. Feelings of previous situations with depression, including many feelings of helplessness, are stimulated within the nurse. As described in Chapter 1, the nurse should autodiagnose her feelings in order to be maximally effective in working with the patient. Some of the feelings nurses may anticipate in working with the depressed person are as follows:

1. At times the nurse feels frustrated because she wants to help but cannot when the patient is not responding. Often motor retardation is evident during severe depressions and this lack of physical or emotional response by the patient may make the nurse feel helpless and frustrated.
2. The bad-tempered hostility and hypercritical attitude of the person is often found in certain kinds of depressions. This patient will try to get the nurse to conclude that his whole family is utterly disagreeable. He will try to have the nurse sympathize with his view of the situation.
3. Some depressed patients display a self-berating quality. The nurse simply cannot talk them out of it because they enjoy playing the role of martyrs. In effect, the patient says, "I am the worst person in the world and there is no one as bad as me." Instead of trying to convince him otherwise, it is more helpful to be supportive and wait it out. Bearing the feeling the patient is expressing will aid in the resolution of the feeling.

ASSESSMENT OF SUICIDAL BEHAVIOR

A major problem confronting nurses is how to identify the person who is a serious suicidal risk. Although it is a fact that suicides will continue, no one has data at present as to what extent suicides are being prevented. Nurses are continually assessing patients for degrees of suicide risk. Strong emphasis is being placed on finding a reliable, quantitative measure of lethality. It is important that nurses guard against dividing people into those who carry out a "serious act" and those who make "gestures." Every suicide attempt is serious; a person must have few alternatives to solving his problems if he puts his life in jeopardy by a self-destructive act. The gesture and the serious attempt and should be seen as points on the continuum of suicidal behavior.

Assessment of behavior: The nature of the intent

A first consideration in the therapeutic approach to the person who has attempted suicide is to listen very carefully to what the person says about the suicide attempt and the nature of the intent. The intensity of the wish to die is an issue that must be directly discussed with the person. If a suicide attempt has already been made, this provides the opening comment by the nurse. The questions to ask may be, "What did you wish would happen when you took the pills?" or "What did you think would happen when you cut your wrists?" or "How do you feel now?" or "What do you wish would happen now?" the nurse can also ask if the person has had previous depressive periods and if there have been previous attempts at suicide.

The nurse may be reluctant to ask about suicide. It has been our experience that the patient is never hurt by direct, respectful questions. The patient generally responds to the questions and understands them as part of the total interview. The patient's impulse control level and how desperate he is regarding self-destruction must be assessed promptly.

As the nurse listens to the patient describe his suicidal act, the nature of the attempt is assessed. Of course, the person who attempts suicide in a severe and self-mutilating fashion is in greater danger of being successful than the person who swallows a relatively minor dose of medication or who superficially cuts his wrist. However, nurses do see someone use a relatively innocuous method of self-injury with the firm conviction that he will succeed. It appears that minor attempts of suicidal behavior may also occur in psychotic or severely depressed people who lack the energy or initiative to act any more aggressively against themselves.

A second high-risk factor is the person who makes a suicidal attempt in an isolated setting. For example, the person who ingests medication in front of a spouse during a family argument is not considered to be at high-risk. It is important, however, to remember that most suicidal behavior is ambivalent, and although the person wishes to escape what appears to be an intolerable reality, at the same time he wishes to be discovered. Farber refers to this aspect of suicidal behavior as a "gamble with death."[5] This feature of suicidal behavior points out the manipulative aspect. However, it is most disquieting to find that the person who commits suicide almost always invariably leaves a warning.[6]

Assessment of the social network

Another important prognostic area lies in assessing the patient's social network, particularly factors that contribute to a loss of hope and to increasing isolation. It is important to know the people who are significantly involved with the patient. The greater the number of people involved, the stronger the support system the patient potentially has.

Attempted suicide is often a sign that significant relationships are under stress, and therapeutic intervention should be directed toward resolution of the conflict. When important relationships are highly disorganized and the people concerned appear unable to cooperate, self-destructive behavior may very possibly recur.

Assessment of current and past history

The nurse may ask the patient to describe his current life situation so that she can evaluate the number and intensity of stress factors. Also, family his-

[5]Maurice Farber, *Theory of Suicide* (New York: Funk & Wagnalls, 1968), p. 7.

[6]Erwin Stengel, *Suicide and Attempted Suicide* (London: MacGibbon and Kee, 1965).

tory, as well as personal history, may be used to assess risk. A history of prior attempts is an indication of heightened suicidal risk.

The presence and nature of past psychiatric treatment are often valuable in establishing the diagnosis and formulating an effective treatment plan. Recurrent hospitalizations are likely to occur with schizophrenia and depression. These clinical syndromes are often treated with phenothiazines (schizophrenia) and electroconvulsive therapy or antidepressants (depression). If the patient is currently in therapy, impending termination or temporary absence of the therapist may provide an important clue to the meaning of the suicide attempt. The extent of prior out-patient therapy may serve as an indication of both past illness and the patient's ability to enter and gain support from a therapeutic relationship.

PSYCHIATRIC DIAGNOSIS

A key prognostic factor in assessing the likelihood of a person's repeating suicidal behavior is the identification of underlying psychiatric illness. The most frequently encountered illnesses will be described as depression, schizophrenia, organic brain syndrome, and certain of the personality disorders.[7]

Depressive syndromes

This group of disorders presents a common clinical picture that is distinguishable from transient mood states. The patient presents a forlorn, generally immobile countenance with varying degrees of psychomotor retardation and/or agitation, with diminished appetite, and almost invariably with insomnia. His thought content is marked by hopelessness, guilt, anger, desperation, loneliness, and feelings of worthlessness. Concomitant suicidal ideas may emerge because he feels that he deserves to be dead, that others would be better off if he were absent, or that suicide is the only escape from what appears to be an intolerable situation. Further progression of the syndrome may be accompanied by evidence of delusion and hallucinations and occasionally by an associated confusional picture and impairment of intellectual functioning.

Diagnosis is made by clinical observation and direct questioning of the patient and relatives. Often, he has a history of depressive episodes that may have responded to antidepressant medication or electroconvulsive therapy and that may have required hospitalization. The organic brain syndromes can generally be ruled out through the history and through tests.

Depression is the pneumonia of psychiatry; if left untreated, it often has high morbidity and mortality. Treatment, however, often leads to complete remission. Attempted suicide in a depressed patient calls for rapid, definitive treatment by psychotherapy, antidepressant medication, and/or elec-

---

[7]This chapter is based in part on Owen S. Surman and Aaron Lazare, "Management of the Attempted Suicide Patient," *Medical Insight,* **4,** July (1972), 14–21. Copyright, Insight Publishing Co., Inc.

troconvulsive treatment. When the depressive symptoms are severe with marked alteration in normal life-style functions or pronounced feelings of hopelessness and guilt, out-patient management is a high risk. The patient may be so convinced of his hopelessness that he is unable to cooperate in an out-patient program; his antidepressant medication may present the temptation of a lethal overdose. And there is often a considerable time lag before treatment takes effect. It is advisable to hospitalize the depressed patient who has attempted suicide when his depressive symptoms are severe, when he is out of contact with reality, or when he presents continuing suicidal ideation.

The schizophrenic syndromes

These are characterized by impairment of the capacity to distinguish reality from fantasy. There is a progressive tendency toward disordered communication, altered emotional responsiveness, and social isolation. The onset of the syndrome may be insidious or sudden. Classically, the patient's presentation is marked by bizarreness in dress, deportment, and speech. There is an air of cold indifference and/or inappropriate outbursts of anger, sadness, or mirth. The stream of talk is generally loosely connected, and its content is marked by bizarre somatic preoccupations, ideas of a grandiose or paranoid nature, fear of thought control, and /or feelings of estrangement and depersonalization. Suicidal thinking may relate to any or all of these thoughts. With progressive decompensation there are frank delusions and hallucinations; suicidal behavior at this point may relate to the delusional system or be dictated by an hallucinated voice.

Diagnosis is made in the same way as in the depressive syndromes – by clinical observation, direct questioning, and a review of the past psychiatric history. There may also be a family history of similar illness.

Although schizophrenia is frequently managed successfully on an out-patient basis by using a combination of phenothiazines and psychotherapy, the schizophrenic patient who has attempted suicide is an extreme risk even when the attempt appears to be a minor one. Because of the patient's impaired cognitive function and tendency toward isolation and disordered communication, suicidal behavior is highly unpredictable.[8] For this reason, hospitalization is almost always indicated.

Organic brain syndromes

These are psychotic reactions of organic etiology which may be reversible (acute brain syndrome) or irreversible (chronic brain syndrome). The nature of the dysfunction may be toxic metabolic, traumatic, hemorrhagic, vascular, or infectious. Attempted suicide may occur in any of the organic psycho-

[8]Edwin S. Shneidman and D. M. Lane (1957) "Psychologic and Social Work Clues to Suicide in a Schizophrenic," in *Clues to Suicide,* eds., E. S. Shneidman and N. L. Farberow (New York: McGraw-Hill Book Company, 1957), pp. 170–87.

ses, but it is most common in the presence of drug and alcohol abuse and more recently in the toxic psychoses induced by hallucinogenic drugs.

The patient with an organic brain syndrome generally appears confused and perplexed. Wide mood swings are classical. His speech may be highly disorganized; his attention, grasp, and memory may be impaired; he is usually disoriented and frequently he has illusions, delusions, and hallucinations. Suicidal behavior tends to result from the combination of confusion, disorientation, and delusional thinking. In alcohol related syndromes, the depressant effects of alcohol are an additional factor.

Diagnosis is made through history, physical examination, and laboratory tests.

Like all persons in psychotic states, these patients are highly unpredictable and require close observation following a suicide attempt. Once medical management has successfully reversed central nervous system impairment, it is necessary to perform a careful psychological reassessment, particularly when the etiology is related to drug or alcohol abuse. The disturbed patient who has limited adaptive resources, whose history is characterized by impulsive behavior, and who deals with stress by resorting to some form of intoxication is likely to repeat the patterns which result in central nervous system impairment and suicidal behavior. In such cases, psychiatric hospitalization is often advisable.

Personality disorders

These consist of a broad group of characterological impairments. Patients who have attempted suicide frequently present life-styles characteristic of three major subgroups: hysterical personality, antisocial personality, and chronic alcoholism.[9]

Although hysterical personality does occur in both sexes, the classic hysteric is young, female, coquettish, and inclined to histrionic behavior. Attempted suicide in these patients is often a dramatic display or the acting out of an interpersonal conflict. Their demanding dependency frequently antagonizes others (especially the medical staff) and evokes an angry response; a power struggle may then ensue in which the patient becomes increasingly willful and intransigent. This struggle is best avoided if one views the suicide attempt objectively, as an inadequate and maladaptive means of dealing with life stress. The major goal in management is to support the patient through the crisis and encourage more healthy and socially appropriate modes of problem solving. This intervention is best initiated by mobilizing support from family and friends and by referral to a mental health professional. Although these patients require a great deal of help and careful follow-up, hospitalization can most often be avoided.

The patient with an antisocial personality is characteristically impulsive, demanding, manipulative, egocentric, and has a history of behavior

[9]Stengel, *Suicide and Attempted Suicide*.

which is injurious to others. Like the hysteric, he is often highly engaging in the absence of stress but meets frustration with frantic attempts to manipulate the social situation. The suicide attempt is often such a desperate maneuver. The patient needs support to get through the crisis, but the patient frequently presents highly unrealistic demands. Again, there is a risk that anger on the part of the nurse will be followed by increasingly willful behavior. Management therefore requires that the nurse support and set firm limits as she offers assistance and requires that she clearly define the reality of the situation and the patient's responsibility. If this approach fails and the patient is unable to cooperate, hospitalization is often advisable.

The alcoholic often exhibits demanding, dependent behavior and disordered interpersonal relationships. The major problem in dealing with him is that ongoing stress often leads to increased alcohol consumption; in turn, intoxication leads to depression and overwhelms the patient's capacity for adaptive behavior. He is then vulnerable to impulsive and self-destructive behavior. It is generally best to encourage withdrawal in a hospital setting. Following withdrawal, the alcoholic must have therapeutic supports that will meet some of his dependency needs and at the same time assist him in developing realistic means of dealing with stress. Anger on the part of the physician increases the alcoholic's belief that the world is hostile and leads to further disorganization and self-destructive behavior.

MANAGEMENT OF SUICIDAL BEHAVIOR

The suicide crisis is a common psychiatric emergency that is seen in outpatient settings such as in emergency departments of general hospitals. Since there is an ever-present danger that the suicide attempt will be repeated with lethal consequences, psychiatric consultation is advisable. When such consultation is not available, the most important decision following treatment for the crisis, is whether to hospitalize the person in a psychiatric facility or refer him for outpatient evaluation.

Patient's attitude about the attempt

When there is no sign of psychosis, severe depression, or a highly disordered personality structure, and when the social situation is relatively stable and the attempt has not been of a highly lethal nature, the nurse can be further reassured if the patient regrets his recent suicidal behavior and ensures that he will return for help if future events threaten to overwhelm him. Alternatively, the nurse should never disregard a patient who states that he is sorry he did not succeed or threatens to try again. This individual is clearly asking for help, however disordered the nature of his communication. The nurse should also be extremely cautious about the patient who has suffered a loss and believes that death will reunite him with a loved one.

Just as the suicide act communicates a wish for escape and at the same time a plea for rescue, so the wish for rescue is frequently associated with a tendency to alienate the helper. The suicide act is often an expression of the patient's rage against the environment turned in against himself, [10] what Shneidman has called "murder in the 180th degree."[11] This is of consequence in management because the patient's anger and hopelessness may evoke similar feelings from even the most empathetic nurse and increase the patient's tendency to see his environment as hostile and unforgiving.

During the initial interview, it is essential to listen very carefully to what the person says about the nature of the suicidal intent. After the information is assessed, it is important to assess the patient's feelings of inadequacy in coping with the immediate and chronic stresses in his life, his level of hope, his view of the situation as being intolerable. The nurse listens and tries to understand the patient's view of his existence at that very moment.

In our experience, people who make suicide attempts are out of a caring system, that is, they are not being cared for by a professional or mental health worker. People who are successful in their suicidal behavior are generally not actively engaged in treatment. They may be involved in situations in which the therapist has terminated or is on vacation or is in the process of leaving, and thus the patient is in transit.

The main intervention in this situation is that someone take responsibility to care and to watch over the patient. A danger for nurses is that they are so busy making referrals for the suicidal person that, in essence, he is getting no care. We caution against this danger of making transfers and referrals because it gives the message that no one in the system really cares. The quality of hopelessness decreases when the patient feels that someone does care in a human way. When the patient feels this, he believes that there is some hope and this feeling may be a life-line at that point in time.

In-patient hospitalization

The risk of repeated suicidal behavior and the indications for hospitalization can be assessed by referring to the psychiatric diagnosis, nature of intent, social matrix, and current and past history. Hospitalization is indicated when there is high risk in any of these areas.

In-patient psychiatric units of hospitals are a major resource for referral of the suicidal person. These units have a dual task: First they have an administrative obligation to prevent suicide and to protect the patient by removing harmful objects such as razor blades and extra medicines; and second, they provide the caring aspects of the therapeutic environment.

SUMMARY   This chapter showed that there are many ways to view depression. Because the nurse works with many mental health people it is important to have an understanding of the four viewpoints: (1) depression viewed as a mood state; (2) depression viewed as a symptom complex; (3) depression viewed as a

[10]Sigmund Freud, "Mourning and Melancholia," in *The Standard Edition of the Complete Psychological Works of Sigmund Freud,* Vol. 14 (London: Hogarth Press, 1957), pp. 243–58.

[11]Edwin S. Shneidman, *On the Nature of Suicide* (San Francisco: Jossey-Bass, 1969), pp. 1–30.

discrete disease entity or diagnostic category; and (4) depression viewed as a complex of psychodynamic mechanisms.

Since there is no single way to treat depression, several nursing approaches were described from which the nurse may select, in order to plan nursing care of the patient. These approaches were identified as bearing painful feelings, resolving feelings, dealing with anger, responding to the dynamic issue, implementing the biologic model, providing controls for the patient, evaluating the symptom cluster, assessing the suicidal patient, and dealing with subjective feelings.

This chapter has also examined some of the assessment factors of suicidal behavior in terms of nature of the intent, affect of the patient, the social network, and current and past history.

REFERENCES AND SUGGESTED READINGS

Beck, Aaron T., Harvey L. P. Resnik, and Dan J. Lettieri (1974). *The Prediction of Suicide*. Bowie, Md.: The Charles Press Publishers, Inc.

Crary, William G., and Gerald C. Creary (1973). "Depression," *American Journal of Nursing,* **73,** No. 3, 472–75.

Farber, Maurice L. (1968). *Theory of Suicide*. New York: Funk & Wagnalls.

Journard, Sidney M. (1970). "Suicide: An Invitation to Die," *American Journal of Nursing,* **70,** No. 2, 269.

Kelly, Holly S. (1969). "The Sense of an Ending," *American Journal of Nursing,* **69,** No. 11, 2378–81.

Kiev, Ari (1974). "Prognostic Factors in Attempted Suicide," *American Journal of Psychiatry,* **131,** No. 9, 987–90.

Lazare, Aaron (1970). "The Difference between Sadness and Depression," *Medical Insight,* **2** No. 23, 23–31.

Provost, Judith (1974). "Intervention in a Schizoaffective Depressive Behavior Pattern: A Behavioral Approach," *Perspectives in Psychiatric Care,* **12,** No. 2, 86–89.

Oast, Samuel P., and Arthur Zitrin (1975). "A Public Health Approach to Suicide Prevention," *American Journal of Public Health,* **65,** No. 2, 144–47.

Redlich, Frederick C., and Daniel Freedman (1966). *The Theory and Practice of Psychiatry*. New York: Basic Books.

Rochlin, Gregory (1965). *Griefs and Discontents: The Forces of Change*. Boston: Little, Brown and Co.

Surman, Owen, and Aaron Lazare (1972). "Management of the Attempted Suicide Patient: Indications for Psychiatric Hospitalization," *Medical Insight,* **4,** No. 7, 14–21.

Vollen, Karen Helm, and Charles G. Watson (1975). "Suicide in Relation to Time of Day and Day of Week," *American Journal of Nursing,* **75,** No. 2, 263.

Westercamp, Twilla M. (1975). "Suicide," *American Journal of Nursing,* **75,** No. 2, 260–62.

NEUROSES AND PERSONALITY DISORDERS

14

Neurotic feelings and behavior are maladaptive reactions that result in a diminished capacity to adjust to the environment and a failure to live up to one's full psychological potential. In viewing the difficulties that people have in adapting to stressful situations, we see that four general areas of maladjustments can be identified: relationships, work productiveness, value problems, and society or cultural patterns.[1]

1. Interpersonal relationships. Problems in this area generally focus on the issue of intimacy. People function well with superficial relationships, but deeper relationships, such as are involved in the marriage relationship, prove difficult. People may try to avoid emotional closeness and involvement with family members. Another example in this area is that of encouraging a member of the opposite sex to the point that success is imminent and then withdrawing to the complete frustration of both parties.

2. Work productiveness. People who have difficulty adjusting to work situations tend to be one of two kinds: the person who changes jobs frequently and thus fails to make the advances commensurate with his abilities or the person who has difficulty producing satisfactorily in the job. The person may have occupational failure resulting from fear of success.

3. Problems with values. The issue of integrity is important in this area. Sometimes the person just does not feel that he is living the kind of life he wishes to live and he feels empty and unhappy. Or the person experiences feelings of guilt and shame for acts he did not commit. The person, for example, a housewife, may have an excessive need for orderliness and cleanliness which leaves her little time and energy for anything else.

4. Cultural patterns. Sometimes people are socialized into roles that have been part of their culture for decades. At some point the person may

[1]Clara Thompson, "An Introduction to Minor Malady Adjustments." in *American Handbook of Psychiatry,* ed., Silvano Areti (New York: Basic Books, Inc., 1959).

step back and ask herself what these values mean to her personally and she may become frustrated within a prescribed role. Women may find that as grown children leave the home they are unprepared to commit themselves to roles in life and this leads to the development of symptoms. Or people may become used to and abuse their use of alcohol and drugs in order to avoid imagined external threats.

Neurotic behavior is rigid, repetitive, and inappropriate. The neurotic person cannot seem to learn from past mistakes. Considerable energy is taken up by worrying and fantasizing. The person has difficulty in distinguishing between wishing and acting. He may feel guilty over fantasies and, consequently, feel the need to be punished. He tries to satisfy his needs in inadequate or forbidden ways. Although the behavior must provide some benefits, it really turns out to be ineffective. It is as if the neurotic person is fighting a battle that no longer exists. The battle is over, but the neurotic person fights on.

Everyone behaves at times in a neurotic manner, and the severity of a neurosis is thus a matter of degree. A person may be regarded as "severely neurotic" to the degree that the neurotic behavior is all pervasive, socially and psychologically incapacitating, and yet totally unrelated to psychological stress.

Neurotic behavior may be distinguished from psychotic behavior by several criteria:

1. The patient is aware that there is a disturbance with his mental functioning.
2. There is no gross distortion of external reality.
3. The loss of adaptation is only partial.

NEUROSES AND PERSONALITY DISORDERS

Neurotic behavior may be divided into the neuroses and the personality disorders. The *neuroses* are characterized by anxiety which is either felt directly or is converted by various mechanisms into other symptoms which distress the patient. He finds these feelings, thoughts, or actions strange, undesirable, unwanted, irritating, or upsetting. In other words, neurotic symptoms are ego-alien.

The feelings, thoughts, and actions of the *personality disorders,* neurotic as they may be, are felt by the person to be part of himself. This behavior is therefore regarded as ego-syntonic. His behavior may be disturbing only to those around him and not to himself. As distorted and constricted as his behavior may be, the person functions in such a way as to minimize psychological tension. This behavior represents lifelong, deeply ingrained, maladaptive habits which have had their onset at or before adolescence.

In clinical practice the distinction between a neurosis and personality disorder is usually blurred. There are times when a person finds his character traits irritating, even to himself. Similarly, a person may become so accustomed to his symptoms that they almost become a part of his character. To further blur the distinction, patients who suffer from neuroses are likely to simultaneously suffer from personality disorders. As a result of this blurring of the neuroses and personality disorders, we refer to these mal-adaptive feelings, thoughts, and actions as *neurotic behavior*. We maintain the distinction because most textbooks make these distinctions.

THE NEUROSES The neuroses are officially classified in the diagnostic nomenclature of the American Psychiatric Association as follows:

> Anxiety neurosis
> Hysterical neurosis, conversion type
> Hysterical neurosis, dissociative type
> Phobic neurosis
> Obsessive compulsive neurosis
> Depressive neurosis
> Neurasthenic neurosis
> Depersonalization neurosis
> Hypochondriacal neurosis
> Other neuroses

A single neurosis rarely exists in pure culture. More often, aspects of several neuroses occur together. We will describe a few of the neuroses listed above with case material.

Anxiety neurosis

This neurosis is characterized by anxiety, acute or chronic, which may be manifested by dry mouth, rapid heartbeat, diarrhea, and hyperventilation. The anxiety tends to fluctuate in intensity and may be unrelated to specific events.

The following excerpt from an interview with a patient suffering from symptoms of anxiety neurosis illustrates the mental anguish these patients experience:

Nurse: "How are you feeling tonight?"

Patient: "The day has been awful. All I do is worry."

Nurse: "What are some of your worries?"

Patient: "I have pains in my chest and a burning in my stomach and chest. Everyone tells me these symptoms are my 'nerves' but I'm worried that it might be cancer or heart disease or an ulcer. I have to be well to care for my sick kids and husband. He can't help me because he's a man and has his job all day.

Then I think about my responsibility at home. I hate the housework part and the kids being sick all the time.

I saw my sister at the doctor's office. She used to take care of me when I was little and I'm afraid I'll be a chronic mentally ill case like her.

Then I worry about the noise, and crowds, and riding in a car. Maybe I should just forget about my kids and the responsibilities. Maybe I'll never be better. Or, maybe I should just go home. I'll just have to force myself to do the things I hate to do."

Hysterical neurosis, conversion type

The conversion reactions are named for the major intrapsychic mechanism. Conversion is an unconscious process through which intrapsychic conflicts find symbolic expression through a variety of body symptoms. The voluntary nervous system is affected and causes such symptoms as paralyses, blindness, deafness, and anesthesias. The person may frequently show a lack of concern about these symptoms which may actually be providing secondary gains by winning the person sympathy or by relieving him of unpleasant responsibilities.

The conversion reactions were the first illnesses of psychogenic origin to be so recognized and the first neurotic reactions to receive intense psychologic study. In the early 1900s conversion symptoms were familiar to physicians. The term *hysteria* was often attached to these symptoms.

Fainting is an example of a conversion reaction (assuming that neurological causes are ruled out). From a psychogenic aspect, it is a defensive reaction that a person uses to shut out the outside perception. Some students in nursing and medicine have been known to faint when they observed certain medical procedures or operations. Some will faint at the sight of blood and others will faint while they await inoculations at a clinic setting or at a military induction center. Fainting at funerals is observed. The unconscious wish to avoid reality situations is obvious and understandable in many situations. It is the mind's way of defending against painful events.

It is important to distinguish this kind of hysterical neurosis from psychophysiologic disorders in which the autonomic nervous system is affected, from malingering which is a conscious act, and from neurological lesions.

Hysterical neurosis, dissociative type

The dissociative reactions are the large group of uncommon, and often bizarre, patterns of defensive reactions to anxiety or stress. In this reaction such symptoms as amnesia, sleepwalking, fugue, and the multiple personality syndrome occur.

The dissociative reactions generally create public interest. The newspapers often publicize amnesia victims, and there are many jokes about somnambulism (sleepwalking). The state of fugue, a type of personality dissociation, often brings people to the police station rather than to a mental health clinic. The strangeness, particularly the phenomenon of semiautomatic, nonconscious behavior, intrigues and fascinates people.

Phobic neurosis

The phobic patient is characterized as having an intense fear of objects, places, or even particular groups of people. The phobia defends against unconscious anxiety by displacement onto the phobia object. In this way, the person now fears an external object rather than an internal and unknown source of distress. Phobias are common experiences in childhood—fear of animals, darkness, lightning, and strangers. In adulthood, a phobia can become a crippling experience.

Common adult phobias are agoraphobia, the fear of or avoidance of open spaces; zoophobias, the fear of animals; aerophobia, the fear of flying; and claustrophobia, the fear of confined places.

Obsessive–compulsive neurosis

This neurosis is characterized by the presence of ego-alien thoughts (obsessions) that the patient cannot control or actions (compulsions) that the patient must perform. Common examples of obsessive thoughts are the urge to recheck whether or not your keys were locked inside your car after you had left the car or to recheck if you have your airplane ticket with you prior to a trip. Examples of compulsive acts include throwing spilled salt over the left shoulder to ward off bad luck or walking back to the car to check whether the lights were left on.

The following is a case example of obsessive–compulsive neurosis:

A 38-year-old married housewife, mother of three is admitted with the chief complaint of uncontrollable, excessive thoughts about wars, destruction, and of Hitler. She has the obsessive thoughts that if she thinks like Adolf Hitler she does not deserve to have sex.

The depressive situation began 6 months previously when her 18-year-old daughter brought home a boyfriend from college for Christmas. The patient began to lose her appetite and had increasing difficulty in sleeping.

The age 18 is significant to her. This is the age at which she herself married. She wishes now she could be 18 and apparently seems quite angry toward those who are 18, including her daughter.

The patient has had obsessive thoughts off and on throughout her life, apparently aggressive wishes breaking through her defenses; for example, at age 16 she thought she was swearing at God and cursing God because the Church was so strict. She had subsequently many obsessive thoughts about death and destruction and whenever she heard about someone ill or dying, she said she wished they would be dead. She says negative things about anything and everything and wishes she could undo this.

Five years ago the patient had a hysterectomy and at present has colitis. For the past 2 years her parents have been living in a basement apartment with her and she has had many severe arguments, with the mother especially, but the secondary gains of her illness have resulted in her parents' being very nice to her.

She said she was quite infatuated with the friend of her present husband, but read in a book that one should marry someone with whom one is comfortable. She felt she was comfortable with the man she did marry because he was madly in love with her. Their marriage, however, has had periods in which she has been negative toward him.

Patient states that her problem is not new to her, but only within the past 2 weeks has it become unbearable She related the 19 years of her marriage: when she married her husband, she was not really sure she loved him. However, they enjoyed each other's company and felt "comfortable" and since he was "crazy about her," she married him. Over the years she has noticed a growing restlessness, a tendency to look at other couples and envy them their happiness. She claims she often goes to the movies to seek the "thrill" that is missing from her marriage. At first she was able to "bury" these feelings, but more recently they have obsessed her although she has "never done anything wrong in her life." These thoughts led her to feelings of guilt, making her consider herself a "bad" person.

She also describes, with vague and confusing half-finished sentences, a "spell" that she has experienced with increasing frequency. She reads headlines of a tragedy (for example, the number killed in the war or in an accident) and dwells on it. The purpose seems to be to convince herself of her relative happiness compared to so much sorrow in the world. Unfortunately, since she wants to feel happy, she welcomes a lot of tragedy with which to contrast it and then feels guilty because she has had pleasure in someone else's misfortune. Lately these spells have become more necessary to her as a means of escape from her own unbearable obsession.

In looking at her problem she, on the one hand, feels that the only way to relieve herself of her obsession would be to separate from her husband; on the other hand, she cannot bear the thought of living without him because he has been very good to her and their life has been "a good one, at least superficially."

PERSONALITY DISORDERS

Personality disorders, like the neuroses, rarely exist in pure culture. More often, personality or character styles form a blend in any given patient.

Character or personality styles are much more important to try to understand than are the symptoms of neurosis. For example, knowing that a person develops blurred vision or faints as hysterical symptoms is of much less importance than being aware of her whole style of life which operates every second of every living day. One specific symptom is only one particular incident in the total context of the person's style of living that deals with life by exaggeration and by the egocentric calling of attention to her behavior.

As previously stated, in Chapter 8, personality traits differentiate one person from another. They determine how one appears, how one behaves, how one is liked and judged by others, and what one accomplishes in life. Character or personality traits neither appear by accident nor are they necessarily inborn. They have evolved over the years of living. Their essential function is defensive. They may be called character defenses. They are a gradual autonomic and unconscious process.

This section will briefly describe the following personality disorders: paranoid personality, schizoid personality, obsessive–compulsive personality, hysterical personality, passive–aggressive personality, antisocial personality, and sexual deviations. Alcoholism and drug dependence are personality disorders which will be covered in separate chapters in Part Five, The Community.

The paranoid personality

The paranoid personality is characterized by a rigid and pervasive sense of suspiciousness. He constantly searches for confirmation of the idea that particular people, or all people, will betray him or otherwise do him harm. Evidence to the contrary is likely to be ignored. In this sense, paranoid individuals, in their most extreme form, suffer from impaired reality testing and may therefore be regarded as among the sickest of the personality disorders. In contrast, less severe paranoid personalities, as well as normal people, have the ability to correct an initial notion that they are being discriminated against or are facing a particular psychological attack. People with paranoid personality styles may either be shy, seclusive, furtive, and frightened of involvement or they may be aggressive, ambitious, outwardly hostile, and arrogant. Whatever variation we see, they spend a great deal of their energy searching for clues that will confirm to them that danger is forever lurking. They seem particularly prone to hurts and humiliations. The above description may help the nurse to understand some of the paranoid behaviors which may be expected in clinical situations. Slight rejections and inadvertent oversights on the part of the nurse as well as the feeling of vulnerability that is part of being a patient may precipitate an array of paranoid behaviors. These may take the form of inappropriate anger, threats of revenge, threats of litigations, claims that the nurse is like "all the others," and proclamations of self-righteousness. In this way, the patient projects all his perceived badness onto the world. Pathologic behaviors of paranoid patients may be minimized by avoiding situations in which the patient feels that his autonomy is threatened or in which he feels trapped. Whenever possible, the nurse should not interfere with his freedom of choice and movement. She should neither argue with nor reassure the patient. Instead, she should strive to be a safe person who does not take sides so that the patient may have the opportunity to begin to break out of his psychological isolation.

Schizoid personality

The schizoid personality is characterized by a tendency to withdraw from others, a chronic sense of loneliness, and a subjective sense of emptiness. These patients may be very aware of their intense need for people and they may fear that their needs, if expressed, will overwhelm and hurt the other person. They maintain distance in order to protect themselves from rejection, to protect the other person from their own aggression, and to protect themselves from the feared aggression of others. Schizoid patients may also describe excruciating feelings of discomfort when someone attempts to be close, kind, warm, or affectionate. Many of these patients never marry. They obtain solitary jobs in which there is barely enough interpersonal contact to sustain them. They may feel comfortable dealing with other people by telephone, correspondence, or through brief and fleeting contacts. Schizoid patients may seek treatment after they have been completely isolated from their few sustaining contacts or after they have been overwhelmed by the intensity of a close relationship. They are likely to present with depressive symptoms characterized by an empty, hungry quality. Often these patients resort to drugs, alcohol, or excess food which may be regarded as depressive equivalents. The nurse must be ever mindful of the schizoid patient's need for human contact on the one hand and his need for respectful distance on the other. A delicate balance must be maintained. Some patients respond to a one-to-one interpersonal contact in which they learn that there is more pleasure than fright in a relationship. For others, group therapies seem to be more useful.

Passive-aggressive personality

This personality disorder is usually divided into two subgroups which include the passive–dependent and passive–aggressive personalities. The passive–dependent personality, hereafter referred to as the *oral character,* relates to others by pleading helplessness, by communicating a special need for care, support, advice, concern, and love. He may make gestures of generosity to others, but he expects even more in return. When his needs are not met, the patient is likely to respond first with feelings of helplessness, depression, and despair and then with feelings of anger and rage. This person is likely to come for treatment after his support system, which has fulfilled these oral needs, has failed. The patient will then both directly and indirectly request that the nurse and other staff provide for him that which was taken away. The nurse may wish to gratify these needs from the outset, only to find that she feels manipulated and controlled into providing more than she can possibly maintain. In the passive–aggressive personality, many of the above clinical features are still pervasive. In addition, however, the patient has learned to express his aggression in a passive and compliant manner. For instance, if he wishes to oppose someone else's suggestion, he may do it by forgetting, by misplacing the instructions, or by procrastinating.

Obsessive–compulsive personality

The obsessive–compulsive personality is characterized by the personality traits of orderliness, rigidity, perfectionism, severe conscience, constriction of affect, perseverance, a tendency to hoard (parsimony), indecision, a critical and self-righteous aggression, and stubbornness. Defense mechanisms associated with this personality are isolation of affect and doing and undoing. In the obsessional patient, one can see neurotic ambivalence in its clearest form. There are always two sides to every feeling and thought. This ambivalence and indecision may significantly impair the patient's ability to act. When it involves others, the behavior can also be extremely provocative and frustrating.

Obsessive personalities may operate at high levels of functioning when they are able to make good use of their orderly manner, frugality, and perseverance. Creativity, however, may be seriously limited. These people have a great need to be in control of their impulses, their feelings, and the world around them. Psychic decompensation often results from a loss of control in these very areas. Depression, obsessional symptoms, or anxiety may result. Effective treatment is fostered by respecting the patient's autonomy and by assisting him to regain control over his world. This may be accomplished by verbal interaction which assists the patient to gain control over overwhelming feelings and impulses. Various occupational tasks requiring detailed efforts are also helpful.

Hysterical personality

The hysterical personality is characterized by a constellation of personality traits which include exhibitionism, egocentricity, suggestibility, sexual provocativeness, and lability of emotions. In addition to these traits, these patients have difficulty in triangular situations, by this, we mean that in a situation with a male and female, the patient becomes competitive with the person of the same sex and seductive to the person of the opposite sex. Although hysterical dynamics occur in both sexes, the literature focuses almost entirely on the hysterical female, probably because most of the literature is written by men. Whether an hysterical patient is a normal, charming person or a severely impaired patient depends on the degree of ego strength (see Chapter 4). In clinical practice, the nurse is likely to see sicker hysterics with considerable ego impairment. These patients usually describe severe deprivation in their early years. Their sexual behavior is deceptive, for it is a masked way of asking for caring. When asking for sexual responses, they are really wishing to be held. Female hysterics behave in a seductive manner toward male personnel and in a competitive manner toward female nurses. The nurse can best help the patient by providing maternal responses to competitive provocations. Similarly, male nurses may be helpful by providing maternal (caring, nonsexualized) responses. These treatment strategies recognize that the primary pathology resides in the relationship between the patient and her mother.

Case history of a patient with hysterical personality and hysterical symptoms

The patient, a 38-year-old married Roman Catholic mother of four, was in her usual state of mental health until December 1973, the 25th anniversary of her mother's suicide. Her mother died at the age of 37 or 38. The patient's husband described a specific event which heralded the onset of psychiatric symptoms. They were attending a party at which most of the guests were intoxicated. The patient walked into a bedroom and found her husband and another man playfully wrestling with another woman. The patient screamed, called the other woman a "slut" and went "absolutely wild, hysterical." Shortly thereafter the patient felt sad and blue and experienced frequent episodes of crying. She noted a decrease in energy and was unable to do her chores at home. She feared being alone and felt "frightened, nervous and shaky." There was a decrease in appetite with an 18-pound weight loss, difficulty in falling asleep, and pains throughout the body. Sexual desires were both heightened and diminished at various times. These symptoms continued for 4 months before the patient came to medical attention. She initially saw an internist because of the arm pains. He referred her to a psychiatrist who, in March 1974, hospitalized the patient and administered 13 electroconvulsive treatments. There was no clinical improvement. In October 1974 the patient began out-patient psychotherapy with a resident psychiatrist at a teaching hospital. She responded neither to psychotherapy nor to therapeutic doses of imipramine and chlordiazepoxide. In February 1975 she was admitted to an inpatient unit under the care of the same therapist. The working diagnosis was depressive reaction in an hysterical personality.

The patient was the eldest of four children born to Roman Catholic parents. Her mother, who became "mentally ill" when the patient was 11 years old, committed suicide with an overdose of sleeping pills two years later. The patient held the father responsible for the death because of his cruelty. She claims she always felt rather distant from her mother, who usually left the care of the children to domestic help. At her mother's funeral, a friend stopped the patient from jumping into the grave. The father was an insurance broker, whom the patient recalled as always being drunk and chasing the maid, his wife or the children about the house. He opposed the patient's marriage because he desired both her physical presence and her wages. She secretly married at age 19 in an attempt to run away from her father, who, 3 years after the marriage, died of gastrointestinal hemorrhage secondary to alcoholism. The patient found it difficult to understand why she was unable to remember where her father is buried.

The patient described her marriage as unhappy, "one constant argument, one long grudge." Her husband had always left clues that he was having extramarital affairs. The patient had rarely enjoyed sex. Orgasm was infrequent. At the time of admission there were four children: aged 19 (female), 15 (male), 12 (female), and 5 (male). The patient voiced no concern over her eldest daughter's sharing the husband's bed during the hospitalization or the joint bathing of the two youngest children.

The patient herself came from a family of four children. There was a 37-year-old sister and two brothers aged 33 and 30. Both brothers had psychiatric care; the younger received electroconvulsive treatments when he was 25.

The patient was a high-school graduate of average intelligence who was raised in the Philadelphia suburbs. She had worked as a saleswoman before marriage. Her personality could be described by the following traits: aggressive, sarcastic, demanding, clinging in her dependence, pessimistic, suggestible, emotionally labile, sexually provocative.

During the first 7 weeks of hospitalization there was a gradual diminution of depressive symptoms. Then suddenly there was an acute exacerbation of the depression following a quarrel with her husband. Simultaneously, the patient was experiencing uncomfortable feelings in her body, especially in the presence of the therapist: "I feel suspended . . . I feel it's absolutely choking me, whatever it is . . . I feel like my whole body tickles, like a raw nerve, a crawling sensation." This interview material was a response to an inquiry about the sexualized transference. The patient visited home the next weekend. During the visit her husband said that he could no longer stand her complaining and that he was "fed up." On the evening of her return to the hospital the patient developed camptocormia (this was the end of the eighth week of hospitalization). She walked with a flexed spine which made an 80° angle with the pelvic girdle. The head and trunk were nearly parallel to the ground. While in bed the patient could maintain her body in a straight line without difficulty. Except for the abnormal posture, the neurological exam was within normal limits. Just prior to the onset of the symptom, with the crisis in therapy and the crisis in the marriage, the depression had reached its greatest depth as measured by the patient's subjective feelings, her general appearance, the sleep disturbance, and the weight loss. The onset of camptocormia heralded an abrupt change in the depressive syndrome. Sadness and anxiety were markedly diminished; appetite and sleep pattern improved. The patient displayed an exhibitionistic joy over her new symptom as she waved cheerfully and triumphantly to onlookers in the halls. Although most depressive symptoms were lessening, there was an increase in somatic concerns, including the conversion symptoms of transitory blindness and paralysis of the hands.

The symptom of camptocormia was unchanged for 2 weeks. During the third week after the onset of this symptom the patient would flex to anthropoid position only when seeing the therapist or hearing his name. During the fourth and fifth weeks after the onset of the symptom the camptocormia subsided. At the end of the thirteenth week of hospitalization the patient was discharged. During the 5-week period from the onset of camptocormia to hospital discharge, important changes occurred in the patient's relationship to her husband and to the therapist. The husband saw the patient as sick and not malingering; the threat of abandonment was therefore temporarily removed. The resident therapist, too, perceived the patient as more ill, partly because of the ease with which incestuous material became available during the interview and partly because of a consultation with a new supervisor. He had been treating her as a fairly healthy neurotic and had overstressed the importance of the sexualized transference. When the therapist altered his approach and became more supportive, the patient commented that he was becoming more like a mother than a father. She appeared relieved.[2]

Antisocial personality

Antisocial personality also may be called *sociopathic behavior*. This disorder tends to be characterized by abnormal behavior rather than subjective discomfort. The seriousness of this disorder is due to the patient's persistent violations of the laws, mores, and customs of the community. These people seek gratification of instinctual needs without the influence of superego values or regard for the demands of society.

In the adult the behavior is manifested by some or all of the following:

1. *Inability to postpone pleasure.* The antisocial person wants what he wants when he wants it.
2. *Inability to tolerate frustration.* There is no evidence in the patient of his ability to tolerate discomfort.
3. *Failure to learn from experience.* The person may repeatedly be punished for similar offenses.
4. *Numerous socially unacceptable activities.* The person will have a history of antisocial conduct.
5. *Promiscuous sexual behavior.* The sexual activity is aimed at immediate physical gratification with a variety of sexual partners.
6. *Alcohol with drug abuse.* A history of episodes of drunkenness or drug habituation is often in evidence.
7. *Poor interpersonal relationships.* The person lacks the ability to make close, lasting relationships with other people.
8. *Relative absence of anxiety and guilt feelings.* Anxiety is usually only seen under external stress situations.

[2]Sections reprinted with permission from Aaron Lazare and Gerald Klerman, "Camptocormia in a Female: A Five-year Study," *British Journal of Medical Psychology,* **43** (1970). 265–70.

9. *Poor judgment.* The judgment used in situations by this person may, at best, be described as poor.

10. *Poor school and employment history.* The ability to conform to standards in school or at work proves frustrating and the person rebels and breaks rules.

Case situation   The following case example presents information on a patient hospitalized with the diagnosis of antisocial personality:

Judy, a 20-year-old single female, is admitted to the psychiatric unit following a 2-week period of progressive inactivity at home. The mother reports that her daughter just sat and watched television and drank vodka all day long.

The patient states that she had completed all high-school courses successfully but because her senior paper was not accepted, she was not graduated. Her I.Q. was stated to be 140.

Family history states mother and father living and well. Patient was adopted at the age of 6 months. One brother, age 17, was adopted at the age of 2 years.

Previous hospitalizations indicate two previous psychiatric admissions. The first admission occurred when the patient was 17 years old. She was hospitalized for 6 months at that time. The second admission came when she was 18 years old and she was hospitalized for 1 year at that time.

Between hospitalizations the patient worked as an aide in a general hospital. She went out with girlfriends but never dated boys. After being discharged from the two previous hospitalizations, she rapidly reverted to inactivity.

The patient's appearance is significant in that she has short, straight hair, continuously wears dungarees and sweat shirts, and assumes masculine posturings and mannerisms.

Her presenting behavior to staff is that of being very demanding of staff attention. She becomes angry at other patients for any attention they receive from staff. She is uninterested in any activity except watching and learning about the personal lives of the staff.

The following are some of the problems that are described in the nursing report:

1. Judy has a swelling on her knee for which she continually requests pain medication. The orthopedic consultant who evaluated her knee condition feels that the swelling was caused by her banging her knee against something in order to bring about the swelling.

2. Judy has been very angry and physically abusive to several patients after the patients had spent time talking with a staff nurse.

3. Judy spends more of her time and energy at this time trying to find out about the personal lives of the staff. She tries to become a close friend of staff members. She plays staff against each other with statements such as, "How come you won't let me do it? The other nurse always lets me do it."

4. Judy appears to have been drinking on two occasions since her arrival on the ward but denies it when asked.

5. Patients are angry with Judy because of her behavior. She avoids other patients for the most part and takes part in ward activities only if some of the staff members are participating. The patients are also afraid of Judy.

6. Discomfort and anger are rising in the staff because information given out by staff members is being "misused."

The above list of nursing concerns is not unusual for patients with antisocial behavior. The management of such behavior and the nursing approaches required are discussed later in this chapter.

SEXUAL DEVIATIONS

Antisocial sexual behavior is classified with the personality disorders. There are various viewpoints on what is considered perverted sexual practice and what is considered deviant sexual behavior. From the clinical view, sexual behavior is considered abnormal when it is a source of concern, discomfort, or of unpleasant consequence to the person indulging in it or when there is no consent from a second person involved in the sexual activity.

A current debate in psychiatric nomenclature involves the classification of homosexual behavior. By definition, a homosexual by choice seeks a sexual partner of the same sex. A decision made in 1973 by the American Psychiatric Association has removed homosexuality per se from the standard official nomenclature and describes a new category, *sexual orientation disturbance,* which is defined as follows: "This is for individuals whose sexual interests are directed primarily toward people of the same sex and who are either disturbed by, in conflict with, or wish to change their sexual orientation."[3]

We believe that the implications for nursing practice regarding the overall issue of sexual deviations are twofold. First, if the person finds his own sexual behavior disturbing and thereby seeks therapy, the issue becomes a treatment concern, unless there is a second party who has been victimized by the sexual activity. In such a case, the victim should also receive treatment. Second, the antisocial component of sexually deviant behavior must be confronted because more often than not the person does not seek help on his own, but only when he is charged with antisocial behavior by another person, for example, the victim or the law. Therefore, the dangerous aspect of sexually deviant behavior concerns the nurse and all health professionals, and it is a responsibility to be met.

Cohen, Groth, and Siegel define the sexually dangerous person as one who has a high probability of inflicting serious bodily injury on another.[4] *Dangerousness,* as a term, refers to a prediction of a future state and the behavior resulting from such a state. In their work with dangerous sexual offenders at the Massachusetts Treatment Center, the staff have identified the following factors as present in the sexual offenders:

1. An extremely inadequate sense of self. Although an occasional presence of a manifest supernormal posture of self-comfort may be noted, there is

[3]Robert L. Spitzer, "In Defense of the New Nomenclature for Homosexuality," *Medical World News Review,* 1 (1974), 16.

[4]Murray L. Cohen, A. Nicholas Groth, and Richard Siegel, "The Clinician's Approach to Dangerousness and Social Policy Issues," paper presented at the annual American Psychological Association Conference, September 4, 1974.

always discerned an underlying feeling of worthlessness, inadequacy, and helplessness. The individual also places a premium on sexuality or aggression as the experiences which could undo, rectify, or reestablish a sense of well-being.

2. There is a major use of projective mechanisms with the experience of being victimized; not in a superficial sense to deny culpability, but in a pervasive dynamic experience of life.

3. There are marked defects in object relationships and no feelings of attachments to other persons or even to possessions that are not eroticized or narcissistic. In order to fend off the resultant sense of aloneness and emptiness, there is a peculiar investment in abstractions, such as courage, motherhood, or independence. This quality of attachment makes him insensitive to the feelings and needs of others, a tendency to experience others as unreal and such qualities as warmth, empathy, and trust are noticeably absent.

4. There is a general inability to tolerate frustration which shows itself in an inability to persist in long-range, goal-oriented actions and in impulse ridden behavior.

5. The general mood state is dysphoric, characterized by a dull depression, feelings of fear bordering on panic, anger, and irritation and an overwhelming sense of purposelessness and hopelessness.

6. The basic attitude toward women reflects a splitting of ambivalence with idealization of a select few and fear and anger toward others. Pain and hurt from the idealized objects are quickly displaced onto the despised others.

7. In general, although perception, judgment, and reasoning are relatively intact, serious impairment occurs under the impact of emotional or motivational arousal.

Sexual deviations have been listed in the official nomenclature as follows:

Sexual orientation disturbance:

VOYEURISM. The "peeping tom" seeks out visual experiences for sexual stimulation.

EXHIBITIONISM. The exhibitionist displays his sexual organ to a person of the opposite sex.

TRANSVESTISM. The transvestite seeks sexual gratification by wearing clothing of the members of the opposite sex.

FETISHISM. The fetishist is sexually stimulated by articles of clothing (such as panties) or by non-erotic parts of the body (such as feet). The fetish is the object or article used by the patient.

SADISM. This is the need to inflict pain in order to achieve sexual gratification.

MASOCHISM. This is the need to have the partner inflict pain in order to obtain sexual gratification.

Case situation The following case example illustrates the mental and physical anguish of a man with a homosexual history. It also includes factors to be evaluated in terms of predicting sexual dangerousness. This case can be used to discuss a treatment plan on an out-patient basis.

Mr. Bar is a 29-year-old single man who explained his problem as "experiencing strange things that frighten me."

Three weeks previous he began feeling hands touch his bed at night and on several occasions pull at his arm. One night in his sleep he felt as though he were being choked. He had not experienced seeing or hearing anything out of the ordinary but "feels the presence of someone." This happens during the hours of 3:45 A.M. until 12:00 noon. His working hours are 3-11 P.M. He is not happy in his work because he often has to work overtime and he must stand in only one place all the time. He is thinking about changing work. Mr. Bar presently lives in a private home; he and two other men live on the second floor. He describes one man as being like a father. The other is a young man who just moved in a few days ago. The married couple who own the house are "very good to him and they understand his difficulties."

He was in prison for 6 years for indecent sexual assault of minors. He is presently on parole. His brother introduced him to homosexuality at age 11. He does not have long-term relationships with any one man. He was accustomed to making contacts every night, usually with younger men. When the nurse asked if he were currently having contacts, Mr. Bar became upset. He said that even though he tried to control himself and though the parole officer had forbidden him to have contacts, he does have them, though less frequently than before.

He explained one reason he comes for professional help. He wants to be able to give up his homosexual life pattern and have "normal" relationships with women. When the nurse asked if he would want this if he were not on parole, Mr. Bar was not able to say that he definitely would.

He feels that he is under a great deal of stress when trying to control his homosexual activities and related that the "hallucinations" may have something to do with the stress since he used to "make contacts" every other night (the first year out of prison) and the hallucinations were occurring every other night.

Mr. Bar expressed fear that the nurse might tell his parole officer about his homosexual activities. This might mean further imprisonment.

Mr. Bar has one brother who is 2 years older than he. This brother gave up his homosexual activities 2 years ago and married a woman 15 years his senior. Mr. Bar spends a great deal of time at the brother's house. He describes his childhood as being a very unhappy one. His alcoholic father and his mother fought continuously about money and his father's drinking. Mr. Bar was never disciplined, even when he stole money, and he felt that his parents really didn't care about him.

Mr. Bar lived at home until his father died from "too much alcohol" 10 years ago. His mother had died 3 years before his father from "heart attack but she also had diabetes, arthritis, and asthma." Mr. Bar never discussed his personal problems with his parents. He describes his reaction to the death of his parents as "horrible." He cried a lot when his mother died and felt like "jumping out a window when he saw his father die in an alcoholic stupor." He explained that he feels very lonely all the time now. He has never dated women and feels uncomfortable with them.

NURSING MANAGEMENT OF NEUROTIC BEHAVIOR

When neurotic people seek treatment, it is often found that their character patterns or their ways of avoiding distress have failed. This situation commonly occurs following severe stress.

The nurse can be therapeutic by assessing the stress factor. Persons in crisis often appear with acute symptomatology. The person may have physical symptoms, have acted in an exaggerated way, or have demonstrated distress through anxiety or tenseness. The nurse should look for a social situation that has triggered the symptom, for it is usually this kind of event that has precipitated an exaggeration of the neurotic behavior. When the person presents with a complaint such as a physical symptom, it is important to find out what has happened in the family or what important person has left the patient. The following example illustrates this situation:

> A 45-year-old married mother of three children was admitted to a psychiatric unit appearing disheveled and angry. She was screaming and hitting her husband as he brought her to the door of the ward. She called him obscene names and said she never wanted to see him again. Alcohol was heavy on her breath and she refused to answer any questions asked of her. Her husband said he brought her to the hospital because he did not know how else to handle her.

> The next day the patient was able to talk of the situation that precipitated her drinking behavior. She and her husband had planned for years to purchase their own home and had just made arrangements for a home of their own. The evening before her admission, the husband had told her he had mismanaged their budget and therefore did not have the money needed for the downpayment of their home. The patient became so angry that she began to drink several glasses of liquor.

> As the nurse was able to explore in detail this situation, the patient was able to talk of her resentment of her husband's mismanagement of the money for the house as well as the money that had been set aside for the children's education.

> In the morning the patient felt remorseful about her impulsive drinking behavior and felt guilty about her behavior.

> Arrangements were made for the husband and wife to be able to talk about this situation, their feelings about it, and plans for the future.

> Over a 3-day period of hospitalization the patient resolved issues sufficiently enough to feel ready to return home and to continue short-term therapy on an out-patient basis.

This case example demonstrates the second step for the nurse to consider in working with neurotic behavior. After the patient has resolved the intense crisis situation, she should be referred to her social network in which the major work must be done in readjusting to the reality setting.

One aid in the assessment process of the various character styles is to see and evaluate how people deal with actions, feelings, and thoughts. For example, the person with hysteric character traits tends to think globally and impressionistically. She does not think in detail. If you ask, "What was your date like last night?" she would answer, "Wow, was it great!"

An obsessional person answers the same question in great detail going into a minute description of all facets of the date and "where they had gone."

The person with hysteric character traits dresses in bright stylistic clothes and behaves in a flirtatious manner. The person with obsessional traits tends to dress conservatively, has restricted behavior and expression of feelings. It is to be stressed that these styles may be well within the range of normal.

"Acting up"

One defense used by some patients to avoid becoming severely neurotic or psychotic is to act up. That is, they deal with the distress in their life through action such as ingesting drugs and alcohol, wrist cutting, or other kinds of antisocial behavior. Some pathological "acting up" incidents involving behavior that occur within a hospital setting are being absent from the ward without permission, returning late to the ward, scratching or slashing wrists or other parts of the skin, medication overdose, attempting suicide or self-assault, damaging property in the hospital or at home, inappropriate sexual behavior (homosexual or heterosexual), assaulting staff, patients, or family, force needed by staff to get patient to the quiet room, to get patient to bed, to get patient out of bed in the morning, to prevent patient from hurting self; disturbing the ward by screaming or throwing tantrums; consuming alcohol in or out of the hospital; possessing unauthorized articles such as weapons; stealing and misbehaving in group activities or meetings.

The function of this behavior is a complicated subject. However, three principles do seem to apply to the acting-up behavior of patients:

1. The acting of psychic distress in the psychotic person is a very different issue from the more ego-syntonic acting out of the young neurotic person.
2. In the nonpsychotic patient the behavior may be a way of dealing with an unbearable affect or issue as an alternative to suffering an affective disorder or a thought disorder.
3. The behavior is often a clear communication translated as:
   a. I am sick, treat me. Give me attention.
   b. I cannot stand it here; throw me out.
   c. Are you going to be like my parents and do nothing?
   d. Punish me. It excites me.
   e. It feels good inside when I cut myself.

Nursing management of acting-up behavior

Full-time hospitalization certainly complicates the therapeutic problems in the management of the acting-up patient. Treating these patients on day care or at the clinic or community center communicates a certain degree of detachment from responsibility which may provide special therapeutic opportunities.

In the community, mental health center (out-patient) staff can communicate this message: "I am here to *talk* with you and to help you understand your behavior and feelings. But I will not attempt to control your behavior. If you get in trouble with the law or decide to slice your arm, you must do it on your own. We can only talk about it."

This approach is not only practical, it is also effective. Once the patient is admitted to the hospital, this message is not and cannot be communicated. The staff becomes responsible. Furthermore, by our listening to the patient, being concerned about the patient, and being close to the patient, the patient then has the family situation recreated in terms of against whom and toward whom to act out. This makes hospitalization both an opportunity for more

valuable therapy in terms of helping the person work through the interpersonal conflict that seems to increase his need to act rather than talk.
However, it also makes hospitalization a challenge to the staff in terms of the
management problems they may be forced to handle.

The patients with behavioral disorders stir up a great deal of staff feelings and create complicated countertransference problems. The incidence of
patients acting up often reflects staff harmony or disharmony. For instance,
when more than two patients act up at one time, there are usually some
unsettled intrastaff conflicts.

In the nursing management of acting-up behavior the following questions should be considered:

1. Does the nurse understand the patient? Is the patient acting on his unconscious thoughts or feelings? Is the patient overwhelmed by any relationships on the ward or with the staff?
2. Are limits being set therapeutically? Are they fair, firm, and consistent?
3. Is there conflict between two or more staff members over the management
   of the patient? Is the patient overwhelmed by this conflict or is she acting
   out the unconscious wishes of one of the team members?
4. Are there intrastaff conflicts such as doctors vs. nurses or social workers
   vs. doctors?
5. Is the patient population of such a composition that staff cannot be in control? Does someone need to be discharged to restore equilibrium?
6. Are therapy groups being used to help patients see how they use each other
   in maladaptive ways? Can they see how they act up and act out through
   others?

Manipulative behavior

Manipulation may be defined in a broad context to mean purposeful activity
to meet needs. The influencing of another person's behavior may be accomplished in subtle as well as overt ways. Behavioral scientists have demonstrated how behavior can be manipulated even without a person's awareness.

Because manipulative behavior occurs in relationships, the nurse
needs to be aware of such patterns in order to promote healthy patterns.
Patricia Wiley[5] defines constructive manipulation as the "application of
one's own capabilities and strengths in interpersonal situations which promote successful relationships with others" and destructive manipulation as
"the wielding of other persons or getting something from others for one's
own purposes, both of which create difficulties in interpersonal relationship
and prevent personal growth in the user."

Manipulative behavior patterns that are common in the ward setting
are:[6]

[5]Patricia L. Wiley, "Manipulation," in *Developing Behavioral Concepts in Nursing,* eds.
Loretta T. Zderod and Helen C. Belcher, Report of the Regional Project in Teaching Psychiatric Nursing in Baccalaureate Programs, Southern Regional Education Board, 1968, p. 51.
[6]Ibid., p. 53.

1. *Vying for leadership and control.* The patient organizes patients to oppose staff by either ignoring staff or making fun of staff, for example, by saying, "What do student nurses know about people's problems?"

2. *Making many demands.* The patient complains about the food, the patients, the environment or says, "Bring me another cup of coffee" or "There is no coffee in the machine" or "Get my doctor for me."

3. *Pressuring a person or forcing an issue.* The patient says, "You are in a mental hospital; why won't you admit it?" (this is said to another patient at a group meeting). Or to staff he says, "You never carry out my requests; what's the matter with you?"

4. *Violating rules, routines, procedures.* The patient has more visitors than hospital policy permits; the patient brings drugs or liquor into the hospital; the patient keeps his light on after ward regulations state they must be out.

5. *Requesting special privileges.* The patient says, "Just this once I'd like to stay out past midnight. It won't hurt just once."

6. *Playing staff and patients off.* The patient says, "Mrs. Smith is always talking about you and how mean you are." To Mrs. Smith the patient says, "I heard the staff talking about how difficult a patient you are."

7. *Threatening.* The patient says, "I'll see my family if you let me play the record player while they visit."

8. *Betraying confidences.* The patient tells about another patient's domestic difficulties to another patient.

9. *Acting up.* The patient stomps around after a limit has been set on his behavior or breaks something on the ward when he has been refused a request.

There are subtle maneuvers that serve as distracting methods of manipulation. Some of these are dawdling, procrastinating, slowness, mumbling, changing the subject, monopolizing the conversation, being overly solicitous or ingratiating ("You're such a kind and understanding nurse and the only person I can talk to."), being helpless or tearful with sobs and cries, pitying oneself ("Why do people say such things about me?").

Nursing management of manipulative behavior

The nurse's emotional reaction to the manipulative behavior is the first consideration when dealing with the patient. Common feelings that the nurse may experience are anger, defensiveness, embarrassment, frustration, helplessness, withdrawal, indifference. As control of one's feelings is accomplished, the nurse can identify and acknowledge the uncomfortable feelings. The nurse can only be therapeutic if she has her own feelings under control. This counteracts the opportunity for the patient to manipulate the nurse.

The next step is to try to understand the meaning of the behavior and also to assess how the patient understands what he does. Validation of the meaning of the behavior comes from staff discussions and case conferences. It is extremely important that all staff understand the dynamics of the patient's behavior. Staff, to be therapeutic, must present a unified approach to the manipulative behavior because disunity and staff conflict will provide more incentive for the patient to manipulate. For example, if a patient is denied off-the-ward privileges until he completes his ward assignment and one staff member, feeling sorry for the patient and seeing this as a punitive limit, allows the patient to go off the ward with a visitor, the action could later be used by the patient to play staff off by saying, "Miss Green let me go; what's the matter with you?"

There are several nursing actions specific to dealing with manipulative behavior.[7]

1. The therapeutic setting of limits implies an attitude of firmness and a communication to the patient of expectations.

2. Asking for clarification, elaboration, and details of the situation implies a concern for the patient. For example, "Tell me what it was like when someone else said 'no' to you?"

3. Encouraging the verbal and nonverbal expression of feelings helps teach new behavior to the patient. The nurse might say, "Rather than hurting your hand by banging it against the wall, can you talk about what is upsetting you?"

4. Changing the subject tells the patient that the nurse is not interested in what he is saying. This is helpful when the patient is on an inappropriate subject and the nurse intervenes by saying, "I have to check something back at the office."

5. Leaving the situation is another way the nurse can imply to the patient that the conversation is not therapeutic. If a patient is especially manipulative with dramatic tears and crying, the nurse can leave the situation by saying she has to return to the office and will discuss the situation later.

6. Encouraging the patient to bring his problem to group therapy or to a therapy appointment helps clarify for him the importance of discussing an issue with specific people. The nurse might say, "If you want to find out why people react to you as they do, bring the subject up at the next group meeting." The nurse should continue to follow up the suggestion to see that the patient does indeed bring it up at a meeting.

Individual needs of patients must be taken into consideration, but generally the therapeutic handling of manipulative behavior depends on the nurse's identifying and controlling her emotional reactions, on the firm, consistent setting of limits on the behavior, on the communication of expectations for a change in behavior to the patient, and on consistency of staff approach and understanding of the dynamics of the behavior.

SUMMARY This chapter described neurotic feelings and behavior as maladaptive reactions resulting in an inability to fully adjust to the environment and a failure to live up to one's full psychological potential. Neurotic behavior was divided into the neuroses and the personality disorders. Symptoms of neurotic conflict and manifestations of personality disorder coexist. Therefore, this blurring over of maladaptive thoughts, feelings, and actions is referred to as *neurotic behavior*. Several of the official categories of neurotic behavior were described with case examples.

Nursing management of neurotic behavior discussed the care of the

[7]Ibid., p. 54.

hospitalized patient with antisocial personality. The special management problems of acting up behavior and manipulative behavior were presented with the nursing approaches.

**REFERENCES
AND SUGGESTED
READINGS**

Braverman, Shirley J. (1973). "Homosexuality," *American Journal of Nursing,* **73,** No. 4, 652–55.

Cullen, Agnes A. (1974). "Labelling Theory and Social Deviance," *Perspectives in Psychiatric Care,* **12,** No. 3.

Davitz, Lois (1971). "Where Did You Grow Up?" *American Journal of Nursing,* **71,** No. 10, 1974–79.

Deutsch, Helene (1965). *Neuroses and Character Types.* New York: Universities International Press.

Roncoli, Marianne (1974). "Bantering: A Therapeutic Strategy with Obsessional Patients," *Perspectives in Psychiatric Care,* 12, No. 4, 171–75.

Stoller, Robert J., Judd Marmor, Irving Bieber, Charles W. Socarides, Robert Spitzer (1973). "A Symposium—Should Homosexuality Be A Diagnosis?," *American Journal of Psychiatry* **130,** No. 11, 1207–16.

Wiley, Patricia L. (1968). "Manipulation," in *Developing Behavioral Concepts in Nursing,* eds. Loretta Zderod and Helen Belcher, report of the Regional Project in Teaching Psychiatric Nursing in Baccalaureate Programs, Southern Regional Educational Board.

Zinberg, Norman (1964). *Psychiatry and Medical Practice in a General Hospital.* New York: International Universities Press.

THE SCHIZOPHRENIC SYNDROME

15

The following quotation is from a psychiatric admission interview with a 21-year-old male. His psychiatric diagnosis is schizophrenia, paranoid type. His words capture the fright, the misery, and the pain he is experiencing.

> I remember seeing the doctor in the emergency ward. He smiled when I shook his hand. I didn't know what was so funny but I went along with him and smiled back. I didn't know this was a mental hospital when I first came here. I thought it was a place for abnormal males. That is what they all looked like—rather feminine. My doctor asked me if I was scared of this place—didn't know what he meant by that. He used to stare at me. He never blinked and he stared at my hands too. I had them down and he kept looking at them.
>
> I could feel the membranes slithering across and back in my head. The doctor didn't say anything when he examined me. When he put the light to my eye, I felt the electricity go through me. He burnt my eyeballs.
>
> The head doctor talked to me; he had a curlicue. I thought he was a communist.
>
> When I went near someone, I would hear the voices saying, "It's time to put the number away and hang up the cleats."
>
> The doctor told me to look at the wall. It was yellow—must have been China. . . .

The person suffering from schizophrenia needs attention, skilled judgment, and respect. The nurse feels that she is seeing mental illness in its most profound state when she talks with the acutely psychotic schizophrenic person.

Schizophrenia continues to be a controversial and baffling subject not only to the clinical professions, but also to society. In spite of increasing research interest and newer therapeutic drugs, many questions still remain unanswered in the area of etiology, diagnosis, and treatment.

Not only is schizophrenia one of the most complex problems in psychiatry, but statistically one-half the population in many mental hospitals has the psychiatric diagnosis of schizophrenia. Many people with schizophrenic symptomatology, however, are able to function within the community without ever needing hospitalization. One speculation is that there are far more people with schizophrenia in the society than there are confined in institutions.

**THE MANIFEST
SYMPTOM-
ATOLOGY**

Schizophrenia is described in varying ways by clinicians. Some see it as a disease in the classical medical sense. Others see it as a maladjustment in living or an aberrant style of life. For our purposes, schizophrenia represents a complex clinical syndrome consisting of various symptoms.

Schizophrenia is one of a group of psychotic reactions, characterized by basic disturbances in the individual's relationships with people and an inability to communicate and think clearly. The person's thoughts, feelings, and behavior are often evidenced by a withdrawal behavior pattern, fluctuating moods, disordered thinking and regressive tendencies.

Researchers are attempting to develop more objective reliable methods of classifying patients and are testing standardized structured interview schedules. Grinker and Holzman,[1] for example, used the Schizophrenia State Inventory (SSI) and identified the following five qualities that distinguish the young schizophrenic from the nonschizophrenic: the presence of a disorder of thinking; a diminished capacity to experience pleasure, particularly in interpersonal relationships; a strong tendency to be dependent on others; a noteworthy impairment in social competence; and an exquisitely vulnerable sense of self-regard.

A symptom classification system has been devised by Dr. Schneider and is widely accepted and used throughout Europe and is gaining popularity in the United States. Schneider's system[2] is based on the presumption that there is a group of easily and reliably observed symptoms that are found only in schizophrenia. These symptoms are grouped into (1) first-rank symptoms (FRS) which are considered pathognomonic of schizophrenia in the absence of organic brain disease; (2) second-rank symptoms which may be used as evidence for the presence of schizophrenia but are less diagnostic than FRSs; and (3) symptoms that may be present but are not diagnostic. Schneider's first-rank symptoms are:

1. Hears voices speaking his thoughts aloud.
2. Experiences himself as the subject of hallucinatory voices, arguments, or discussions.
3. Hears hallucinatory voices describing his activity as it takes place.
4. Experiences delusional percept.
5. Experiences somatic passivity.
6. Experiences thought insertion.
7. Experiences thought withdrawal.

[1] Roy R. Grinker and Philip S. Holzman, "Schizophrenic Pathology in Young Adults," *Archives of General Psychiatry, 28,* No. 2, (1973), 168–75.

[2] John G. Gunderson, Joseph H. Autry, Loren R. Mosher, and Sherry Buchsbaum, "Special Report: Schizophrenia, 1974, *Schizophrenia Bulletin,* No. 9 (1974), 21.

8. Experiences thought broadcast.
9. Experiences externally controlled or imposed affect.
10. Experiences externally controlled or imposed impulses.
11. Experiences externally controlled or imposed motor activity.

The person who experiences these symptoms shifts his interest and attention from other people to himself. This change in his relationships with others generally results in the loss of social encounters, friendships, and goal-directed behavior. The person becomes totally absorbed in himself, his thoughts, and experiences; he withdraws from people; he loses his grasp of communication with the world or with what we experience as reality. Because of this impairment, nurse and patient have difficulty talking with each other; neither understands the other when the patient is hearing or experiencing the voices or thoughts. However, there are times in the conversation when the patient does make sense and responds to the nurse. For example, the patient says, "I can't go out for a walk today . . . . The television is broadcasting my thoughts." In another example, the patient says, "I can't go to group therapy. Dr. Karl is sending nerve gas to my brain and killing my brain cells." In each case, the patient responds rationally to the question in part of the dialogue, but he then gives an example of a psychotic symptom as the reason he cannot meet the request of going for a walk or going to group therapy.

The following is an example of how a person can slip in and out of levels of communication between psychotic statements and rational statements. This dialogue was between a nurse and an 18-year-old man on his admission to a psychiatric unit of a general hospital.

The nurse sits down to talk with the patient who is working on a model airplane. The patient says, "I know what I'd like to be doing."

The nurse says, "What is that?"

Patient replies: "Just enough to keep them happy. I can keep on an even balance. I know what I want."

The nurse says, "You are the only person who knows?"

The patient says, "A few other people; only the ones I want to know."

The nurse replies, "Certain people you trust?

The patient says, "You are going around in circles."

The nurse begins to feel confused and says, "I am going around in circles."

The patient continues, "They all have complexes; keeps them mixed up and gets them crazy. We give them complexes. I am going from jazz bop to be-bop. Does all this sound crazy? I don't know. Sometimes I get carried away. You know what I mean?"

The nurse says, "You are trying to tell me your thoughts confuse you and send you in circles."

During this conversation the nurse could sense the times when the patient himself knew he was going off the subject. He slipped in and out of the levels considered normal, reality-oriented, understandable conversation. The nurse defined the times she felt confused in an attempt to get the patient back to the subject.

The phenomenon of multiple levels of communication can be readily witnessed in ourselves when we become distracted. This experience may have some similarity to that of the schizophrenic patient. For example, as we are listening to a lecture, we can feel our minds wander as we become preoccupied with other thoughts or daydreams. A word or question can often bring us sharply back to the level of the lecture, but sometimes the wanderings into our fantasies become so complex that we are unable to get back to the precise level of the subject of the conversation. Then we may say, "You have lost me" or "I missed that point." By having a point reclarified we can find our way back to the lecture. Similarly, it is helpful to the schizophrenic patient to reclarify reality points and situations. In the example cited above the nurse could say, "I do feel as though I am going in circles. Could we go back over your first statement in which you said that you knew what you would like to be doing?

Fundamental symptoms of schizophrenia

In the attempt to confine a cluster of symptoms that have distinguished schizophrenia from other emotional disturbances, Eugen Bleuler's classical "four A's" denoting the fundamental symptoms are generally observed. These symptoms are ambivalence, associative disturbance, autism, and affective impairment. The signs of perceptual disturbance such as ideas of reference, delusions and hallucinations, and illusions can also be experienced in the psychotic situation. The defense mechanisms of denial and projection are prominent. Negativistic behavior may also be a major sign of the syndrome.

There are some aspects of human behavior within normal limits in which the person does have a sense of losing contact with reality. These examples may give the reader an idea of what some of the subjective states may, in fact, be like. They are the feelings of unrealness (or dreamy states, as in adolescent experiences) or even the state of being in love. In these phases we are experiencing the uncanny, sometimes frightening and sometimes idyllic feelings of dissociation and of being completely removed from the situation. To be awakened suddenly from a sound sleep can be an unreal experience; having to deal with unpleasant realities, for example, taking exams, studying, or working can tempt us to dreamy states in which we prefer the pleasures of our fantasies to the immediate reality scene.

Watch a child play in his make-believe world. Although the people in his world are not real, the child treats them as if they are real. Observe a brother and sister playing the roles of mother and father. In the "game" their wishes of how they would like to be treated, as well as how they are treated, come through. The use of thought in the child tends to be part creative and part a testing process. The games help the child learn to deal with the reality of living.

The state of being in love may be likened, in a sense, to the "psychotic" state. When one is completely preoccupied with the thoughts of the beloved person, daydreaming is chronic and the perception of the loved person may be distorted. Unlike the psychotic state, however, the perfunctory reality details of living, such as eating, working, and sleeping, are usually managed. From the thought standpoint, there is a focus and a preoccupation with one theme. The creative, expressive aspect of the thoughts is usually documented through letters, poems, and other signs of endearments.

These examples point out that a thought alteration is not a sufficient condition for a diagnosis of schizophrenia. Other signs and symptoms (to be discussed below) will be necessary in order to establish this diagnosis.

Ambivalence

As discussed in Chapter 9, ambivalent feelings are present in all relationships. The normal person has to constantly deal with the contradictory feelings he has within himself. The schizophrenic person experiences ambivalence, but it is greatly exaggerated and has a special unrealistic nature toward a given object, person, or situation. For instance, the person may make glaringly opposite statements such as "I wish my mother would drop dead. I love her so much."

In an interview when a patient asked, "Mind if I open the window?" the nurse replied, "No." The patient then said, "I opened it because I was going to jump. I want to live my life." This patient was psychotically ambivalent about his wish to live.

Knowledge of this ambivalence provided the nurse with clues to the kind of thoughts the patient was having. This patient was having self-destructive thoughts and the nurse had to carefully evaluate and make a judgment about whether or not the patient was also hearing voices that might command him to jump out the window. The nurse applied external controls when the patient was unable to control his actions. For this patient, the control by constant observation by a member of the nursing staff was indicated.

*Associative
disturbance*

Association is the term used to identify the progression of thoughts one has as he talks. Normally, one thought logically leads to another thought. When this logical association progression does not occur, the listener feels lost or confused. The person's thinking comes through to the listener as illogical, chaotic, and bizarre. For example,

> "I'm not in the hospital. It is the White House; a college campus. I'm trying to tell you the situation. I was shaving and getting my father's hairs. I was relaxed. Didn't jump or anything. A few hairs under the razor every day. I saw six nuns having breakfast at the automat; dinner at Joe and Nemo's."

These associations are not logical. The listener cannot make adequate sense out of one thought before the patient is speaking the next thought. Generally, the illogical thoughts increase as the patient's anxiety increases. The listener has difficulty understanding the talk because the associations do not follow any logical progression of one thought to another thought.

Another patient said:

"I was standing by the window with my arms folded and a flash of blue hit my side. We're sneaking in just like the commies. Let's get down to brass tacks. Feel off and on again. Going to throw another curve."

The nurse can best help the patient who has these dissociated thoughts by talking about concrete realities such as the ward environment, his eating or sleeping, or how he is feeling in the hospital.

Autism   *Autism* is the extreme retreat into fantasy. The person is continually pre-occupied with daydreams, fantasies, or psychotic thoughts such as are experienced in delusions and hallucinations.

Sometimes the patient coins his own words (*neologisms*). For example, one patient coined the word "atmospherets" and when he was angry, he would say "those atmospherets are doing it." He felt these little things called atmospherets were making him do the things that he did not want to do.

The symbolism of the schizophrenic can be seen in his autistic thinking. To understand what the patient is trying to communicate through his symbolic thought is one of the nurse's goals in talking with the patient. The following is an example:

"I am a ball bearing; just need to get some oil and get rolling. Get down to a low level and build up slowly to go up the hill . . . . Cut out the malarky. You give me some answers. When do I go to the slave camp? I should have gone last year at this time. How long does a congressional term go? Eight years? What are you waiting for? Me to cry? They can put it on tape. I had a dream. Who runs Washington? They are going to shoot me. Those pigs (bangs head against wall).

They're pushing me. I'm the class clown in school except in one class. The only school around a monument. White onyx rings. Let's go by Air Force One. They're making a lot of noise. Bomb shaft open. You're beginning to dislike me. I'me getting discouraged (bangs chair). I woke you up (screaming). All my new clothes. Don't interrupt me so I can get my story straight."

A ball bearing, slave camp, congress, president, white onyx ring, and airplane are symbols for the schizophrenic patient's feelings of inadequacy and isolation. The symbols all have meanings.

Affective   *Affect* refers to feelings and emotions. In the normal state these generally
impairment   synchronize with the content of thoughts. When there is impairment of affect, this synchronization does not occur. The emotional response to what the person is saying is inappropriate and it does not match. The mood of the person may appear exaggerated, inconsistent, indifferent, flat, or blunt.

Other symptoms of schizophrenia

Ideas of   *Ideas of reference* occur when the person has the impression that he is the
reference   subject of a conversation. In general, the patient interprets cues in the environment as having reference to him. For example,

"At the dance I felt everyone was staring at me."

"There was a new group of nursing students walking down the hall and I heard one say, "There are lots of young kids in the hospital. I knew she was talking about me."

These ideas may symbolize feelings of guilt, insecurity, and alienation. The nurse can deal more realistically with these feelings by helping the patient feel secure within the ward or community setting.

The following are ideas of reference that later developed into a psychotic episode and delusional ideation:

The patient, a 19-year-old college student and ice hockey player, had begun to withdraw from people and school in a subtle way. His parents, not aware of this, began nagging him about his falling school grades, the coach began pushing him for his laziness on the ice, his roommate began picking at him for not keeping the room cleaned up, and his girl friend said she was interested in another boy. Following an unsuccessful hockey game in which his performance was poor, the team lost, and the coach yelled at all the players, Charlie had many paranoid thoughts about the team members. He thought they were talking about him on the bus ride home and that they were either going to throw him in the shower or kill him.

Delusions   A *delusion* is a false, fixed belief that cannot be corrected by logic. Delusions often develop as a defense against intolerable feelings, impulses, or ideas that cause anxiety. The belief, although false in nature, becomes very real to the patient and nothing can challenge his belief. It is a favorable prognostic sign when the delusional material begins to lose its solid detail and firmness of conviction.

A 17-year-old boy developed the delusion that he was wanted by a national baseball team as a bat boy. He would say:

"I was going to be bat boy for the Red Sox. I've let everyone down because I didn't go with them. When the Red Sox took off for spring training, everyone was at the airport waiting for me. I know they were all there. I told Father Murphy about wanting to be a bat boy and he said he would help me. That was 2 months ago. Everyone is laughing at me. If I go with the Red Sox, everything will be OK. I'll get straightened out; not here in the hospital."

This delusion started out as his natural wish and it was a subject that people naturally responded to with the 17-year-old boy. Since he was never able to follow through or to test out the idea, the unreal wish that the Red Sox wanted him in Florida for spring training with them increased. When a topic of conversation that would make him uncomfortable came up, he would revert to the Red Sox bat boy talk.

When he was under stress, the delusional material reappeared in the dialogue. This was the clue for the nurse to back off the issue and to understand how uncomfortable the patient was feeling.

One could speculate that the meaning of the delusion could be that the Red Sox, who symbolize authority and idealized males, would give him strength and care for him, a boy who never had a father or any male figure in his home. Another aspect is that the status of being bat boy might mean that people would like him better as a bat boy than as a boy in a mental hospital.

Hallucinations   *Hallucinations* are spontaneous, unwilled sense perceptions for which there is no reality basis. Some examples are:

> AUDITORY: "When I went near someone, I would hear the voices. They said, 'It's time to put the number away and hang up the cleats.' "

> TASTE: "No matter what you give me to eat, it tastes like horse manure." The patient interprets everything he eats as horse manure.

Depersonalization   *Depersonalization* is feeling not quite real. This state is not necessarily psychotic. In depersonalization the person feels alienated from himself. He finds it hard to distinguish himself from others and often his own body has a strange and unreal quality to it. Psychotic examples of depersonalization are seen in the first example in this chapter when the patient says, "I could feel the membranes slithering across and back in my head." This statement indicates the unreal feeling the patient had in his head.

Another example is a patient who says, "My head felt like it took off on a pigeon." This statement describes the unreal quality of the patient's feeling about his head.

Projection   *Projection* is a defense mechanism and is used at times by everyone. In psychosis the patient is unable to distinguish between what is real and what is projected. For example, the patient says, "My mother said I had to come to the hospital. She is the nutty one. She started crying." This example would not necessarily indicate projection unless the nurse had witnessed the situation or had verification from the mother that it was the patient who had been crying.

Later this patient said to the nurse, "Have you been crying? There are tears in your eyes." The nurse, realizing that the patient was projecting, tried to encourage the patient to express his feelings by saying, "When people are upset, they can cry. Have you known people to cry?" To directly state reality would probably make the patient feel that he had to deny the fact that he was crying. If the nurse were to say to the patient, "No, I am not crying. Why do you ask?" might cause the patient to feel that he had to defend himself and to say he was not crying.

By expressing the awareness that people do cry, which supports the feelings of the patient, and then asking if he has known someone to cry allows him to make the decision on whom he can select to talk about, his mother or even himself.

Illusions   We have described delusions and hallucinations which are commonly seen in schizophrenia. These are to be differentiated from illusions that may occur in nonpsychotic as well as psychotic states.

An *illusion* is a misinterpretation of an actual sensory experience.

Unlike hallucinations, illusions usually can be corrected by supplementary information, unless the person is psychotic.

Some conditions that can cause illusions to occur are as follows:

ANXIETY: A toy gun is used in a bank holdup and is interpreted as a real gun because of the extreme anxiety surrounding the circumstances.

FATIGUE: Driving in a car on a long monotonous road, without a car radio or companions and after long periods without rest, can provoke illusions of obstacles in the road that are not there. Or walking in the desert without water or rest can stimulate the mind to see mirages of water.

INTOXICATION: Alcohol and drugs can induce a person to misinterpret objects.

GERIATRICS: Elderly patients who have to stay in bed without benefit of sensory stimulation are prone to illusions. Often the nurse may be mistaken for a family member.

BLIND/DEAF: People who have lost hearing or sight may be prone to illusions because of the diminished sensory perception skills.

Negativistic behavior The schizophrenic patient often shows negativistic behavior. The negativistic defense is generally used to cover feelings of inadequacy and unworthiness. A patient behaving in a negativistic way usually will speak to no one, go about his own business, and answer no one. Because of this behavior, he is often ignored or left alone. For example,

Lorraine is a shy, withdrawn 29-year-old woman who looks 16. She has been on the continued care ward of a large state hospital for 5 years. Her childhood history cites examples of her bearing the brunt of an antagonistic foster mother's hostility. The mother constantly beat her physically and mentally shamed the girl regardless of anything she would try to do.

The history was obtained from an older sister who stated that Lorraine was always the scapegoat, the littlest and youngest of the family who was always picked on.

A nurse tried to establish contact with Lorraine daily over a 2-week period. During this time Lorraine would seek all available places to avoid the nurse. She stayed in the bathroom, would lie on her bed with her eyes closed, would select a chair in the middle of the large day room with nothing else available to sit on, would walk very fast between the beds and chairs making it impossible for the nurse to walk with her or talk to her in any way.

In the third week Lorraine stopped long enough to say to the nurse, "I don't talk. I don't go out. I don't have anything to do." This was the first verbal communication between the nurse and the patient. In the ensuing 3-month period, Lorraine was talking about painful issues regarding her unhappy marriage and having to give up her three children to foster homes.

A symptom picture of schizophrenia

The following is a portrayal of the general description that a patient or family gives of the clinical symptoms of schizophrenia.

The patient often becomes ill for the first time between the ages of 17 and 27. Personality difficulties prior to this early onset tend to go unnoticed, although a careful investigation of the patient's history may indicate early problem areas such as withdrawal behavior, the inability to mix with groups, and angry and unpredictable behavior.

Gradually the person becomes less involved with his daily life in general and becomes obsessed with ideas in particular. At this point he usually expresses verbally some ideas that seem unusual and illogical to his family and community. He thinks that these ideas have special meaning and are related specifically to him (ideas of reference). For example, an uncle may come to visit the family and the patient thinks he is there solely to spy on him. He might also feel that the static or interference one occasionally hears on the telephone is someone listening in or wiretapping the conversation. More and more frequently this kind of behavior is in evidence. The patient may then feel that the whole house is bugged, the television is speaking directly to him, and the FBI is pursuing him. These are false beliefs and delusions that tend to be negative in nature in the beginning with the feeling that people or some outside forces are intending to hurt him. Later on these delusions may become positive to the person and acquire a grandiose content. The person feels that he is Christ or the Virgin Mary. For example, one woman watched David Brinkley on television and felt that he was in love with her and could not proclaim this publicly but would send messages to her through the medium of television. Every gesture the newscaster made had special meaning to her. Another patient, a young boy, said, "Did you watch the TV press conference? The President said, 'We need the kid here in Washington.' "

The person experiences difficulty in perception. He may develop hallucinations which means he can see, hear, smell, taste, or feel things in a distorted way. For example, one patient said, "Before I came here, I went to a fire and felt I was going crazy. The voices told me I was."

Another patient said, "I can't eat the food here because it is poisoned." Another patient said, "The air in here is polluted. You are trying to kill us with the gas that comes in through the ventilating system."

At times the schizophrenic patient misidentifies things that are illusions. The patient says, "I was watching TV and everyone turned white." Another patient said, "The headlines of the newspaper said, "This boy will die. The ship will sink off the Florida Keys.' "

Often the behavior may be seen as normal. The only abnormality is connected with the thoughts and ideas, but closer scrutiny of the behavior often discloses gestures, stereotyped mannerisms, or actions that seem odd. This behavior is often in response to the hallucinations and delusional thoughts.

The mood and affect are usually altered. The person is withdrawn and suspicious or he might be showing a blunting of affect. He may seem more involved with something personal that no one is aware of. His physical appearance and dress may be affected or he may have lost interest in his personal grooming. Regressive behavior might be observed. This is often how we perceive the patient in a general way in the symptom picture of schizophrenia. A specific example of how a patient is perceived follows. The admission interview with the nurse and a 22-year-old patient shows the loosening of thoughts and feelings of the young man.

Nurse: Can you tell me how things have been going for you?

Patient: Trying to get my mind off myself. I'd like to get going. I'd like to play some softball. I asked my mother to bring in my low-cut sneakers and she brought in my high-cut sneakers.... Aren't I getting better? Pause ... can't sit in the chair (moves to a chair behind the nurse). Where do we go from here? I feel I have lived 50 years already. Maybe I have. What should we talk about? Seems like a lifetime. But when I see my mother, it's okay. Why talk to other people? They are not involved in it. (Silence.)

Nurse: What are you doing? (Turns chair to face him.)

Patient: Watching you and what you are doing. It means something and not good. You are rubbing your face (nurse was not). I've got to start somewhere. Feel like crying sometimes.

Nurse: What have you been thinking?

Patient: I'm ashamed of myself. I'm sick. It's hereditary. I'm trying to comfort you but you are still scared. You have the cards. I'm scared. I want to get straightened out and I can't get going. It's been 2 years.

Nurse: I want to hear how you are feeling.

Patient: This is the silent crisis. I was swimming in the pool and I cut my knee. The police took me to the hospital. Walking by the police station I was limping and my knee hurt and I wanted a ride. I'm 9 years old now. I think I am riding in a truck. Can I tell you this too? He was driving a truck. There was a newspaper between us. I got scared when I saw the headlines. Another time I got lost in the zoo. I'm lost now but I'm in a state hospital trying to get myself straightened out. I'm just a kid . . . 15 years old and I'm scared of myself and what's going to happen. Somebody has to get the clamps . . . I scare you; you rubbed your eye. I'm living a farce. I wish I were 30 years old when this happened. It's pathetic and very evil. Do you mind if I stand up and walk around? You turn colors when I look at you.

In this admission conference the patient talks very freely and it is difficult to ask any of the usual admission questions. The nurse's role would be to spend time with him helping to adjust to the unit and feel more comfortable. As his discomfort decreases, he is in a better position to talk about what really hurts him.

CLINICAL TYPES OF SCHIZO-PHRENIA

There has been an increased focus on developing more precise diagnostic techniques for schizophrenia in order to more accurately predict outcome and to formulate treatment plans. One method, previously described, is to develop and use standardized structured interview guides, symptom checklists and a scoring system, and computer programs for psychiatric diagnosis. Each of these three symptom based approaches demonstrates the systematization rationale necessary for research practice.

Following Kraepelin and Bleuler, many diagnosticians group schizophrenia into the five types described on the following pages. Because many institutions classify in this manner, we include the four descriptive types of paranoid, catatonic, simple, and hebephrenic schizophrenia and also the undifferentiated type.

Paranoid type

The major presenting symptoms of paranoid schizophrenia are delusions and extreme suspiciousness. These characteristics may be seen in the patient's relationships with others. For example, the patient may feel that people are against him and do not like him or that they are plotting against him. Auditory hallucinations are frequent, and the voices heard may be very threatening and may command him to do specific acts. Ideas may be bizarre, for example, the person may believe that he is God or an important political figure.

The following case illustrates this clinical type:

> The patient was brought to the hospital by the police who had received a complaint that a "man was disruptive and making a scene in a public place." On interview, the man said that he believed he was telepathically in contact with several political leaders. He felt that his own actions had a direct effect on the actions of the political leaders. He said that he was being locked up because of the cosmic knowledge that he had, that because he knew the truth about the conspiracy against those political leaders, the conspirators had to keep him locked up in order to protect themselves.

Several weeks later the patient was able to say that he no longer believed he was psychic. He said that he had also thought he could control the world in a good way and not the bad way in which it was going. The nurse asked him when he had first started noticing this kind of thinking. The patient said that he believed he changed when he was 13. Exploration of this issue revealed that when he was 13 he was happy and enjoying being 13. During the fall he was at a football game with his grandfather and his grandfather fell over dead with a heart attack right in front of him. He said, "All of a sudden I had to be a man." He said no one expressed his feelings about grandfather's death—that even his grandmother controlled her feelings. The patient said, "Since then I get very frightened when my thoughts begin to drift and I cannot control them."

This case illustrates not only psychotic symptoms but also an unresolved grief reaction that lasted 11 years. Part of the therapy was to help the patient resolve his feelings about grandfather's death instead of keeping them so tightly controlled.

Catatonic type

The most obvious symptom in catatonic schizophrenia is the abnormal and postural movements. In some cases, the patient becomes so inactive that he cannot move, take care of himself, talk, or eat. He looks paralyzed and acts as if he is in a stupor. When the behavior reaches this point, some treatment approaches suggest tube feeding as a life-saving device to ensure adequate fluid balance; other approaches suggest electroconvulsive treatments. Currently, because of early intervention, many patients do not reach this stage of deterioration and regression.

At the other behavior end of the spectrum, the patient may become extremely agitated and show excessive motor activity. This is called catatonic excitement and is characterized by stereotyped motion, impulsivity, and unpredictable purpose. The patient may neither eat nor sleep and thus become dehydrated and exhausted. Negativistic behavior, or doing the opposite of what is requested, may present itself. When asking a question, the patient may keep repeating the question. Mannerisms, grimaces, and bizarre acts may be part of the symptom picture.

The more classical textbook symptoms of the stupor and waxy flexibility of the musculature, in which the patient would stay in statuesque positions for hours, has become a rarity. A possible explanation is that people seek treatment earlier and therefore chemotherapy is effective in preventing the regression to this phase. The following case cites this clinical type:

> Mary, a 27-year-old single woman, was admitted to the psychiatric unit from the emergency ward. She posed her hands and arms at times for brief periods during the admission interview. She could be brought back from periods of staring and standing motionless by short questions such as, "How old are you?" She volunteered that her 18-month-old baby was being cared for by her mother.
>
> In her room she had to be directed how to put clothes away in the bureau drawer. She would stop talking in the middle of a sentence but would continue when a question was asked of her. She laughed inappropriately and said things out of context such as, "I'm a bastard." She could give no further explanation for the comment.
>
> She said she was at the hospital because her brother was killed in a fire 4 months previously. She kept asking for cigarettes and then would say, "I'm not supposed to smoke." When asked if she had upsetting thoughts, she answered, "Yes, of burning myself with matches and going out a window."

Simple type

The main symptom of the simple schizophrenia syndrome is the total lack of any substantial relationships and a complete poverty of the thought process. Overt symptomatology of delusions, hallucinations, and ideas of reference are totally absent. Feelings of apathy and indifference pervade and the person is so lacking in social skills that the rehabilitation of the person becomes a serious problem.

Simple schizophrenia is not often seen in the hospital but rather in people who live aimless existences and move from one area to another. They have few goals in life and seem to wander from place to place, being employed as migratory workers or living meager existences. This diagnostic type of schizophrenia is to be differentiated from the schizoid personality type.

Psychotherapy is of limited value because of difficulties in aiding the person with relationships. The main goal is to try to help the person back into his community and with his family and to strengthen existing social network ties.

Hebephrenic type

The main symptom in this syndrome is the inappropriate affect of the person. Giggling, unrelated smiling, and laughter tend to predominate and are undoubtedly responsible for the adjective "silly" being given to this behavior.

People with this disorder can have delusions that are usually grandiose in nature. Also, the hallucinations tend to be pleasant ones (the smiling and laughing attest to that fact).

The prognosis is poor because regression is generally present. One is struck with the rapid deterioration of the personality. The person often has complete disregard for social restrictions. He eats as he chooses, urinates and defecates at will and wherever he chooses, and masturbates openly. Personal grooming, especially in the female, denotes excessive emphasis. The person may wear odd clothing, for example, blouses buttoned wrong side out, and heavy theatrical makeup. Hair styles tend to be representative of the years prior to their illness.

The following case illustrates this clinical type in which the patient has been hospitalized over a 20-year-period in a state hospital. The following dialogue was recorded by a nursing student in her first interview with this 54-year-old woman:

> I approached this woman and observed her to be slightly unkempt with a state hospital dress that was too short and ankle socks in two unmatched shoes. Her face was marked with a skin disorder and she sounded as though she had a speech impediment until I realized she had no teeth.
>
> I introduced myself and then asked how she felt about being here in the hospital.
>
> She said, "Could you please write to my mother?"
>
> I repeated my question and she started dictating, "Dear Mother. I had to go back this morning. God will take care of you. He is the power."
>
> I asked how she felt about her mother.
>
> She said, "I feel wonderful. God takes care of the good ones and the bad ones."
>
> I decided to try once again and I asked her why she lived here at the hospital.
>
> She said, "I have to live here because I didn't eat my supper."
>
> *Student:* What supper was that?
>
> *Patient:* Yesterday, I tear up my clothes too, you know, yes I do.
>
> *Student:* Why do you do that?
>
> *Patient:* They tie me up you know, but I am not going to do that anymore.

Student: Why do you tear your clothes?

Patient: Because I am not going to lunch. I threw my hot dogs down the hopper, I did. I'm always yelling and screaming. Then they tie me up. Yes, I have to be tied up.

Student: Do you like being tied up?

Patient: Yes, yes, I do. But I won't do it anymore.

Student: Do you really like being tied up?

Patient: I'm not hungry. I'm not going to lunch. I feel terrible.

Student: Is there anything I can get for you?

Patient: No, I have freckles (points to her arm and then abruptly gets up and leaves).

This interaction between student and patient illustrates a stall situation. The student stalled the dialogue by continuing direct questioning of the patient's behavior rather than focusing on the feelings of the patient about either being in the hospital (original question) or about her mother (patient request to student). This example also illustrates some of the difficulties in establishing dialogue with the chronically ill schizophrenic patient.

There has been a marked decline in the number of patients suffering from this disorder, in terms of either new cases being diagnosed or schizophrenics deteriorating to that level within the hospital setting. The explanations are that early intervention and comprehensive treatment prevent regression to a deteriorated stage.

Undifferentiated type

More frequently seen on admission to a psychiatric unit is a mixed or undifferentiated clinical type. Varying symptoms are observed. This is seen in the following example:

Dick, a 23-year-old college graduate and an analysis engineer was admitted directly to the psychiatric unit. He sat slumped in the chair with his coat completely covering his face and head. His mother sat next to him looking quite upset and anxious. Dick was reluctant to walk to the ward but when encouraged with, "Would you like to get better?" he came in the door.

During the initial interview Dick said that he had been hearing voices for a long time. He said his eyes seemed funny to him, expressed fear that he was bald, and worried because he was sallow, pale, and his eyes were too red.

Later that day Dick was observed dancing around the ward humming and whistling. He would wave his hand and foot in the air in a spiral motion which ended with his falling on the floor. He replied to questions with grunts and groans. His actions were infantile; he made strange noises with his lips and mouth.

At one point in the afternoon Dick was observed crawling down the hall on his hands and knees. When asked what he was doing, he said he was smelling the flowers.

Prognosis of schizophrenia

A major effort to refine diagnostic categories has been in trying to predict outcome. There are varying opinions, on this matter. Some diagnosticians talk of acute vs. chronic schizophrenia; they say that acute schizophrenia and chronic schizophrenia may be qualitatively different entities. However, one often sees acute schizophrenics go on to become chronic schizophrenics; this implies similarity rather than differences between the two stages.[3] One textbook on psychiatric diagnosis has suggested that schizophrenia be divided into categories of either good or poor prognosis.[4] Woodruff and his colleagues suggest that the labels schizophrenia, chronic schizophrenia, process schizophrenia, nuclear schizophrenia, and nonremitting schizophrenia be applied to poor prognosis cases. They suggest that the labels schizophreniform, schizoaffective, acute schizophrenia, reactive schizophrenia, and remitting schizophrenia be applied to good prognosis. The following chart illustrates how the authors have categorized the nomenclature and diagnostic criteria for schizophrenia and schizophreniform illness.[5]

Diagnostic Terms	Poor Prognosis	Good Prognosis
	Schizophrenia	Schizophreniform illness
	Chronic schizophrenia	Schizoaffective schizophrenia
	Process schizophrenia	
	Nuclear schizophrenia	Acute schizophrenia
	Nonremitting schizophrenia	Reactive schizophrenia
		Remitting schizophrenia
Criteria		
Precipitating events	Usually not reported	Frequently reported
Mode of onset	Insidious	Acute
Pre-psychotic history	Poor, many symptoms, such as social isolation, aloofness	Good, few symptoms
Affective symptoms	Usually absent	Often present and prominent
Confusion	Usually absent	Usually present
Marital status	Often single, often male	Usually married
Family history of schizophrenia	Increased	Absent or rare
Family history of depression	Less likely present	Often present

[3] Ibid., p. 27.
[4] R. A. Woodruff, D. W. Goodwin, S. B. Guze, *Psychiatric Diagnosis* (New York: Oxford University Press, 1974), p. 25.
[5] Ibid., p. 32.

Research on prognostic indicators has focused on two major categories[6] of variables as outcome predictors — symptom patterns and social factors.

Symptom patterns

A research project involving nine countries (Columbia, Czechoslovakia, Denmark, India, Nigeria, Republic of China, USSR, United Kingdom, and the United States) has been undertaken to examine the cross-cultural aspects of schizophrenia.[7] In all field centers the following symptoms have been identified among schizophrenic patients as poor prognostic factors: lack of insight, pre-delusional signs, flatness of affect, experiences of external control, and auditory hallucinations. Also noted was a similarity in the proportion of patients having delusions, derealization, and disturbance of mood. One study proposed that the longer the duration of the symptoms, the less favorable for a remission of symptoms.

Social factors

Another group of researchers[8] concluded from their work that the current status of the patient's life provided the most valid prognostic clues. For example, strengths within the social environment, such as family interest and participation in treatment, were positively related to patient improvement.

Etiology

Many theories exist and considerable research is being conducted on the etiology of schizophrenia, that is, what causes the syndrome.

Genetics

In the early 1960s a major research focused on the study of whether or not heredity plays a role in causing schizophrenia. By the early 1970s studies were beginning to show that there was strong evidence of a genetic mechanism playing an etiological role in at least some forms of schizophrenia. Studies then focused on whether it was familial genes or familial rearing and thus looked at the mental health of adopted-away offspring of one or more schizophrenic parents with that of control adoptees whose biologic parents had no history of mental illness.

Seymour Kety and associates have recently completed a study of biological and adoptive relatives of 33 index schizophrenics and 33 control adoptees in which they found the following:[9]

> The prevalence of psychiatric disorder both within and outside the schizophrenic spectrum in the relatives was about triple that found from the records of psychiatric hospitals.

[6]Gunderson, Autry, Mosher, and Buchsbaum, "Special Report," p. 19.

[7]Ibid., p. 20.

[8]R. Helene Klein, Tyler Person, and Turan Itil, "Family and Environmental Variables as Predictors of Social Outcome in Chronic Schizophrenia," *Comprehensive Psychiatry,* **13,** No. 4 (1972), 317–34.

[9]Seymour S. Kety, "Mental Illness in Adopted Schizophrenics' Families" (MH 15602), Psychiatric Research Laboratories, Massachusetts General Hospital, Boston.

Whereas psychiatric diagnoses outside the schizophrenia spectrum were not higher in the biological relatives of the adopted schizophrenics than in the controls, the schizophrenia spectrum disorders (especially borderline or latent schizophrenia) were significantly concentrated in the biological relatives.

The diagnosis of schizoid or inadequate personality was made equally among the biological relatives of the schizophrenic and control adoptees.

The adoptive relatives of the schizophrenic probands did not differ significantly from the adoptive relatives of controls with respect to any of the diagnoses in the schizophrenia spectrum or other psychiatric diagnoses.

Seventeen of 33 biological families or the adopted schizophrenics showed one or more cases of definite or uncertain schizophrenia as compared with 5 of 34 biological control families.

Parental influence There have been many research studies on the characteristics of children of psychotic parents. One of the major research studies in the area of mentally ill mothers and their children has been led by a psychiatric nurse, Dr. Carol Hartman.[10] The findings are based on joint admission of child and mother to the hospital, and they show that the early development of children of psychotic mothers did not deviate uniformly with children of nonjoint admission normal mothers. However, concern remains high for these children identified as high risk, and intervention programs have been proposed (see later section of this chapter).

Biochemical research A biological theory of schizophrenia is proposed on the belief that an etiologically significant biological difference exists between schizophrenics and others. Current studies are looking at multifactors in an attempt to correlate specific symptomatology with biological and/or pyschophysiological findings.

The "model psychosis" approach is being increasingly used by biochemical investigators. This method looks at biochemical abnormalities from a variety of psychotic conditions, for example, acute schizophrenia, amphetamine psychosis, and LSD reactions. The investigators hypothesize that drug reactions to the brain will provide clues to how the brain reacts to schizophrenia and the similarities.

Various studies of neurotransmitters are being made, for example, indolamine studies, catecholamine studies, protein abnormalities, enzyme studies, and trace minerals, as well as psychophysiological studies on EEG readings of schizophrenic people.

Prevention studies

High-risk people The population felt to be of high risk or vulnerable to schizophrenia are usually the children of schizophrenics. One study has reported how to distin-

---

[10]Henry Grunebaum, Bertram Cohler, Justin Weiss, Carol Hartman, and David Gallant, *Mentally Ill Mothers and Their Children* (Chicago: University of Chicago Press, 1974), p. 211.

guish high-risk children from low-risk children.[11] High-risk factors include:
(1) inattention, withdrawal, and lack of positive affect in the preschool age;
(2) psychiatric referral; (3) unsocialized aggression among boys and over-
inhibited hyperconformity among girls during high school; (4) absence of
intimate peer relationships during early adolescence; (5) evidence of neuro-
pathology under age 11; (6) frequent ill health during childhood; (7) disorganized disruptive families, including parental loss.

Professionals have been increasingly concerned about how children of
psychotic parents react to their parents. There has been little research on
this. A study by Anthony[12] reports how children describe their feelings and
thoughts. One child states:

> She is quite a nice mother, really. She doesn't do anything bad. She doesn't hit
> or anything. She just sits . . . . When I give her a lot of candy she just sucks it up
> like a vacuum cleaner. She doesn't comb her hair and her dress has spots on it.
> Sometimes she laughs at me and I am not making any jokes . . . . I don't like it
> when she laughs like that. It's not like ordinary laughing. She never used to be
> like that when I was little. She was just ordinary.

Intervention strategies

Although relatively little has been done in the area of prevention with high-
risk children, a start has been made by Anthony[13] to encourage coping mechanisms in children. One strategy is to strengthen the child's affective style by
facilitating attachment, trust, and contact with an emphathetic adult.
Another strategy is to strengthen the cognitive skills and to provide the child
with coping skills of thought with which he can better deal with the aberrant
behavior of the parent. The strategy is divided into precrisis measures and
crisis measures as follows:

*Precrisis
measures*
The precrisis period occurs in between psychotic episodes when parental
behaviors are essentially normal, although the structure of the family may
still be strange, unique, and eccentric. Compensatory measures include ego-
building devices such as establishing relationships with professional staff;
the classical measures of individual or group therapy; contact measures
which focus on close body contact in order to overcome the child's fear of
closeness; corrective measures aimed at counteracting identification with
the sick parent; family reorganization that involves family meetings; and
causal training that focuses on helping the child see and understand the biol-
ogy and psychology of mental disorder.

Crisis measures
The crisis period occurs when the parent is intensely upset and generates a
crisis for the child. Measures during this time include discussions in which

[11]Loren R. Mosher, John G. Gunderson, and Sherry Buchsbaum, "Special Report: Schizophrenia, 1972," *Schizophrenia Bulletin,* No. 7 (1973), 12–52.

[12]E. James Anthony, "A Clinical Evaluation of Children with Psychotic Parents," *American
Journal of Psychiatry,* **126,** No. 2 (1969), 445.

[13]E. James Anthony, "Primary Prevention with School Children," in *Progress in Community
Mental Health,* Vol. II, eds. Harvey H. Barten and Leopold Bellak (New York: Grune & Stratton, Inc., 1972), pp. 131–58.

therapist and child talk about the stressful experience of the parental psychosis; reality conversations that focus on everyday events in order to provide reality contact with a reliable adult; demystification of the parental behavior; home-leaving and home-coming support that provides additional support when the child fears the parent's coming and going; mental health consultation with the school to make the school aware of the situation within the home; and medication if the child is especially anxious and if other interventions have failed.

Intervention with families is receiving more attention as community mental health services are increasing. Some of the suggestions for intervention with families in which there is a mentally ill parent are:

1. Extended day-care facilities to relieve pressures on the mother and child.
2. Prompt intervention when a parent is known to be ill or having difficulty.
3. Day centers for mothers with opportunities for job training, counseling, and medical and psychiatric services designated to facilitate the mother's return to the community.
4. Shift in client responsibility for initiating and asking for services. Professional mental health workers should take the initiative in crisis situations.

The course of schizophrenia

The course of schizophrenia is as difficult to define as is its diagnosis, its symptoms, or its etiology. Some courses progress rapidly, others slowly, and others are static. Some may run the entire gamut and are called *chronic syndromes*. These people tend to spend their days on the wards of state hospitals. Others may become arrested at earlier stages and only under heavy stress will the symptoms become manifest again.

The clinical picture of the patient long hospitalized in a mental hospital is often thought to be related to schizophrenia. It is currently thought, however, to be a result of a social breakdown rather than the disease of schizophrenia. The fact that these patients can be rehabilitated leads to the view that they suffer from a social breakdown syndrome. That is, what is seen in the continued care wards of state hospitals is not a phenomenon of the disease schizophrenia but is what happens when someone is put in a situation in which sensory deprivation exists. The nature of the disorder encourages these patients not to converse or socialize, and hence they are socially isolated.

NURSING ASSESSMENT When a person is suspected of having a thought disorder or schizophrenia, a careful assessment should be taken to provide data for diagnosis, to confirm a diagnosis, or to help formulate a treatment plan. The progress of the patient must be continually assessed in order to update the nursing care plan. We suggest the following format, which includes the four conceptual models of care.

TARGET OR CHIEF COMPLAINT: Is there a precipitant event that triggered the onset of symptoms? Was the onset of symptoms acute or insidious? Who are the important people involved?

GOAL: What does the patient state as his goal?

FEAR: What does the patient fear about his situation?

REQUEST: What does the patient wish the hospital could do to help meet his goal?

BIOLOGICAL DATA: Are there any physical signs and symptoms? Previous medical problems? Current medical problems? Does he take drugs, alcohol?

PSYCHOLOGICAL DATA: What thoughts does the patient describe? Are his thoughts confused? Does his mind race? What is his mood? What are his feelings? What is the level of ego functioning? Is he in a developmental crisis? What is the dynamic meaning of the precipitating event?

SOCIAL DATA: What significant family history is there? What is the patient's social matrix? What are his social supports?

BEHAVIORAL DATA: Does he have difficulty with his behavior or actions? What is his usual life-style in terms of behavior?

STRENGTHS: What is his school and work history? What positive factors are present in his life?

CASE FORMULATION: A summary of the collected data.

Illustration of assessment interview

A 24-year-old white male is interviewed by the nursing instructor for the nursing students and the ward staff. The goal of the conference is to design a nursing care plan for this young man. The following is taken from one of the nursing student's reports on the conference:

TARGET COMPLAINT: "I feel a lot of energy in me." This young man has been brought to the hospital by the police, who had been called to investigate a call that a man was "wandering around by the stores." The police found out that the man was confused and resistive and that he lived in the Halfway House apartment connected with the state hospital. Thus, they brought him to the hospital.

GOAL: "I want to return to my job at the battery factory — the job is waiting for me when I get out."

REQUEST: "My mind races and I go up and down." "Help me control my mind."

FEARS: "I feel I'll be here forever."

BIOLOGICAL DATA: No reported previous or present medical problems. He appears in good physical condition. Played tackle for a semi-professional football team and looks in good shape. He has taken LSD and describes his trips as "going in circles, bouncing off things."

PSYCHOLOGICAL DATA: "I hear myself think — get backed up thoughts. I take waves and thoughts and they go into a laser beam and become alpha rays. Also hear other voices such as Abby Hoffman." Feels that people watch him — like at work — and that he gets too involved with his work. When this happens, he "blows a fuse." Talked about ITT and IBM and industrial spying and business could not be trusted. Said he was in the hospital because Nixon was also. Believes he can project his thoughts: "Like I can take a pyramid and function at various points."

SOCIAL DATA: Father is a football coach and has tried to encourage his son in sports, but his son really likes music and wants to play the flute but knows this would not please his father. He has a younger brother and sister. States that his mother is overbearing as were all mothers. Talks of one special friend who has not visited him in the hospital. Was doing well at the Halfway House apartment, but it was noticed he had not been taking his medications.

BEHAVIORAL DATA: Brought a pencil and tablet to interview and frequently would draw electronic related figures. He said he felt vibrations from his environment and drew them as oscillating lines being recorded on a machine. At another point he said he was receiving a message and had to write it down. The message was political in nature and referred to Kissinger, the USSR, and the USA.

STRENGTHS: Completed high school. Played football for 2 years. Has a responsible job and the employer wants him back. His parents would be available for family therapy. Has done well at the co-op apartments. Has some friends—talks of a previous girl friend. Staff responds positively to this young man.

CASE FORMULATION: This 24-year-old young man presents in good physical condition and a semi-unkempt appearance, is currently socially isolated from family and friends, but was working at a nearby factory until admission; demonstrates auditory hallucinations during the interview and is suspicious that all students present are really not nursing students; writes frequently on his pad of paper and laughs inappropriately as he does this; described previous drug involvement. Has been diagnosed as a schizophrenic, paranoid type.

Nursing care plan

The main nursing concern is controlling his impulsive behavior when he hears voices and responds to them. He is also verbally abusive to the staff. Medications have been started. Staff is making short, frequent contacts with him; he is on one-to-one when off the ward for dining room and recreational activities. One nurse is assigned each shift to spend time in talking therapy in order to assess how troublesome the voices are and the logic of his thought. Family will be contacted for possible therapy and the supervisor of the co-op apartment will be contacted by the community mental health nurse for the state hospital.

It may be difficult to talk with someone who is psychotic, but it is important to obtain valuable data on how severe the thought disorder is and how troublesome the voices or thought projections are to the person. These data are often obtained by a staff member who has established some degree of trust with the patient.

The patient might be asked if he feels that he has control over the voices, for if he does not, the nurse can tell him she will help with controls either by medication, one-to-one support, or some kind of physical restraint so that he does not have to act in a self-destructive manner.

The case formulation is similiar to that described in Chapter 7, and often the medical diagnosis can be obtained from the chart. Nursing diagnosis will focus on patient problems that develop during hospitalization. For ex-

ample, the patient who breaks windows or strikes other people needs immediate nursing attention in order to control his behavior so that he does not
endanger himself or others.

Milieu management

The role of the psychiatric nurse in the care and milieu management of a
person who has a thought disorder must be flexible. Because the person
communicates at various levels and is in control of himself at various times,
the nurse, by necessity, has to be able to adjust the nursing care as the situation demands.

The nursing management skills may vary from defining reality for one
patient, handling patient control, strengthening the patient's self-image, and
strengthening interpersonal relationships. Specific goals might be:

1. Establishing dialogue or communication with the patient in order to be able
   to talk with, feel comfortable with, and listen to the patient.
2. Once communication has been established, understanding of the patient
   becomes the next goal.
3. Once the patient feels that he is understood, he tends to feel confident in
   the nurse. Then the work toward establishing the patient in his community
   begins.

It is also important to realize that the patient has his goals (we discussed this previously in Chapter 8). This point is exemplified in the following interview:

Patient: (Looking hard at the nurse.) "So you are a nursing student?"

Nurse: "Yes. You look as though you want to ask me something."

Patient: "What is your goal?"

Nurse: "To finish the nursing program."

Patient: "No, I want to know what your life goal is."

Nurse: "Yes, that is an important question everyone asks himself. I'm sure
you have thought a lot about it yourself."

Patient: "I'm always thinking about it."

This dialogue now allows the nurse to talk with the patient about the
wishes and hopes he has for himself. The nurse can help the patient to reality
test his ideas without her being judgmental as his family might well have
been. As an interview goal, the nurse can be extremely helpful in talking
over alternatives and realistic aspects of the patient's hopes for himself.

The therapeutic concepts of listening and understanding will enable the
nurse to look at the levels of communication and begin to interpret the symbolism for her own understanding of the patient. The meaning of the
patient's communication is discussed in supervision and staff meetings.
Making the interpretation to the patient would not be done unless it was part
of the supervised psychotherapy.

The following is an example of a patient's using symbolism and the nurse's response:

Patient: It's Operation Water Moccasin.

Nurse: What was so scary about the situation?

Patient: So many watching. I feel closely screened in now. Everyone watches how I walk, wash, eat, the bathroom. One wrong move and someone will strike.

This patient was so frightened and suspicious of the hospital that the routine aspects terrified him. As he was able to talk of "Operation Water Moccasin" the nurse became aware of his fright and this then became the therapeutic issue. Once his feelings were expressed, he was able to relax a bit and settle into a therapeutic treatment plan.

A second example of levels of communication and listening in between the lines to try to interpret what the patient is endeavoring to say follows:

A 29-year-old female patient states, "I can't do anything. I'm no social worker."

What she was expressing were her feelings of not being socially adept. This patient had been confined to the continued care ward of a state hospital for 5 years. She had neither been off the grounds nor had any visitors during that period. She was right in saying that she did not know the usual social amenities because she had been completely alienated from society.

Define reality

One of the specific functional roles of the psychiatric nurse is to *define reality*. One aspect of the schizophrenic disturbance is in the person's inability to reality test. The person thinks primarily in his own world or within his own frame of reference. Therefore, basic to the nursing treatment of this disturbance in reality testing is the need for the nurse to understand the patient's world and what it means to him and why he has to retreat into it. Being able to understand will help gain the patient's confidence which in turn allows the patient to share with the nurse the pain he is experiencing. The nurse lets the patient know when she understands him and when she does not. As the nurse learns to understand the patient and helps him bridge the gap, reality becomes the attainable goal.

The nursing care must address itself to the different levels of the patient's communication. When the patient is acutely psychotic, the nurse must be concrete in her statements and help him with what is real. She tells him her name and that this is a hospital and that she is a nursing student. Following is an example:

Patient: "The doctor said to one of the nurses, 'He is getting worse.'"

The nurse understood this statement to be an idea of reference. In other words, the doctor had talked with the nurse, but he did not make the statement regarding the patient. To merely correct the patient would not deal with the patient's reason for making the statement to the nurse. His reason in reality was caused by anxiety or feelings of discomfort. Therefore, the more helpful statement back to the patient would be to focus on the first part of the remark and say:

> *Nurse:* "You saw the doctor talk to the nurse. This happened today?"

To explore the reality aspect of the doctor-nurse talking and what this means to the patient will be the therapeutic and reality focus. Deal with the reality. To deal with the idea of reference (he's getting worse) would be supporting an unreal statement.

Part of defining reality is *responding to the thought disturbance.* Often nurses are confused themselves about what and how to respond to the thinking disorder of the patient. The basic concept to keep in mind when having to verbally react to symptomatology and communication that the patient displays is that underlying his acute and pressing problems are his feelings of being overwhelmed. The anxiety and discomfort he feels give rise and credence to the distorted thinking. If the nurse understands this, her next step is to look for the reality stimuli creating the stress. The following examples of varying symptomatology show possible nursing approaches in response:

Symbolism

> *Patient:* "My mother brings me hard candy. I must be getting worse."
>
> *Nurse:* "Your mother was in to visit?"
>
> *Patient:* "Yes, she hasn't been here for a while."
>
> *Nurse:* "How long has it been?" (determining patient's concept of time)
>
> *Patient:* "Can't remember if it was a week or days."
>
> *Nurse:* "Seems long in between her visits."

Delusion

The following example shows some of the pitfalls of talking with a patient about his delusion:

> *Patient:* "People in Washington are looking for me. I can't stay here."
>
> *Nurse:* "Who is looking for you?"
>
> *Patient:* "The President."
>
> *Nurse:* "What does he want?"
>
> *Patient:* "I have to go before the nine judges of the Supreme Court."
>
> *Nurse:* "What for?"

It is nontherapeutic to let the patient get more and more out of control. The nurse must provide limits for him when he is unable to provide them himself. The analogy can be made to the child. The child is told to be in at a certain hour. He becomes terrified and frightened if the mature ego (the parent) lets him get out of control. One does for the child, or the patient, what he cannot do for himself. When he can assume more of his own control, the parent (or nurse) removes the controls. This is very important in the healing process. The patient will not be able to trust the nurse unless she shows him that she understands him enough to prevent him from doing himself harm when he is overwhelmed and not in control of his behavior.

Various methods may be used to help patients get back into control. A quiet room, which has an unlocked door, can be used for resting when the patient is being too stimulated by all the usual ward activities. Medication is another control for overactive behavior. A staff member's talking or walking with the patient can be a quieting method.

The following example describes the patient's losing control and telling the nurse:

> *Patient:* "The voices say, run, jump, do this, do that. Sometimes it is my own voice telling me to do things and I may start."
>
> *Nurse:* "We don't want you doing what the voices tell you to do. We won't let them control you."
>
> *Patient:* "Why do they bother me so?"
>
> *Nurse:* "Come to us when they bother you. The medicine should help and we will either stay with you or talk with you so the voices aren't so troublesome."

Setting the reality terms of the need to control helps to make the patient feel secure. The nurse makes sure that this is communicated to all nursing shifts.

Nurses help patients regain self-control. The nursing staff and team deal with the patient's feelings about limits being set within the hospital setting. This is part of the therapeutic process.

Tolerant firmness is essential in setting limits and helping the patient to reestablish his own capacity for self-management and self-control. The issue of defining reality and setting reasonable limits can produce a variety of responses by the patient who often tries the patience of the nurse. The analogy of setting limits on the child may again be used. When the child is denied candy just before mealtime, he may try many techniques to get the candy. It is not unusual to find that the parent gives in because the will and the stamina required to be firm and consistent are lacking at the moment of the child's testing.

Strengthening the self-image of the patient

Another approach of the psychiatric nurse working with the schizophrenic patient is *to strengthen the self-image* of the patient. The patient has a serious disturbance in his sense of self. Causing him to feel good about himself and his body is one of the aims of those working with him. Research on the use of music and rhythm in facilitating the growth of self-image has been done and found successful. Psychomotor therapy, whereby the patient relates to some experience he has had with role-playing feelings in his life, has been successfully done. Joint family meetings are useful in helping the patient clarify himself within his family.

Emotional support is an important factor in this area. Sometimes the patient can admit his inability to accomplish direction in his life, as, for example, the patient who described his fragility in the hands of another person by saying, "I am like a feather and you say poof."

It is important to realize how vulnerable the patient is and how fragile he can be as he faces the realities of life again. By respecting the patient and giving emotional support so that he can incorporate positive feelings and feel good about himself, he will have a stronger chance to be able to return to the community and to normal living again.

The patient often becomes very clear in displaying his need for the fostering of self-confidence and esteem. When he feels that he is not being understood, he in turn does not think much of himself. This fact points again to the importance of trying to understand the patient. The following example shows this:

> *Patient:* "This place is making me worse. I wish someone would talk straight. You talk in riddles. I want someone to talk my language. They say my talk is a delusion."
>
> *Nurse:* "You want to talk to someone whom you will understand and who will understand you."
>
> *Patient:* "Yes, but I don't know how to do it."

Here the patient clearly states his dilemma (this is not unusual for the schizophrenic patient). Patients can tell nurses their problems and it is the nurses' role to intervene and to help them to communicate. Stressing the importance for the patient's talking with other patients at the unit or other staff members will help to keep the interview here-and-now focused as opposed to having him talk about his problems at home or with his family. That aspect of therapy can be meaningful when the family is together after the patient has learned to communicate at the unit. Part of the patient's difficulty is his inability to trust people and understand their styles of talking. It is appropriate for nurses to talk about these issues with the patients in order to pave the way for a clearer understanding and the solving of lifetime difficulties.

Strengthening interpersonal relationships

The schizophrenic person has difficulty relating to people. Therefore, one of the roles of the nurse is to try to *strengthen interpersonal relationships* of the patient. Individual therapy via the transference phenomenon helps. The patient transfers the same feelings he has had for significant people in his life to the nurse. The following example shows this:

> *Nurse:* "What will you do during your day home?"
>
> *Patient:* "Jesus, you are just like my old lady. You are blocking me from something. You are using me as a guinea pig. You don't understand me. My mother didn't understand my father."
>
> *Nurse:* "My asking you about your time at home reminded you of your mother's doing the same thing?"
>
> *Patient:* "She was always on his back about what he was doing and where he was going."
>
> *Nurse:* "You feel I am on your back and just like your mother."
>
> *Patient:* "Just your saying it at that moment did—almost the same tone of voice and such. I can hear her saying it to my father now and he would scream and storm out of the house."

This example shows how the nurse can use the transference or sub-jective feeling to help the patient take a look at his feelings. The dialogue continued so that the patient could see that he was acting the same way his father did when he felt like storming out of the interview. Together they looked at the situation and the patient realized that he was not his father and the nurse was not his mother. This dialogue helped the patient be objective on an issue that had considerable meaning for him.

Another example pointing out the patient's need for clarification of an interpersonal relationship issue dealt with the patient's feeling that he could not trust the nurse:

Patient: (Mumbling to himself and then saying to the nurse), "Isn't that right?"

Nurse: "I can't hear what you said."

Patient: "You heard but you don't understand."

Nurse: "I have the feeling you don't want me to understand."

Patient: "The people I want to hear do."

The approach in the above example is for the nurse to help clarify the interpersonal relationship issue through the nurse–patient dialogue. The nurse can follow up the issue that she didn't hear, but it is more important to learn just what this means to the patient. Instead of arguing over whether or not the nurse could hear the question, it is more therapeutic to point up the patient's difficulty in dealing with people. The patient is not ready to have the nurse hear him, but he is testing to see if she would hear him. Her role remains to help establish a communication link between them.

It is important to remember that the defenses of the schizophrenic are not working adequately for him and that they are producing an intolerable and overwhelming situation for him.

The schizophrenic who feels he is falling apart needs immediate first aid. This is a crisis situation and all the forces must be mobilized to help him heal his wounds. The following example shows this need:

Patient: "I see you turning colors: white, pink, and all. Your eyes are popping out."

Nurse: "You felt your eyes just popped out?"

Patient: "Yes. They came out of my head. I didn't mean to upset you."

Nurse: "You feel you are upsetting me?"

Patient "You are turning white."

Nurse: "You are upset."

Patient: "Everyone turns colors. This is a revolting situation. I don't know what to do; where to sit; what to say. I can't think right."

Nurse: "That is why you are here and we will help you to know what to do and get your thinking straightened out. It isn't helpful for you to be so upset. We have a schedule we follow every day and we want you to go by it. We want to help stop those bothersome thoughts, and as they decrease, we will stop turning colors to you and you will feel better."

It is important to be real and factual with this patient who is in the acute phase. When he is able to deal with concrete issues or with the reality details, he will then be ready for more abstract thinking, for example, what his future plans will be.

Diagnosing stall situations

Autodiagnosis

The nurse should avoid putting herself in the position of being terrified of the patient. If she is afraid, she should acknowledge her fright. For example, if patients dare her to go in a room with them and if that would frighten her, she should not do it. As she becomes more familiar with the therapeutic tools of psychiatric nursing, some of these fears will dissipate. However, even experienced psychiatric nurses still feel frightened by some patients and they must autodiagnose their feelings to best know how to deal with the situation.

With the patient who feels out of control, help him understand that the symptom is part of his illness. For example, a patient with sexual delusions is best handled by a staff member who does not frighten the patient and who will therefore help decrease the panic.

Avoid crowding the suspicious, paranoid patient either verbally or physically. The less said, the less misinterpretation the patient may make. Having him know that the nurse is available when he asks for her is therapeutic.

The nurse should avoid verbal encounters with the paranoid patient that could lead to her having to contradict him. For example, a patient on Day Care was suspected of having a gun in her pocketbook. This information was obtained by another nurse in another setting talking with the patient socially. The problem of how to confront the patient with this information then arose. If the patient is doing something to frighten the nurse (is there a gun in the pocketbook?), the nurse should merely say to the patient, "You have said something to people that has made us all worried and afraid that you have a gun. I hope you do not have it, but it is important for your protection and for our protection that we look and we must do it."

It is an open and clear statement and the patient will be relieved that you are going to act on it. If someone had successfully sneaked a look in the woman's pocketbook, she might have been disturbed because she never would have known that anyone had looked (if there was no gun in the pocketbook). It would have been a difficult situation if someone had sneaked a look and found a gun. How would the staff explain its behavior to the patient?

The concept of honesty

Patients are most perceptive of hypocrisy. The nurse should aim to talk clearly and honestly with the patient. For example, if the nurse is going to be away for a few days or on vacation, she should say that she is going on vacation. She should not say, "I think it is best for you to spend the last two weeks of August without me to help you be independent." In concluding a conversation with a patient she should say, "It is three o'clock now and I am leaving the ward because it is time for me to go home." If the patient asks the nurse if he frightens her, she should answer, "Yes, you do frighten me sometimes." Honesty in explaining her behavior is essential.

If the nurse thinks that the patient cannot be trusted in controlling his actions, she should say, "I don't feel I can trust you now and I don't feel you can trust yourself now because you are out of control." It would be wise to give the patient medicine to quiet him until he is in better control of himself. The paranoid patient says, "You are destroying my mind or you are taking my brain out." Probably he feels he is right in saying that because symbolically the nurse is doing something noxious to him. It should not be chalked up to irrational thinking; the nurse must always pay attention to what the patient says to her.

For example, a patient following admission is given medication and says, "I don't want the pills. They are bad for me." The nurse says, "No, it is in your best interest to take medication. It is important for your well-being." The patient says, "You're destroying my mind."

It would have been much better if in the above example the nurse had been honest and said, "The doctor has ordered this medication for you. We believe this will help to make your thoughts more clear and help you feel more calm." It is better to explain and give the reality reason than merely tell the patient it was for his own good.

Biologic model of care

The prominent medical treatment of schizophrenia is prescribing phenothiazine medication. Delusions, hallucinations, and bizzare behavior are often partially controlled by adequate doses of phenothiazines. Medical research is looking for the proper dosage schedule (i.e., rapidly increasing dosage until side effects become bothersome vs. gradually increasing dosage), the pros and cons of prophylactic or maintenance anti-Parkinson drugs, and at what point, if ever, maintenance phenothiazines should be discontinued.[14]

The nurse's role is to dispense the prescribed medication and to be responsible for knowing the reactions and the side effects of the drug dosage. The nurse must watch for Parkinsonian symptoms, skin rashes, bone marrow toxicity, photosensitivity, and all other reactions described in Chapter 11.

Patients must know the drugs they are receiving and they must know how to report the side effects. This should be part of the negotiations for the nursing care plan. Teaching patients about their medications is an important service that the nurse provides during in-patient treatment as well as when the patient is an out-patient.

[14]John G. Gunderson, John H. Autry, III, Loren Mosher, and Sherry Buchsbaum, "Special Report: Schizophrenia, 1974," *Schizophrenia Bulletin,* No. 9 (1974), p. 45.

Psychological model

There are two main talking therapies that the nurse may select for intervention with the schizophrenic patient: the primary therapist role and the one-to-one therapy relationship.

Primary therapist

The role of primary therapist does not differ from that used in clinical diagnostic situations. The nurse uses the skills and techniques appropriate to the specific therapy of crisis or issue-oriented therapy, psychotherapy, or other models for which the nurse has been educated. Training to practice psychotherapy generally requires additional clinical and academic experience at the masters level and is equivalent to other professional discipline training in psychological therapies.

One-to-one relationship

The one-to-one relationship is indicated for patients who are acutely psychotic or who have been hospitalized for a long period of time. They need a one-to-one relationship as a prelude to other psychological interventions. Many of these people do not begin to mix in and socialize until they experience a one-to-one relationship with a reliable professional. It helps to integrate the patient into the ward or group through the experience of being able to relate to one person. They begin to reach out to another human being and do not feel so threatened. They have some support and positive experiences that make them less likely to be frightened of other people. Many schizophrenic people are hospitalized because they cannot get along with people and most of the significant relationships outside have deteriorated. If the therapeutic relationship is continued long enough, many of the problems the patient has in dealing with people will eventually come out in the treatment situation. Learning that they are being treated differently from before can serve as a corrective emotional experience. These patients come expecting to be rejected or to be hurt or to hurt someone emotionally. The therapeutic relationship should teach a new, healthier way of interacting with another human being.

Below are the steps that are usually followed in initiating, developing, and terminating a one-to-one relationship. A case illustration follows this outline of steps.

Establishing an Alliance

Explain to the patient who you are, why you want to talk, and for how long (weeks or months, see Chapter 10).

Negotiate a therapeutic contract: patient request and nurse's services.

Diagnose needs that you can meet and that won't frighten the patient.

Collaborate with psychiatrist or staff to ensure this therapy is compatible with the overall treatment plans.

Go slowly in the beginning both in time spent with the patient and content of sessions, especially in terms of talking about patient problems because nobody talks to you until they know you.

Keep detailed notes for supervision. Take down as much detail on what you say and what the patient says and then what you do. By reviewing this with your supervisor you both can get a picture of the dynamics of the therapy.

Developing the Relationship

Watch for things that might drive the patient away, for example, certain topics or issues. You are dealing with persons whose biggest problem is people and they are easily frightened and threatened.

Listen to what the patient wants to talk about.

Listen for themes. As the patient feels more comfortable, she will talk about more meaningful issues. The nurse's role is to help the patient see an issue clearly enough so that she can make up her own mind. A stall can occur during this phase if you give advice because you will be controlling someone who is agreeing in order to please you.

Use the therapeutic relationship to support looking at issues in depth. This is an indicator of the patient's ability to respond to psychotherapy. If the patient moves to this point, psychotherapy might be a treatment model of choice.

Termination

Allow adequate time to talk about your separation and termination of the relationship. At least 3 weeks are necessary for a 3-month relationship. New symptoms and regression may occur, as well as the painful memory of previous losses. The patient and nurse need to talk about this as a reality issue.

The following case illustrates the one-to-one relationship with a severely withdrawn chronic schizophrenic patient:

Lorraine S. is a 29-year-old woman who physically looks about 16 years old. She is a shy, withdrawn young woman who has been hospitalized at a large state hospital for the past 5 years. Very little data have been gathered on her family, although one part of the history cites examples of her bearing the brunt of a foster mother's anger. She was abused both physically and verbally. The history was obtained from an older sister who stated that "Lorraine was always the scapegoat—the littlest and youngest in our family who was always picked on."

Lorraine's retreat to isolation and feelings of unworthiness were so deep-rooted that it took a 2-week period for her to accept any kind of communication from the nurse. The following is taken from the nurse's supervision notes on the one-to-one relationship:

Prior to my entry on the ward, Lorraine spoke to no one, answered no one spontaneously, but was able to respond to commands of the ward staff and function as they requested. She never answered back or displayed any anger, but she unquestioningly performed whatever was asked of her.

During my first three meetings with Lorraine, I repeated each time that I would be with her for a specific time period and all three times Lorraine shook her head no and then proceeded to go through a series of nonverbal communications telling me to go away and leave her alone. She would seek all available places to keep me away, such as going into the bathroom, lying on her bed with her eyes closed, selecting a chair in the middle of the room with nothing near it for me to sit in, and walking very fast between the beds and chairs of the ward making it impossible for me to follow next to her.

On the fourth visit, Lorraine spoke her first words to me. I asked her if she had gone out with the patients the day previous. Lorraine looked at me and shook her head no. She did, however, look as though she wanted me to continue talking because she did not make her usual movements to get away from me. She then said, "I don't go out for walks. I can't go." I asked why not. She said, "No, I get lost. I don't go anywhere."

The fifth visit proved to be the initial breakthrough in establishing an alliance for communicating. This day as I went up to her, she was able to stand in front of me and pace in step. Her feet kept moving the whole time and she began an inspection of me. She looked at me very carefully, first at my face and told me I had pretty lipstick. Then she pointed to a pin and asked me what it was. Then she asked me what time it was and took hold of my wrist to see my watch and put the watch to her ear. I took my watch off, handed it to her, and said she could listen to it tick. Lorraine did exactly as I requested and then gave the watch back to me. She paced a little faster and then asked me my name. I had repeated my name each time I went to visit her and this time she repeated my name back after I told her once more. She then wanted to know where I came from—what town. I asked where she came from and she told me "no place." At this point Lorraine began to walk and I walked with her. It was a leisurely pace and I could keep up with her.

At this point in the relationship, the patient is reaching out to the nurse and is able to ask questions of the nurse, but she is not able to cope with the questions she is asked. The next 2 weeks were characterized by this kind of dialogue. Lorraine asked the nurse questions, but in return she was negative to each of the nurse's questions. She said there was no where to go, that she never went anywhere, that she didn't do anything, that she didn't like television, that she didn't like to walk, that she didn't know anyone. One day during the third week the nurse said that it was a nice day out and asked Lorraine to walk outside with her. Immediately Lorraine said that she didn't go outside. Then suddenly she grabbed the nurse's hand and started down the stairs. The relationship continued with many walks outside. Lorraine was now able to verbalize freely, but her talk was so jumbled and symbolic that the nurse could not easily understand the content. Lorraine, however, just wanted to talk and did not want the nurse to say anything. During one of the early walks outside, Lorraine indicated her need to be listened to and to be accepted. Lorraine said that she did not have a boyfriend but she did have a sister. She said that she never hears from her husband and that she has two daughters, ages 7 and 2.

The next week Lorraine presented more material which seemed to be testing whether or not the nurse would be able to accept her and her past. She repeatedly had been asking the nurse if she was a "bad girl." Finally, she mumbled something about "not a virgin—a prostitute—oh, I don't know." She continued to mumble something about the law and then she started to cry. This was the first time that human emotion appropriate to the content of the interview was expressed. It seemed that Lorraine felt very distressed that she had had a baby when she was not married, that the law defined the child as illegitimate, and that people called her bad names.

Lorraine was able to continue to talk about the sadness and loss in her life. She told of her parents' deaths and her husband's loss of desire for her. She worried about her daughters being in a foster home. She said that neither her brother nor her sister wanted her to live with them and that "no one wants me." Lorraine was able to cry at length when she talked of this part of her life and the nurse helped to bear the feelings of loneliness and rejection. Gradually, she was able to talk more about doing something. Again, the initial presentation was a negative one. In the third month of the relationship, Lorraine said, "I don't know what to do. I don't want a job. I don't have anyone to talk with." At this point the nurse and Lorraine were sitting on a bench in the day hall of the hospital ward where another patient came along and sat down, but first she gave Lorraine a little push. Lorraine became overtly angry for the first time and said loudly, "Quit pushing me around." She then turned to the nurse and said, "Let's go." As she walked past the other patient, she said very distinctly, "Go to hell." Lorraine was beginning to feel secure in expressing both negative and positive feelings and was able to take a stand for herself. She also was able to say she had been thinking about work.

It became an appropriate time for the nurse to begin to set limits on some of Lorraine's behavior, for she was becoming very demanding of the nurse's attention and time. This example of holding firm and being consistent can be seen in the following example in which Lorraine tried seven different ways to maneuver the nurse into taking her out for a walk. The patient had a bad cold, the weather was cool and rainy, and therefore, the decision was made that the patient would be seen for the therapy interview inside.

Patient: "Take me outside, please take me outside today."

Nurse: "We can't go outside because of your cold. We will be able to go outside when your cold is better. Today we will stay inside."

Patient: "I don't have any cold." (Pauses for about 4 minutes.) "Come on, let's go outside."

Nurse: "I have told you we can't go outside."

Patient: Loudly states, "I don't have any cold. Oh, what's the use of talking." (Very disgusted tone of voice.)

Nurse: "You don't feel like talking if we can't go outside?"

Patient: Walks away angrily. "Everything is useless."

Nurse: "Useless?"

Patient: Silence.

Nurse: "I can't take you for a walk; what can we do today?"

Patient: Relief is shown. "What are you supposed to do?"

Nurse: "Let's talk about it."

Patient: Mumbles softly and then bursts out, "Help me."

Nurse: "Yes, I want to help you."

Patient: "Please take me out (takes nurse's hand and pulls her toward the door).

Nurse: "We can walk up and down the ward and we can talk, but I can't take you out."

Patient: "Why can't you?"

Nurse: "I like being able to see you and talk to you."

Patient: "There is nothing to talk about. Why can't you take me out?" (Becomes increasingly angry and loud.)

Nurse: "Seems like I can do nothing."

Patient: Outburst of anger with arms thrashing and aimed at the nurse. "This is all useless." Patient starts away from the nurse.

Nurse: Nurse catches up with the patient. "You are angry with me."

Patient: Patient starts to cry, "I want a cigarette."

Nurse: "I don't have any."

Patient: Patient stops still and looks at the nurse. "I haven't heard one word you have said today" and stamps away.

In this situation there are at least seven different ways in which the patient dealt with the limit set by the nurse: persistently requesting to go out, denying the rational reason, crying, indirectly asking with the request for a cigarette, acting stubborn and saying, why talk, using physical force, and by withdrawing.

Helping the patient to learn to accept the denial of wishes is not easy for the nurse. If the nurse can remain consistent and accepting through all the patient's testing maneuvers, the greater will be the therapeutic gains that can be made.

It was shortly after this session that the nurse brought up the issue of separation and termination of the relationship. The last 3 weeks of the 4-month relationship were spent working on the problem of separation which had created an upsurge of feelings of rejection and unworthiness. However, Lorraine had shown positive growth, and the hospital staff had starting noticing her more and commenting on her in a positive manner. She was seeking out staff and making requests of them. Lorraine was presented at a staff conference and plans were made to help her become involved in an activities group and to encourage her to take a hospital job. One of the hospital nurses said that she would continue to meet with Lorraine to talk about her work, her leaving the hospital, and her living in a co-op apartment.

Social model

Various aftercare programs have been developed to help the patient during the transition from the hospital back into the community. Following are some of the programs in which nurses have been most involved.

Group therapy Patients come back for supportive group sessions on a once weekly, biweekly, or monthly basis. One of the goals is the enhancement of social functioning and participation. Patients are able to discuss the problems they encounter in their adjustment to normal social responsibilities.

Co-operative apartments For patients who have been hospitalized for a long period of time and are homeless, a program to move long-term patients into apartments that are supervised by a landlord-supervisor is proving successful. Initially, the landlord-supervisor oversees the everyday tasks of the person and gradually the person is encouraged to gain autonomy. Studies have shown that this kind of aftercare has a positive effect on ex-patients. The programs cost considerably less than alternative community aftercare facilities such as halfway houses, family-care homes, and nursing homes.

Indigenous
community
workers

In another project, indigenous members of the community were trained to help discharged patients deal with the daily activities of living in the community. Some workers took patients into their own homes; other workers regularly visited the patients in their apartments.

All these methods are ways to strengthen community resources to enable the discharged patient to move out of the hospital and back into the community. Inherent in this progressive movement is the importance of safeguarding that all this is not done in order to transfer the problem of caring for the mentally ill to the community. It is hoped that all community planning considers the person's wishes; that is, the person with schizophrenia should be free to live alone when he wishes, live with his family when he wishes and can, live with similar persons when he wishes in a communal social setting that is cohesive enough to give support yet casual enough not to be too demanding. It is also essential that supervised care be given when it is necessary.

Community
assessment

The community mental health nurse has an important role in working with the previously hospitalized or the disturbed person in the community. When a person presents himself to the clinic, one of the first things to do is differentiate the chronic state from the acute state of emotional disturbance. The chronic patient who has increased psychotic symptoms because of a loss of an important member in his social network is different from the patient who is experiencing schizophrenic symptoms for the first time. For example, in the chronic patient's situation the treatment might be the social model to help restructure his social milieu. If the patient's brother, for instance, left home because he was drafted or because he was going away to college, or if this brother who was the only one to understand him died, then the question to ask is, "What does this person need to best manage at the level he was accustomed to?" There must be a substitute available to the patient for him to readjust to the missing brother.

The stable level of social adjustment is important to look at when assessing the patient in the community. Is he working or fitting into some kind of social matrix by his living arrangements? Where is he psychologically in general? Is he going to hurt himself or someone else? What is his ability to function outside a hospital? It is important to know whether or not the behavior takes antisocial forms and whether or not it bothers other people. How ill is the patient considered by the people around him in the community? The nurse can use the group process in initiating group activities for discussions about living and adjusting to the community.

Interdisciplinary collaboration

An essential component of community work is collaboration and planning between various health disciplines. Standard VIII emphasizes this aspect of the nursing process.[15]

STANDARD VIII

NURSING PARTICIPATES WITH INTERDISCIPLINARY TEAMS IN ASSESSING, PLANNING, IMPLEMENTING AND EVALUATING PROGRAMS AND OTHER MENTAL HEALTH ACTIVITIES.

RATIONALE: In addition to the nurse, the number and variety of people working with clients in the mental health field today make it imperative that efforts be coordinated to provide the best total program. Communication planning, problem solving and evaluation are required of all those who work with a particular client or program.

Assessment Factors:

1. Specific knowledge, skills and activities are identified and articulated so these may be coordinated with the contributions of others working with a client or a program.
2. The value of nursing and team member contributions are recognized and respected.
3. Consultation with other team members is utilized as needed.
4. Nursing participates in the formulating of overall goals, plans and decisions.
5. Skills are developed in small group process for maximum team effectiveness.

SUMMARY   In this chapter schizophrenia was discussed as a complex clinical syndrome consisting of various symptoms. The manifest symptomatology was described in terms of the fundamental symptoms of ambivalence, associative disturbance, autism, and affective impairment. Other symptoms described were ideas of reference, delusions, hallucinations, depersonalization, projection, illusions, and negativistic behavior. The clinical types of schizophrenia (paranoid, catatonic, simple, hebephrenic, and undifferentiated) were discussed.

The prognosis, etiology, prevention studies, and course of schizophrenia were covered. The nursing process of the schizophrenic person identified and described the milieu model and specific nursing approaches as defining reality, responding to the thought disturbance, handling patient control, strengthening the self-image of the patient, and strengthening interpersonal

[15]Congress for Nursing Practice, *Standards of Psychiatric-Mental Health Nursing* (Kansas City, Mo.: American Nurses' Association, 1973), p. 5.

relationships of the patient. The psychological model included the nurse as primary therapist and the one-to-one relationship; the biologic and social model and the community assessment by the community health nurse were described.

**REFERENCES
AND SUGGESTED
READINGS**

Burkett, Alice D. (1974). "A Way to Communicate," *American Journal of Nursing*, **74**, No. 12, 2185–87.

Field, William E., and Wylma Ruelke (1973). "Hallucinations and How to Deal with Them," *American Journal of Nursing*, **73**, No. 4, 638–40.

Geach, Barbara, and James C. White (1974). "Empathetic Resonance: A Counter-Transference Phenomenon," *American Journal of Nursing*, **74**, No. 7, 1282–85.

Green, Hannah (1964). *I Never Promised You a Rose Garden*. New York: Holt, Rinehart & Winston, Inc.

Grunebaum, Henry, Justin L. Weiss, Bertram J. Cohler, Carol R. Hartman, and David H. Gallant (1974). *Mentally Ill Mothers and Their Children*. Chicago: University of Chicago Press.

Hoover, Carl, and Juliana Frantz (1972). "Siblings in the Families of Schizophrenics," *Archives of General Psychiatry*, **26**, No. 4, 334–42.

Kety, Seymour, David Rosenthal, Paul Wender, and Fini Schulsinger (1971). "Mental Illness in the Biological and Adoptive Families of Adopted Schizophrenics," *American Journal of Psychiatry*, **128**, No. 3, 302–6.

McArdle, Karen (1974). "Dialogue in Thought," *American Journal of Nursing*, **74**, No. 6, 1075–77.

Opler, Marvin (1967). *Culture and Social Psychiatry*. New York: Atherton Press.

Phinney, Richard P. (1970). "The Student of Nursing and the Schizophrenic Patient," *American Journal of Nursing*, **70**, No. 4, 790–92.

Rosenhan, D. L. (1973). "On Being Sane in Insane Places," *Science*, **179**, No. 4070, 250–58.

Rubin, Theodore I. (1962). *Jordi: Lisa and David*. New York: Ballantine Books.

Schwing, Gertrud (1954). *A Way to the Soul of the Mentally Ill*. New York: International Universities Press.

Sechehaye, Marguerite (1951). *Autobiography of a Schizophrenic Girl*. New York: Grune & Stratton.

———— (1951). *Symbolic Realization*. New York: International Universities Press.

THE BORDERLINE SYNDROME

16

There are a group of patients, referred to as *borderline*, who lie on the diagnostic continuum between neurosis and schizophrenia. From one perspective they have many strengths of the neurotic patient, but on more careful examination they appear sicker. From another perspective these patients may appear at times to be as seriously ill as the schizophrenic patient, only to surprise the observer with many strengths. Because of these apparent contradictions, these patients have troubled clinicians from both a diagnostic and treatment standpoint.

During the past two decades, there has been a resurgence of interest in the borderline patient. We can only speculate on the reasons why: (1) recent advances in psychoanalytic theory (ego psychology) provide the conceptual tools which enable the clinician to understand behavior that he previously ignored and (2) a much broader group of patients is currently seeking psychiatric care than ever before.

Whatever the reason for the upsurge in interest, we feel that it is important for nurses to understand the concept and to be able to identify the borderline patient so that she can provide the appropriate clinical management.

CHARACTER-ISTICS OF THE BORDERLINE PATIENT

From a broad clinical perspective, borderline patients may differ from neurotic and schizophrenic patients in the following ways:

1. When there is regression to psychosis, the regression is relatively brief (a few days to a few weeks) and the patient then returns to his usual normal level of functioning.
2. There is a stability to the chaotic nature of the patient's functioning. In other words, what appears to be chaos is a part of the patient's life-style.
3. The patient is usually very demanding in interpersonal relationships and has exaggerated disappointment reactions to relatively minor frustrations.
4. The depression and anger are not usually a part of an acute depressive reaction but are a pervasive part of the patient's character.

In 1959 a research team began a study on the ego functions of borderline patients at the Illinois State Psychiatric Institute. In this study the overall characteristics of the borderline syndrome were defined as follows:[1]

1. Anger constitutes the main affect that the border patient experiences. This affect is directed at a variety of targets.
2. The border patient characteristically has difficulty in his social and personal relationships.
3. There is an absence of consistent and positive self-identity. This trait is probably related to the lack of consistent and affectional relationships. Anger tends to be a defense against closeness in a relationship.
4. Depression and feelings of loneliness are present. The difficulty in achieving satisfactory interpersonal relationships make the patient prone to loneliness.

CLINICAL TYPES OF THE BORDERLINE SYNDROME

The following are four types of the borderline syndrome as identified and described in the research study:[2]

The border with neurosis

These people are often misdiagnosed as depressive because they are similar to the neurotic, chronic depressive-type personality. The depression communicates a dull dejection, bland loneliness, and hopelessness. These patients seem defeated, discouraged, and apathetically accepting of their state.

These people react with whining, crying, and sadness when dependent needs are not satisfied. They reveal more overt positive affect than the other three diagnostic groups. They lack a consistent self-identity and they have minimal capacity to give emotionally to others. Their clinging to people is for satisfaction of their own needs rather than for a reciprocity of human needs in a relationship.

Clinical characteristics are:

1. Childlike clinging depression not associated with anger or guilt feelings.
2. Anxiety.
3. Lack of self-esteem and confidence.

The core borderline syndrome

Patients in this group have a vacillating involvement with others. Their feeling of anger is usually overt and acted out in various ways. They fail to achieve their own identity and they actively search for companionship and affection from others. They move emotionally toward someone but then become anxious, lonely, and depressed. The resultant picture is often labeled an ambivalent pattern, but in reality there is little real affection, only anger and loneliness.

These patients do not become psychotic, although the fluctuating patterns are confusing to the observer.

[1]Roy R. Grinker, Sr., Beatrice Werble, and Robert C. Drye, *The Borderline Syndrome* (New York: Basic Books, Inc.,1968), pp. 90–91.
[2]Ibid., pp. 83–90.

Clinical characteristics are:

1. Vacillating involvement with others.
2. Overt or acted-out expressions of anger.
3. Depression.
4. Lack of consistent self-identity.

The adaptive, affectless, defended, "as if" borders

Patients in this group show bland, nondescript, and adaptive behavior. Negative and positive affect is missing and behavior generally is appropriate. These people are isolated and withdrawn. They take cues from other people in an attempt to relate by assuming complimentary roles. They behave as expected; the role vacillates depending on the other person to whom they adapt. They live in a world in which they feel no personal identity. The defense mechanisms most frequently used are withdrawal and intellectualizing.

Clinical characteristics are:

1. Adaptive and appropriate behavior.
2. "As if" relationship—no real sense of identity.
3. Little positive affect or spontaneity in response to situations.
4. Use of withdrawal and intellectualizing as ego defenses.

The following case example deals more with the type of personality style presenting a bland, nondescript, "as if" behavior:

A young man presented himself at a Walk-In Clinic with the complaint that he felt he was going to fail in his college courses. This graduate student was the nephew of a prominent bishop and came from a famous family of religious people. Whenever he was asked in therapy how he felt, he would say, "My uncle, the Bishop, said this or someone said that." The question of his feelings would never be answered because he really did not know how he felt about himself.

Following college he went into the ministry. He did not let anyone know that he was related to any religious person, but 4 months later someone found out this fact. The young man was so upset about this that he almost jumped off a tower of the school. The young man was just beginning to identify himself as an individual. When that was taken away from him, he felt great despair.

In effect, this person saw himself as a donut because he felt like the center of the donut with his relatives being the circle around him. He felt there was nothing real about himself.

The border with psychosis

Under stress the patient will become psychotic. Generally, one can see the psychosis on admission or when the person is in the stressful situation (during an interview; family therapy). Patients in this group show inappropriate and negative behavior toward other people. They may sleep and eat erratically and become careless about their personal grooming. Anger comes out in explosive ways and depression is present.

This patient presents the closest picture of psychotic behavior and therefore he is at the psychotic border of the borderline.

Clinical characteristics are:

1. Inappropriate and nonadaptive behavior.
2. Minimal sense of self-identity and sense of reality.
3. Negative behavior and anger toward people.
4. Depression.

The following case example describes this diagnostic category:

Nan, an 18-year-old secretarial student, was admitted to an in-patient psychiatric unit with the chief complaint, "I'm all messed up; I need to straighten out my thoughts."

She isolated herself from the staff and patients during the first few days of admission and seemed catatonic in posture. She stated hearing voices, the voices being from her lectures at school.

Diagnostic conference revealed the following: Nan was the second of four children of a closely knit family who placed high values on "being good, work productivity, and scholarship." The family lived at a summer island resort community where activity was seasonal and pressures minimal during the fall, winter, and spring. Nan received a scholarship to a school in Boston. The city environment was exactly opposite her previous environment. Similarly, academic competition and values in living were decidedly different. Nan came from a social environment in which she was in control of herself. When she became upset or under pressure, she could to to the beach, lie in the sand, and think through her thoughts. She had no alternatives in the city where pressures built up for a period of 6 months prior to her hospitalization.

During her 10-day hospitalization she was most concerned about (1) how long she had to stay in the hospital, (2) how she was letting people down, and (3) what she would do with her future.

Her family wanted her home. Her mother was also extremely anxious in the environment of a big city. For example, she could hardly find a parking spot in the hospital parking lot when she came to visit.

Under the stress of hospitalization the "as if" behavioral style defended her against her feelings of helplessness in the unfamiliar hospital setting. Nan could cope with the realities of living when she felt in control. Previously when she was out of control she would seek the solace of the beach; in the hospital she withdrew and seemed an island in the community milieu. No one could reach her; she did not seek others out.

NURSING MANAGEMENT OF THE BORDERLINE PATIENT

Borderline patients are often more difficult to manage than either neurotic or schizophrenic patients. They may, at first, be socially engaging with the nurse, but as soon as their wishes are frustrated, they become enraged, petulant, or hurt. They may threaten to terminate the relationship, leave the hospital, or commit suicide.

The demands of these patients seem endless. And when any need is frustrated, they demonstrate their expertise in provoking guilt. For example, one patient said, "Doctor, give me a pill for my anxiety." The physician suggested she wait for 10 minutes to discuss her feelings, during her scheduled therapy appointment. Within 2 minutes the patient returned to the physician with bleeding wrists extended out to him. "Now see! See what you have done." With maneuvers such as this, the patient first makes the staff want to help, then she makes the staff helpless, then she provokes guilt. To complete the clinical picture, the patient often tries to play one staff member off against another staff member. The staff is angry at each other; the patient begins to act up on the ward, insuring that she is the center of attention. She has successfully recreated her own family dynamics.

Discharge from the hospital or termination from out-patient treatment is a very stressful time to the borderline patient who may act out in various ways. Sometimes the acting out is an attempt to get the physician or nurse to postpone the discharge.

At other times, the acting out is designed to force the staff to terminate the hospitalization. One example was a young female with rheumatoid arthritis who knew the time for her discharge had arrived, but she continued to stall. One day she swung her cane at several windows and at a nurse's back. She screamed, "Now I'll bet I'll be discharged." The physician was persuaded by the staff to give this girl another chance, especially since she had not yet found a room to live. One week later, the incident was repeated. She said, "Now I'm sure I'll be discharged." She was.

Many of these patients consciously realize that their place is out of the hospital and that they must be discharged. Nevertheless, they do not want to take responsibility for their discharge from a ward that has been warm and comforting. That part of the ambivalence that wants to stay and be dependent can express anger and righteous indignation at being discharged. The anger they insist on creating in their termination is also a part of an attempt to sever the therapeutic relationship completely. In effect, they are saying, "If you will not care for me completely, I want nothing to do with you."

The angry parting often recapitulates both the patient's family history and previous therapeutic efforts. To allow this kind of parting to occur is to miss the opportunity to deal therapeutically with a major therapeutic problem. The general management principles in the discharge from treatment of these patients is as follows:

1. The nurse must first deal with her own omnipotent fantasies. She cannot be mother, father, or friend to the patient.
2. She must set reasonable goals with the patient and be careful not to promise what she cannot give.
3. In the push and pull of the therapeutic relationship, the patient will want to deal by action, such as wrist cutting, sexual promiscuity, running, asking for discharge. Limits and controls must be set to prevent this discharge of anxiety by action.
4. Limits are lifted according to how the patient handles responsibility. The patient has to learn to bear the uncomfortable feelings. This is accomplished by blocking the route to action, by helping the patient to verbalize the feeling in as much detail as possible, and by the support which comes from the presence of the nurse.

5. The patient's attempts to make the nurse feel helpless, angry, and guilty must be seen as the patient's problem. It can easily be shown how this is a pattern of her relating to subsequent people in her life and how this leads to a great deal of psychic pain. These issues recur every few days, but, if handled successfully, with diminishing intensity. It is common to see an increase in hypochondriasis and depressive symptomatology if the nurse is successful in dealing with the patient's characterological way of dealing with anxiety.

When the nurse is careful in setting goals, when she sets limits judiciously, when she can deal through transference with the patient's pathological way of interacting, and when she is clear as to whose problem is whose, the termination becomes relatively simple. When two people are neither guilty nor angry, it is always easier to say goodbye. When the pitfalls of the therapeutic relationship are avoided, the nurse can show the patient that she owes it to herself and her growth as a more mature person to leave properly.

SUMMARY   The concept of the borderline syndrome as a clinical entity is receiving increasing attention by mental health professionals. This chapter described the characteristics of the borderline patient, the clinical types of the borderline syndrome, and the nursing management of the borderline patient.

PSYCHOPHYSIOLOGIC DISORDERS

17

T he psychophysiologic disorders are those diseases of various organs and systems in which psychological factors play an important role. An older, nonofficial term used for the psychophysiologic disorder is *psychosomatic*.

Psychophysiologic disorders involve physiological changes in a single organ system such as the skin, the musculoskeletal system, the respiratory system, or the cardiovascular system. The majority of organs involved are usually under the control of the autonomic nervous system.

It has not been established that psychological factors cause the psychophysiologic disorders. Nevertheless, it is generally felt that psychological factors have an important role in the etiology and certainly in the expression of the illness. In other words, a pathological emotional state may precipitate or aggravate the illness while a more satisfactory psychological state may facilitate the healing process.

We shall describe several psychophysiologic disorders to illustrate how the nurse can facilitate the healing process by psychological or social means.

CARDIO-VASCULAR DISEASES Emotional stress influences cardiovascular function and produces tachycardia or bradycardia, a rise or fall in blood pressure, vasoconstriction, or vasodilation. It is not known whether or not emotional factors are initial causes of cardiovascular problems, but it is known that they do influence the course of the illness.

Hypertension

Some clinicians believe that hypertension itself and perhaps some of the associated symptoms are related to difficulties with feelings of anxiety, anger, and conflicts over aggressive and dependent needs.

The following case example illustrates some of the psycho-social factors of a patient who has hypertension:

Mr. G. L., a married policeman with three children, has been on the medical ward for 5 days with the diagnosis of hypertension. Since his admission he has been on hypertensive medications and bed rest. He appears tense but denies he is really sick or needs to be in a hospital. He is considerably overweight and is on a 1500 calorie diet. He has found bed rest difficult and at times impossible to tolerate.

While talking to Mr. G. L. you learn that he has never felt sick nor does he now. He went to see the doctor only because his wife thought he was nervous and nagged him continuously. If he has high-blood pressure, and he is not sure that he does, he feels it has been caused by his 12-1/2-year-old daughter. Lately she has been arguing so much with her 11-year-old brother that he no longer can stand it. Mr. G. L. states he never gets angry or "blows off steam." He states he is not worried about finances because he has accumulated so much sick pay.

He does not object to being in the hospital as much as he thought he would and he says, "I needed the rest anyway." Although he admits to some frustration, he states he has learned to accept everything. He wishes he could lose weight but thinks it will be difficult because he loves to eat.

You notice that when his wife and children come in, the children begin to argue. Father soon gets out of bed and one of the children takes his place on the bed.

After the nursing assessment, a formulation for a patient care plan might be made as follows:

Nursing Assessment for Mr. G. L.	Patient Care Plan
1. How patient comes to hospital: Advised by wife to see a doctor.	1. Encourage patient to talk about family.
2. Patient's perception of illness: "Never felt sick. If I have high-blood pressure, it is caused by arguments between daughter and son."	2. Be supportive and listen to his feelings about being in the hospital.
3. Family's perception of illness: Wife feels husband is nervous.	3. Social service referral for mother and daughter about issue of adolescence. Support for the mother.
4. Patient's goal for treatment: "Need the rest."	4. The rest will aid in the healing process— meet his needs to be cared for.
5. Family's goal for treatment: Wife wants him less nervous.	5. Encourage patient to express his feelings; help him feel in control of situations and be independent.
6. Patient's request: "Wish I would lose weight."	6. Negotiate about diet plans.
7. Psychological assessment: Dynamic issue: to be in control, to be strong.	7. Involve him in diet selection; discuss the limits set by the physician to see if he can help negotiate certain limits.
8. Social assessment: Patient does not know how to deal with daughter.	8. Encourage patient to talk about what it is like to have a daughter approaching adolescence.

9. Medical assessment:
   Patient is overweight and loves to eat. Wants to be active.

9. Physician prescribes anti-hypertensive meds, 1500 calorie diet, and bed rest.

10. Strengths of the patient:
    Dedicated to his work; has accumulated sick pay from consistent work record.

10. Encourage patient to talk about his work.

The beginning therapeutic task for the nurse would be to encourage the patient to talk. Since he admits that he does not blow off steam, it can be speculated that some feelings remain submerged and unexpressed. An important issue for the patient is to talk about his feelings about having a teen-age daughter and what he anticipates the next years to be like with her growing up. Also, how does he feel about the son who is also close to the teen years? After the patient talks about these feelings, he may be inclined to talk about how he and his wife see this situation of the children's growing up. Perhaps they disagree on how to deal with the children.

Another therapeutic task is to be supportive. If the nurse is supportive, the patient will feel more in control of himself and the situation (which is a basic issue with him) and more inclined to give up his defense of denial or displacement. The nursing care plan should be aimed toward establishing subgoals by which this patient could feel more in control and independent. A meeting with the physician to deal with this issue would prove beneficial to the patient. Negotiation of the diet and bed rest limits in which the patient could actively be involved in his health care planning might be all that is needed.

The nurse should intervene when the children start arguing while they are visiting their father. It is upsetting to the patient and the nurse is naturally concerned with any outside factor that unduly upsets the patient. The best approach would be to try to take the children aside at some point during the visit so that they can discuss with the nurse their feelings about what it is like to have their father in the hospital. Talking with them before or after their visit but not in the presence of the father would be helpful. To directly handle and control the arguing at the bedside would not be an easy task. To tell the children that they should or should not argue would probably set up feelings in the father that his children were bad or that he was not exercising adequate control. It would be more helpful to try to distract them, for example, by asking if they had seen some piece of equipment that happened to be outside the room or by asking them if they would like to go to the coffee shop so that their mother could visit with their father. Distracting them from arguing is the goal.

The dynamics of the arguing might also include the tactics of vying for attention. One speculation is that the 12-1/2-year-old daughter is starting to assert herself but since she cannot as yet deal directly with the parents, she asserts herself with the brother over whom she has more authority and control. The father finds it difficult to tolerate the arguing.

It might be helpful to explore the possibilities of a social service referral to work with the mother and the 12-1/2-year-old daughter. There is little information on the husband-wife relationship. Since the wife has been nagging her husband so much, one wonders what their communication is like. Father does not feel that he is in control and comes to the hospital. The wife nags her husband and the daughter, who is more assertive and aggressive than her younger brother, picks fights with him. In this respect, mother and daughter are similar. The wife may be very upset because her husband is ill and in the hospital. She may need to talk about her feelings about the hospitalization.

The stall to this situation would come if the patient were forced into an uncompromising position. If the nurse failed to encourage the expression of feelings and continued to enforce the medical limits (bed rest and the diet), which the patient already finds intolerable, the patient might well try to discharge himself against advice.

The stall warning occurs when the nurse sees that the patient is not complying with the treatment of bed rest or finds him eating extra food. To correct the stall means to renegotiate goals and help the patient be a part of his treatment.

Myocardial infarction

A myocardial infarction is a trauma to the heart and a serious threat to life itself. Faced with this threat, the individual needs to use some psychological defenses, the most common one being denial.

In caring for patients with myocardial infarctions nurses have become aware of the patient's use of denial. For example, some patients completely deny the need for restriction and refuse to stay in bed, to be bathed, or to have monitor leads strapped to them. Other patients tolerate the restrictions but with obvious emotional strain and with determination to ignore any limits placed on them after they are discharged. Still others joke, tease, and attempt to impress the nurse with their masculinity and virility. Occasionally, some patients become extremely dependent on nursing personnel and equipment and are too frightened to assume responsibility for personal care when it is allowed.

Some of the identified reactions of patients suffering a myocardial infarction are to ask questions and express feelings, the need for specific information, the fear of enforced dependency, a feeling of threat to one's adequacy and one's role within the family and community, and the fear of the return of the illness.

The nurse plays an important role in meeting immediate physical needs during the critical phase of the illness and assumes a major role in helping the patient gain awareness of his illness.

The readjustment phase for the patient is generally accomplished during the period immediately following the discharge of the patient from the hospital. Nurse-led groups have been found to be most effective for the discharged patient. Focusing on the feelings and concerns of the patient allows the patient an opportunity to express himself as well as to provide information that the nurse will assess for further care.

Some of the statements made by one "heart club group" of discharged patients led by a psychiatric nurse follow:

"You know as soon as you feel lousy you say, 'Oh, oh' it's the ticker.' "

"All my buddies say, 'Forget your heart attack. The less you talk about it the better you will feel.' "

"I was in the store today and there I am a big young strapping man and my wife says to the store clerk, 'Don't make those bags too heavy.'"

"At work I lifted the lift of the machine a little and the girls and the gang yelled to me, 'What the hell are you doing on that machine? We'll call your wife.' "

"My granddaughter is only a little thing and she looks at everything I eat during the day and at night she tells the old lady everything I've eaten."

"My wife asked me to write a will . . . . I said, 'The hell with you; let them fight over it. That will give you something to worry about.' "

"They put me on another diet last Friday . . . low animal fat, low carbohydrate . . . on top of low salt. I'm starving to death."

"The doctor says he can't emphasize how bad smoking is but I see doctors smoking. They say no intercourse, no smoking, no eating. Cripes, what the hell are you supposed to do? You know you've got another 25-30 years. They go by the book, but I'm only human."

"I'm trying to give up smoking but I'm not doing very well and I'm very grouchy. I don't think I had better stop."

"I feel I want to live. I don't want to come back here a second time."

"Look, I'm telling you I intend to live until I'm 90. I'm not going to do any hard work."

"If I have a second heart attack, I'm not coming back to this hospital because I wouldn't be able to face all these people."

"Heart attacks are number one killers, so what's our chances of dying now?"

"By the way, how do they take dead people out of this hospital?"

"It's the name 'heart attack.' People figure your're ready for the grave."

"You're going to die sooner or later."

"I asked the nurse at work how long I had to live."

The group meetings in which patients who have all experienced a similar medical situation gather together to compare reactions and feelings are a therapeutic experience. By coordinating the meetings and helping the patients focus and explore common issues, the nurse meets many emotional needs of the patient in one setting.

Changes in respiration are a sensitive index to emotion. Such changes as the pacing of one's breathing (either increased or decreased), laughing, yawning, crying, sighing, and holding one's breath can easily be observed. The counting and observing of respirations are generally one of the first tasks a nurse learns to do. If changes from the norm are noted, the nurse must look for a logical explanation to tie in with the physical and emotional component.

The common cold

One theory cited to explain the common cold is that certain psychological stresses lower one's resistance to the organisms conducive to colds. Some psychiatrists hold that the common cold is a symptom of depression. Certainly a lowered mood is noted in people suffering from colds, and it can be noted that colds often will follow disappointments, interpersonal conflicts, slights, and humiliations.

Hyperventilation

This rather frequently noted disorder is often seen in the emergency room of a hospital. It may cause fainting, grayouts, and blackouts. When patients are unable to stop breathing deeply and rapidly, there is a sudden fall of blood CO^2 that causes dizziness, anxiety, and faintness. It is not uncommon to observe hysterical features in the character structure in these people.

One suggested way of dealing with these difficulties is to tell the person that he is, in fact, overbreathing or swallowing air. Bringing this to his attention may help him to control it. It is also possible to investigate what is causing the patient's hyperventilation.

Bronchial asthma

The emotional factor that is felt to have some pertinent relationship in asthma attacks has been described as involving the dynamic issue of being cared for. Feelings of inconsistency and ambivalence are heightened in the bronchial asthmatic patient, and they seem to evoke the fear of emotional closeness and the fear caused by the threat of a loss or separation.

The following case illustrates this illness.

Miss E. W., a 20-year-old single girl, was admitted to the medical ward in an acute asthma attack. In the past she had been treated on an out-patient basis or in the overnight unit. Since admission she has been receiving adrenalin every 3 or 4 hours. She is now receiving an intravenous infusion with aminophyllin and has a medihaler at her bedside for p.r.n. use. The nursing report states she slept poorly, was very restless, and has had considerable trouble breathing. She is said to have emotional problems.

When talking with Miss E. W. the nurse learned that she has six brothers and two sisters and lives at home with her parents. She and one sister like her father; the others hate him because he used to drink and beat them. She feels sorry for him. Two brothers have asthma and she is jealous of them because they have milder attacks. Her boyfriend is in the army but she cannot stand being lonely so she continues to date. She said her parents would "kill her if they knew she was dating a Jewish boy" because she is Catholic. She states she has no intentions of getting serious.

She referred frequently to her mother; she misses her and wonders why she is not with her in the hospital and why she went right home after bringing her to the hospital. Whenever she has an asthmatic attack, she wants her mother with her. Whenever she has difficulty breathing, she thinks about dying. However, she is too "chicken" and thinks she would give her mother a heart attack. She has never acted on her thoughts but cannot picture herself going through life with asthma. She describes herself as a stubborn Irishman like her father, she is a worrier and wishes she did not worry so much.

The nursing assessment and formulated patient care plan might be designed as follows:

Nursing Assessment of Miss E. W.	Patient Care Plan
1. How patient comes to hospital: Brought to hospital by mother in acute asthma attack.	1. Encourage her to talk about mother.
2. Patient's perception of illness: "Does not want to go through life with asthma."	2. Protect patient from disturbing stimuli; aid in the healing process after an acute attack.
3. Family's perception of illness: Mother brings daughter to hospital and leaves.	3. Observe family when they visit to see how they perceive the situation.
4. Patient's goals for treatment: "Wants to be rid of the illness."	4. Encourage patient to express feelings; be supportive; help bear painful feelings.
5. Family's goals for treatment: Not stated.	5. Talk with family about their goals for the patient.
6. Patient's request: "Wish I did not worry so much."	6. Encourage patient to talk of fears.
7. Psychological assessment: Dynamic issue: to be cared for and protected, especially by mother. Defense: denial.	7. Encourage patient to express conflict she feels between herself and parents over dating issue.
8. Social assessment: Eight siblings; boy friends; father had drinking problem and used to beat children.	8. Social service referral for mother to help her with separation issue from daughter.
9. Medical assessment: Sleeps poorly, trouble breathing, restless.	9. IV infusion with aminophyllin; medi-haler; adrenalin.
10. Strengths of the patient: Has boy friends.	10. Need to find out whether she works or attends school; her interests.

The dynamic issue of being cared for is important with this patient. She also needs to be protected from disturbing stimuli. The nurse's aims are to set up a situation in which the patient may talk about her feelings; for example, allowing her to cry during an acute asthma attack or letting her confess something, for example, her feelings about dating the Jewish boy. In telling this she expects to be rejected in the same way that her mother rejected her. She needs to talk openly about her feelings and not to be rejected nor have a big scene made of the situation.

The patient needs a solid structure of her activities. The nurse should respond to the structure set by being available whenever the patient rings for her. Nurses can help meet many of the initial dependency needs in the hospital. As these needs are met, the patient will become more secure and less dependent.

It was observed that the patient behaved as a small child and did better when mother was present. Encouraging the mother to come in and work with the daughter would be a first step. In the acute attack it is not important whether or not the relationship is pathological (whether the daughter is too dependent on the mother, for example), for what is important is what is life saving to the patient right then. After the attack the nurse might want to explore the separation issue with the girl and to help her to have other alternatives and people available to her during stressful times. The mother would need support and help in separating from the daughter and to have other people available to her also.

GASTRO-INTESTINAL DISEASES

A direct relationship between emotions and the gastrointestinal tract has been generally acknowledged. For example, anger and anxiety are known to decrease one's appetite, but depression may cause either an increase or a decrease in eating. Anxious anticipation and sustained stress may produce either diarrhea or constipation.

Many current popular sayings show how the world is viewed through our mouths, stomachs, or intestines: the way to a man's heart is through his stomach; don't put your foot in your mouth; my stomach is tied up in knots; my stomach feels as though my throat has been cut.

The positive feelings of love, security, pleasure, and gratification in the early years center around being fed. For many people this continues throughout life. When one considers the amount of time, activity, and effort spent on gastrointestinal functions every day, one can understand why adverse symptoms develop when stress occurs.

Peptic ulcer

The ulcer prone person is often characterized as being hard working, strong, and driving, as one who keeps feelings to himself, and one who is unable to acknowledge dependency needs.

The denial of dependent needs is often strong in men because of the fear of appearing passive and submissive. Many people do not express feelings so that they will appear strong.

The following case illustrates some of the psycho-social difficulties with peptic ulcers:

Mr. C. T., a 57-year-old Italian-American, was admitted by ambulance with a bleeding ulcer. Despite a rigid medical regimen, including frequent feedings of milk and Maalox, his hospital course has been erratic and he still has four plus guiac in his stools. Mr. C. T. has a permanent tracheostomy from previous cancer surgery. The staff feels he is unhappy; he does not always take his milk and Maalox, frequently turns his back to them, and faces the wall.

Mr. C. T. has an appliance that assists him in using esophageal speech so that he can verbally communicate, but he speaks slowly. He states he has been married for 26 years and his wife has left him. His slapping his wife apparently precipitated both his wife and his daughter's leaving the apartment and now his wife is seeking a divorce. The case came up in court 6 days before his admission to the hospital and it will be continued. He does not like living alone in the apartment and has no interest in cooking or eating. His two sons who do not live at home come to visit him but he says this angers his wife because she thinks the boys are siding against her. After the cancer surgery he had to give up his welding job and he now lives on his pension plus odd jobs. He expressed sadness that he had had so much hard luck and that he cannot communicate as well as he wishes he could.

The following nursing assessment and patient care plan might be made:

Nursing Assessment of Mr. C. T.	Patient Care Plan
1. How patient comes to hospital: Brought by ambulance.	1. Encourage patient to express feelings about the sudden need to come to the hospital.
2. Patient's perception of illness: Is ambivalent about his illness; turns his back; does not take milk and Maalox.	2. Encourage patient to talk of previous illness and how he views this illness.
3. Family's perception of illness: Family is not presently involved in this illness.	3. Check on family's intent to be involved, especially the sons.
4. Patient's goals for treatment: Not known at present.	4. Explore with the patient his expectations while in the hospital.
5. Family's goals for treatment: Not known at this time.	5. Explore with family their expectations for the patient.
6. Patient's request: "Wish I could communicate better."	6. Explore with patient other forms of communication such as writing or sign language.
7. Psychological assessment: Dynamic issue: to be strong. Defense: denial and withdrawal.	7. Physical presence of the nurse to help with the feelings; be supportive; bear his painful feelings.

8. Social assessment:
   Divorce pending court decision. Living alone. Wife resents husband; wants children with her. Daughter sides with mother.

8. Social service referral to find out details of the divorce. Community health nurse to coordinate transition between hospital and community.

9. Medical assessment:
   Guiac in stools. Permanent tracheostomy. Esophageal speech. Medical hospital course erratic.

9. Assess physical symptoms continuously. Be patient when he is trying to speak.

10. Strengths:
    Works at odd jobs. Can express his sadness.

10. Establish a community link to encourage more relationships.

The general nursing approaches of providing physical comfort and frequent feedings combined with the psychological approach of listening, understanding, being supportive, and bearing painful feelings are the therapeutic tasks. Mr. C. T. can hear, understand, and perceive what is going on despite his surgery. The nurse must have patience and take time with him. She should neither set difficult situations nor ask him questions that will take time and energy for him to answer if she does not have the time. Phrasing questions that can be answered briefly will be helpful. Other forms of communication can be explored.

This man's sadness cannot be eliminated; it can only be eased. Not only is he dealing with a physical illness, but there is also the family situation in which the family has moved out and left him. The family situation and his reluctance to go home have produced serious conflict within him. The nurse must help him bear this and must help him plan for his future goals.

The patient should not be left to deal with going home alone. The nurse can explore the community or hospital resources that are available, for example, the Visiting Nurse Association. Is sending him home alone to his apartment the best plan now? Will the diet be adequate and will medication needs be met? Alternatives for the nurse to consider are:

1. An extended care facility where rehabilitation for long-term support is possible, along with the opportunity to develop new kinds of relationships.
2. Community resources of a homemaking service or home health care that would give him regularly supervised nursing care in his own apartment.
3. The Visiting Nurse Coordinator in the hospital could make an assessment while the patient is in the hospital. Or the hospital might have a liaison person from its transfer office make these arrangements.

The nurse can see if someone is working with his wife and children. One issue to be explored is whether or not his wife's leaving him is just the "last straw" or just what are her reasons for leaving him. Can the marriage be salvaged? Could a third party help with their problems and feelings?

The nurse can check previous hospital records to see if social service has tried to work with the family. It is important to review the old records for information. It would be reasonable for social service to work with this family and with community resources in the follow-up phase of his health care.

Ulcerative colitis

Colitis is an inflammation of the large intestine and is often the result of an organic disorder. The etiology of the overactive colon is associated with external stress factors and with the person's difficulty in expressing negative or angry feelings. The dynamic issues of control and being good are often of major importance to the person suffering from ulcerative colitis.

These patients need strong and consistent emotional support. If surgery is required, thorough pre-operative psychological preparation is essential. The patient should know if a colostomy is to be performed, and his feelings about this should be discussed. After an understanding has been reached, a carefully planned post-operative course follows.

DIFFERENCES BETWEEN PSYCHO-PHYSIOLOGIC DISORDERS AND PSYCHO-NEUROTIC REACTIONS

The distinction between psychophysiologic and psychoneurotic disorders may be illustrated by the following comparison:

	System	Symptom	Severity
Psychophysiologic	Autonomic nervous system	Organic dysfunction	Life threatening
Hysterical neurosis, conversion type	Voluntary and sensory systems	Symbolic solution to anxiety	Generally nonlife threatening

It is important to distinguish between two different kinds of physical disorders which seem to be related to psychological factors. They are the psychophysiological disorders and the hysterical neurosis, conversion type.

In the hysterical neurosis, the voluntary and sensory nervous systems are involved. Hence, blindness, paralysis, and anesthesias, if psychologically induced, would be hysterical. In addition, the hysterical symptom provides a symbolic solution to anxiety; in this way, for example, hysterical blindness protects the patient from a painful sight and paralysis of the arm may protect the patient from his own aggression. The hysterical symptom is not life threatening.

In the psychophysiologic disorder, the involuntary autonomic nervous system is involved, there may be gross pathology in the organ system (ulcers, colitis), there is no symbolic solution to anxiety, and the condition may be life threatening.

SUMMARY The psychophysiologic disorders are those diseases in which psychological factors are felt to influence the course of an illness. Three case illustrations (hypertension, bronchial asthma, and peptic ulcer) were cited to discuss both general and psychological nursing management principles. The nursing assessment and patient care plan were included in the discussions.

The differences between psychophysiologic disorders and hysterical neurosis, conversion type were also stated in the chapter.

PSYCHOLOGICAL DISTURBANCES RESULTING FROM PHARMACOLOGICAL, MEDICAL, SURGICAL, AND NEUROLOGICAL CONDITIONS

18

Nurses whose daily work involves the caring for psychiatric patients with neurotic, depressive, and schizophrenic conditions must be ever alert to abnormal behavior caused by organic conditions. This awareness is extremely important since organic conditions may appear like the functional disorders described in the previous chapters.

There are particular settings in which the nurse is likely to encounter abnormal behavior resulting from organic conditions:

1. In community work in which the patient may not have had previous medical evaluation.
2. In working with people who are part of the drug culture.
3. In geriatric work in which the nurse is likely to encounter patients with senile changes.

SUSPECTING ORGANIC ILLNESS The psychiatric nurse need not *diagnose* organic illness since this is a medical function which may require neurological consultation and a series of special tests such as electroencephalograms, skull X-rays, blood chemistries, and the like. The nurse should, however, learn to suspect organic illness.

A great deal can be learned from observing the behavior itself. There are certain behaviors that are so commonly associated with organic brain disease that their observation should lead to the "diagnosis" of suspected organic illness.

These behaviors include:

1. The inability to retain and recall information.
2. Disorientation as to time, place, and person. (The patient does not know the date, where he is, or who he is.) These aspects of disorientation do not necessarily occur together.
3. Difficulty in the ability to abstract.
4. Intellectual deterioration.
5. Fluctuating state of consciousness.
6. Visual hallucinations.
7. Episodic behavioral disturbance (seizure disorders).

In a patient suffering from an organic condition, the above symptoms and behaviors do not occur alone but are likely to be accompanied by other behaviors such as paranoid delusions and depressed mood state which also occur in functional psychiatric disorders.

The nurse must also be aware that none of the seven behaviors described above may be apparent in a patient with a behavioral disorder resulting from an organic condition. For example, cancer of the pancreas, brain tumor, and hypothyroidism can all present as a functional depression. For any behavioral disorder, therefore, the nurse should consider the possibility of organic syndromes as well as the functional psychiatric disorders.

This chapter will discuss the four general conditions (pharmacological, medical, surgical, and neurological) that can lead to behavioral disturbances.

PHARMACO-LOGICAL CONDITIONS

It would take too long to list all the various pharmacological agents that can cause psychiatric side effects. For example, the nurse needs to know that hallucinogens can cause thought disorders, psychiatric medications taken in wrong doses can cause psychiatric disturbances, amphetamines can cause a paranoid pyschosis. There are also many medical drugs that can cause side effects, for example, steroids can cause a psychosis.

Drug ingestion is a prevalent cause of behavior disturbance. Common drugs include: barbiturates, bromides, meprobamate, benzodiazepines, and other sedative-hypnotic drugs; opium derivatives, marijuana; the psychedelic drugs.

Delirium, convulsions, and death may occur following rapid withdrawal of the alcohol-barbiturate group of sedative-hypnotic agents.

Many of the drugs are toxins to the brain and are capable of producing a clinical picture similar to schizophrenia. Alcohol is also a toxin to brain tissue and can cause delirium and acute alcoholic hallucinosis.

MEDICAL CONDITIONS

Behavior disorders can result from temporary, reversible, diffuse impairment of brain function such as occurs in infections, circulatory disturbances, disturbances of metabolism, growth or nutrition, endocrine disturbances. These will be briefly described.

Infections

Intercranial infections such as viral meningitis have symptoms of fever, headache, vomiting, stiff neck, and backache. The coma that may follow is most frequently seen in children.

Behavior disturbances may be produced by systematic infections, the most common of which are pneumonia, pyelitis, malaria, septicemia, typhoid fever, and acute rheumatic fever.

The toxins of diphtheria and gas gangrene can cause confusion. High fever with dehydration and electrolyte imbalance can also cause a state of confusion.

319

Psychological
Disturbances
Resulting from
Pharmacological,
Medical, Surgical,
and Neurological
Conditions

Nutritional deficiencies

The relationship of general malnutrition to psychotic reactions is difficult to assess. These states usually occur under extreme conditions, for example, in economically deprived areas, prisons, war environments in which both psychological and biological stresses are great.

A niacin deficiency, associated with the clinical entity pellagra, was responsible for 10% of the admissions to state hospitals in southern United States before preventive dietary measures were taken. This deficiency is characterized by erythematous and pigmented skin, stomatitis, diarrhea, and mental symptoms ranging from anxiety and depression to severe delirium. Hallucinations and schizophrenic-like symptoms have also been reported. Treatment consists of therapeutic doses of 500 mg of nicotinic acid per day orally and Vitamin B complex, thiamine and trytophan combined with a high caloric-balanced diet. A prompt and positive response to this regime is generally seen.

The thiamine (B_1) deficiency (beriberi) is still endemic in Southeast Asia. Symptoms of a mild disorder are irritability, fatigability, anorexia, and insomnia. Severe cases develop neurological manifestations of numbness of the toes, calf tenderness, muscular atrophy. Encephalopathy may follow. This disorder is also seen in alcoholic patients who have a vitamin deficiency and in patients with gastric carcinoma and pernicious anemia in which poor intestinal absorption is present.

Vitamin C deficiencies, as seen in scurvy, may show depression as an early symptom. Depression is also a symptom of kwashiorkor, a tropical protein deficiency disease in young children. Children suffering from this disease die unless they are treated with a high protein, high vitamin diet. Even if the metabolic deficiency is corrected, the children are prone to mental retardation.

A number of metabolic diseases associated with mental deficiency and disease have been described. Although they do not constitute a clinical problem in the usual psychiatric nursing practice, they point up important areas for prevention and education that community health nurses should be aware of. If prevention cannot be accomplished, then early case findings can be instrumental in early treatment.

Internal diseases

Symptomatic psychosis can occur in severe cardiac, hepatic, pancreatic, renal, and metabolic diseases. Hypoglycemia in diabetes is usually caused by an overdose of insulin. It is important to differentiate the confusion, agitation, or lethargy caused by acidosis from that caused by hypoglycemia so that convulsions, coma, irreversible brain damage, and even death can be prevented. In an emergency situation in which there is question of hypoglycemia and a blood sugar determination cannot be done, 10–50 ml of 50% dextrose solution intravenously is generally administered.

Hepatic failure is thought to be caused by such factors as hypoxia and fluid, electrolyte, and pH changes within the brain. The signs and symptoms range from emotional lability, intellectual deficits, and psychotic ideation in impending hepatic coma to stupor and coma.

Characteristics of impending hepatic failure are decrease in consciousness, psychomotor activity, speech, and muscle strength; presence of a slow tremor and perhaps jaundice; absence of anxiety, hallucinations, autonomic imbalance, or disturbance of sleep and appetite. Treatment consists of protein-free diet and purgation.

Characteristics of delirium tremens are increased consciousness, psychomotor activity, anxiety, and muscle strength; presence of fine tremor, rapid speech, hallucinations, and autonomic imbalance; absence of jaundice; and disturbance of normal sleep and appetite. Treatment consists of high-protein diet, hydration, and sedation.

Renal insufficiency may produce apathy, depression, confusion, agitation, convulsions, stupor, and coma. Facial paralysis, nystagmus, and lower cranial nerve dysfunction are common. Symptoms may be noted in dialysis treatment because of the rapid alteration of fluid and electrolyte balance.

In certain decompensated cardiac diseases, particularly aortic stenosis and mitral insufficiency, psychotic reactions are noted. Hypoxia, along with the psycho-social factors, is undoubtedly an important factor. The stressful stimuli that produce general anxiety, specific fear of death or feelings of being incapacitated, humiliated, provoked, or deserted contribute to delirious episodes for patients. Behavior disorder of circulatory disturbances, as in arteriosclerosis and hypertensive disease, are included in this list of potential psychotic reactions.

Endocrine disease

The characteristic symptoms of hyperthyroidism are high anxiety, oversensitivity, irritability, emotional lability, and suspicious and paranoid feelings. Some hyperthyroid patients may develop psychoses. The psychotic symptoms include manic excitement with delusions and hallucinations.

Hypothyroidism or thyroid hormone deficiency in small children causes cretinism which is characterized by dwarfism and severe mental and physical retardation. Early detection and prompt regular administration of thyroid hormone prevent the progression of the disease.

The thyroid deficiency in adults may produce myxedema. Paranoid and depressive symptoms are common. Mental changes progress from mild mental dullness, poor emotional control, apathy, drowsiness, anxiety, irritability, and memory defects to overt psychosis. Generally, the premorbid personality is a major factor in the psychotic symptomatology. Corrective hormonal therapy will produce a return to normal balance.

Behavior disorders in pituitary diseases range from mild to severe syndromes. Patients with Simmond's disease or pituitary cachexia usually show depressive symptoms and apathy.

Diseases of the adrenal cortex often produce marked personality changes in patients. They become irritable and moody, and they alternate between being lethargic and impulsive.

SURGICAL CONDITIONS Many surgical illnesses and procedures produce delirium, hallucinations, and paranoid reactions. Two basic reactions are noted: (1) symptomatic psychosis associated with cerebral dysfunction, for example, cerebral damage occurring during surgery and (2) surgery that produces extreme anxiety.

Symptomatic psychosis may be more frequent after brain surgery, cardiac surgery, surgery of male and female reproductive organs, and ophthalmic surgery. In cerebral operations the direct trauma to the brain produces edema, swelling, hemorrhages, and thromboses.

Other factors that contribute to the psychological stress are surgery with prolonged anesthesia that may cause possible brain damage, loss of blood, and infection. Post-operative psychosis is higher in children and elderly patients.

The psychological stress of surgery is often intensified because the patient has not been properly prepared for surgery. The nurse is a key person in helping the patient deal with his fears about the surgery. Some hospitals send the operating room nurses to the patient's room prior to surgery to ensure adequate teaching and preparation for the procedure. These nurses work closely with the ward staff on the floor to which the patient will return. Since the meaning of organ dysfunction, fantasies of death, mutilation, and dependency may be worrying the patient, it is essential for him to have the opportunity to express his thoughts.

NEUROLOGICAL CONDITIONS There are several neurological conditions that may produce behavioral disturbances, such as trauma or head injuries, epilepsies, congenital brain dysfunctions, intracranial neoplasms, cerebral anoxia, senile and pre-senile brain diseases.

Trauma or head injuries

Cranial injuries are generally divided into closed and open injuries. Closed injuries indicate no fracture or only a linear fracture of the skull. Open injuries indicate compound and depressed fractures.

In both open and closed injuries the brain and its covering membranes may be damaged. Three divisions of acute cerebral injuries are (1) concussion, (2) contusion and laceration, and (3) subdural and epidural hematoma.

Concussion A blow or fall, or both, usually causes a concussion. A short loss of consciousness follows. Car accidents and sports activities are common situations for such trauma.

The next symptom the patient complains of is a diffuse headache which is generally very severe. Patients will be dizzy and often feel nauseated after which they will vomit. With a simple concussion, patients are stunned, confused, and disoriented when they wake up. They cannot tell where they are, how they arrived there, and they are confused about the time and sequence of events. They respond slowly and have great difficulty identifying persons they see.

Retrograde amnesia is usually present. The patient suffers amnesia for the immediate period preceding the blow and the accident itself.

Anterograde amnesia also is present. The patient has memory lapses during the time he is awakening from the coma. During this period of awakening the patient often seems upset, anxious, and suspicious. He is likely to cry or to try to defend himself. These symptoms generally persist for a period of from a few days to a week. If they do increase in severity, a post-traumatic psychosis may develop.

Nursing management consists of careful observation of the patient for possible development of neurological and psychiatric complications. A calm attitude is important in order not to increase the anxiety of the patient.

Medication for the headache, anxiety, or insomnia should be as mild as possible with aspirin being the safest choice. Heavy medication is contra-indicated because it will mask symptoms.

The patient should be encouraged to talk about the accident and to express his feelings about it.

Contusions and lacerations

This condition of the brain is usually associated with compound or depressed fractures of the skull with bleeding from skull openings, especially ears and nose. Tearing and crushing of tissue are usually the results of local injury to the brain.

Coma following these injuries and the periods of anterograde and retrograde amnesia are more prolonged than in simple concussions. The length of the coma is significant for the prognosis. Prolonged coma produces longer lasting symptoms. Convulsions and signs of cranial nerve injury are generally present.

Nursing management is accomplished by nurses who have had neurological training. The use of opiates for sedation is contra-indicated. Strict attention must be paid to the possibility of a serious rise of the intracranial pressure. Signs of this are increased dullness, apathy, and somnolence.

An *acute post-traumatic psychosis* that may follow contusions and lacerations is very similar to the clinical picture of other symptomatic psychoses.

The symptoms of confusion and delirium predominate. Catatonic or manic–depressive symptoms are frequent. Intellectual and characterological changes are common.

Nursing management follows the principles of the symptomatic psychoses. Careful supervision is necessary for the confused or agitated patient who is likely to hurt himself or wander off the ward.

Subdural and epidural hematoma

Venous bleeding into the subdural space generally occurs when fractures of the skull are found. However, subdural hematoma may occur in very ill senile patients who have no history of trauma.

323

Psychological
Disturbances
Resulting from
Pharmacological,
Medical, Surgical,
and Neurological
Conditions

The typical pattern in acute subdural hematoma is head injury, coma, and anterograde and retrograde amnesia. There may be a temporary return of consciousness after which the patient lapses into deepening coma.

This course is also characteristic for epidural hematoma that is caused by arterial bleeding from the middle meningeal artery. Upon awakening, the patient usually shows unresponsiveness, dullness, apathy, irritability, and antagonism. Delirium and confused states similar to other acute traumatic psychoses occur. The patient complains of headache and the most frequent signs are hemiplegia, hemianesthesia, and hemianopsia. Aphasic symptoms develop if the lesion is on the dormant side.

Treatment consists of operative removal of the clot. Patients in good general health have the best chance for successful surgery and recovery.

The epilepsies

Grand mal seizures   Grand mal seizures are a tonic–clonic attack with a loss of consciousness. Many grand mal seizures have warning symptoms of vague, uncomfortable, and anxious feelings, mood changes such as depression, elation or lability of mood, headaches, minor gastrointestinal difficulties, sweating, and hot and cold sensations.

These symptoms are different from the aura that is part of the seizure. The most frequent kinds of aura are epigastric discomfort, dizziness, fainting, sensory phenomena such as seeing bright dots and lines, hearing sounds, and experiencing strange and unusually disagreeable odors and tastes.

The tonic phase consists of extreme rigidity of the muscles of the head, neck, trunk, and extremities. The extremities are in maximal extension, the trunk is opisthotonus, and the head and neck are thrown back. Respirations may stop for as long as a minute. Contraction of the respiratory muscle usually causes cyanosis. When the patient loses consciousness and falls in a rigid position, he is likely to hurt himself. The tonic phase ends with general trembling of the muscles that initiates the violent contraction of the clonic phase.

During the clonic phase the patient may bite his tongue and lose control of sphincter muscles. At the end of the clonic phase the patient is in deep coma, the eyes are turned upward, and the pupils are dilated and do not react to light. Often the patient sweats profusely. Almost all patients wake up dazed and are slow to recognize their environment. They complain about sleepiness, haziness, headaches, and amnesia. Recovery may take from 1 to 4 hours.

Petit mal attacks   The petit mal attacks may be one of three types: (1) a slight lapse of consciousness for 15–30 seconds with minimal twitching of facial muscles, a vacant stare, and subsequent amnesia for the attack; (2) a similiar lapse of consciousness with myoclonic twitches; and (3) an episode of sudden loss of muscular tone and consciousness.

These seizures often begin in childhood and persist into adult years. It is unusual for them to begin in adult years.

Psychomotor epilepsy

The term *psychomotor epilepsy* is used broadly and includes (1) increase tonicity of muscles with adversive movements of head and swallowing movements; (2) autonomic behavior such as unbuttoning of clothing, walking, or running with complete amnesia, although consciousness may be preserved.

Psychic seizures

The diagnosis is made with clinical and electroencephalogram confirmation of abnormal waves. Often the experiences are vague and bizarre and the patient reports them as trancelike and dreamlike. The unreal character of the experience is marked. Some patients are unable to distinguish between fantasy and reality and suffer from hallucinations, illusions, and delusions.

Another type of psychic seizure is a feeling of depersonalization with extreme anxiety and intense feelings of displeasure. These patients are not completely amnesic but show partial memory defect. The aggressive and antisocial nature of the episode can be marked.

Focal discharge

Focal or partial discharges are classified according to the localization of the seizure focus. The focal motor seizure begins with a twitching of a muscle, such as face or lips, and then spreads to the extremities. When skin sensations are involved in focal seizures, they are referred to as sensory seizures. Patients report tingling in a localized region of the body.

Congenital brain dysfunction

Prenatal factors may cause congenital brain damage. Syphilis during pregnancy was formerly a major cause of mental retardation and progressive mental deterioration (juvenile general paresis). Laboratory blood testing has assisted in preventive measures for this problem.

The virus rubella in German measles has been identified as a major cause of congenital malformation. Pregnant women contracting this disease in the first 4 months of pregnancy are in the high-risk category of delivering infants who may have cataracts, congenital heart disease, deafness, mental retardation, and other neurological problems. Prevention in the form of immunization 3 months prior to any conception is advised for all women.

Other prenatal sources such as hepatitis, pneumonia, influenza, cold virus, and urinary tract infection are currently being researched in the etiology of mental retardation.

Brain damage resulting in cerebral palsy may be caused by prenatal, natal, and post-natal factors. Characteristics of this disorder are weakness, incoordination, ataxia, dystonia, paralysis, visual and hearing defects, mental retardation, and emotional disturbances.

Birth traumas include all forms of brain damage resulting from complications of labor or delivery. Brain damage may result from mechanical trauma, for example, the use of forceps, breech delivery, cephalopelvic dis-

325

Psychological
Disturbances
Resulting from
Pharmacological,
Medical, Surgical,
and Neurological
Conditions

proportion and prolonged labor or hypoxia due to Caesarean section, brady-cardia, respiratory difficulties, and anesthesia. Mechanical damage may also produce subarachnoid and intraventricular hemorrhage.

Intracranial neoplasms

Brain tumors are found in 2% of all autopsied cases regardless of the primary cause of death. Brain neoplasms that cause signs and symptoms are most frequently (40% of all tumors) gliomas. Metastatic brain tumors account for 15–20% of brain tumors and they commonly arise from carcinoma of the lungs and breast.

The most important neurological symptoms are convulsions, visual disturbances such as double or blurred vision, headaches, nausea, and vomiting. Convulsions occur in 50–80% of patients and are of the grand mal type. Headaches are severe though intermittent and are usually frontal or occipital.

The person with a brain tumor may be referred to a mental health facility because of psychiatric disturbances that may be the only presenting symptoms. The nurse can be alert to this possibility if she knows the signs and symptoms. If a brain tumor is in question, the patient should be referred for a complete neurological examination. The general symptoms of a brain tumor caused by increased intracranial pressure are: intellectual deterioration; defects of memory, recall, and attention; sleepiness and stupor; coarsening of personality; appearance of asocial and antisocial traits; and apathetic or euphoric reactions. Delirious and confused episodes and disturbances of consciousness are usually the result of rapid changes leading to cerebral edema or swelling, hemorrhages in the tumor, or sudden rises of intracranial pressure.

In many patients the symptoms are not that pronounced. Misinterpretation of symptoms, such as headaches and dizziness and the presence of severe anxiety, may lead to the diagnosis of hysterical or hypochondriacal reactions.

Cerebral anoxia

The cells of the central nervous system are exceedingly sensitive to even brief periods of decreased oxygen supply. Cerebral anoxia, caused by sudden decrease in blood flow as in some cardiac and vascular diseases, by the labor and delivery process, or by decrease of oxygen in the atmosphere rapidly produce a necrosis of cerebral tissue.

Situations (other than described above) in which this disturbance may occur is excessive bleeding, prolonged anesthesia, carbon monoxide poisoning, attempts by hanging or strangulation, altitude sickness, and decompensation illness. Lack of oxygen while flying at certain altitudes without pressurized equipment or in scuba diving accounts for a certain percentage of accidental fatalities. The complex hazards of the space projects have become the subject of the specialty of space medicine.

Symptoms patients complain of are dyspnea, headache, fatigue, sleepiness, anxiety, and irritability. A coma that may result in intellectual deficit may develop.

Senile and presenile brain diseases

In senile dementia, also referred to as *senile brain disease,* the symptomatology may vary from mild to severe. It is characterized by a chronic and progressive organic deficit (*mental deterioration*), usually occurring between 60 and 90 years of age. There is no sufficiently supported scientific evidence to explain this disease. Factors believed to strongly influence the development of this condition are metabolic, endocrine, vascular, and genetic determinants.

Senile dementia is generally accompanied by other evidence of progressive aging affecting the entire body. There is a general wasting of muscles, loss of elasticity of the skin, shrinkage of the soft tissue, unsteady gait, speech disturbances, and easy fatigability. Because of the body's aging process, the person is apt to fall and complicate his difficulties by a fracture, especially of the femur.

The cardinal symptoms of senile dementia are dysmnesia, disorientation, and difficulty with abstract reasoning. The most prominent symptom, *dysmnesia,* is an impairment in the ability to retain and recall information. The mildest kind of memory disturbance consists of lowered ability to absorb and retain new information. Initially, this symptom may appear to be absent-mindedness. In more severe cases, the person will have difficulty remembering events of *recent* past. Incidents experienced or things learned before this period of memory failure began may still be recalled at this stage, but as the dysmnesia becomes more severe, it invades the person's memory of the time period before he was ill. This symptom progressively extends further into the person's *remote* past until it is finally global in the sense that the person neither understands the present nor remembers any part of the past.

The symptom of *disorientation* is closely related to the symptom of dysmnesia. Orientation means knowing what time it is, being able to tell where one is, and identifying the person one is dealing with. This ability is closely related to a person's memory. Thus, disorientation is rare without an appreciable memory impairment. This symptom also becomes progressively more intense. The mildest impairment usually consists of an impaired *time* sense. Initially, the person will be unable to recall when or in what order the current or previous day's events occurred, although he will still be able to describe the events. Thereafter, he may be unable to tell the day of the month, month of the year, or day of the week or year. He will also become disoriented as to *place.* For example, in the beginning of this symptom, he will have difficulty identifying a particular place, and in more severe deterioration, he will be unable to remember his own address or where he is currently. As the deterioration continues, he will have difficulty identifying *persons* around him, forgetting their names and thereafter their relationship to him. It is not until almost every other intellectual function is impaired that

327

Psychological
Disturbances
Resulting from
Pharmacological,
Medical, Surgical,
and Neurological
Conditions

the person will have difficulty identifying himself or remembering his own name. This fact can be important when distinguishing between an amnesia or dissociative state.[1]

The third symptom, *difficulty in abstract reasoning,* is determined through asking the person to explain or rephrase a proverb (mental status exam) or by asking him to repeat five numbers in reverse order.

An assessment of these symptoms provides some uniformity in the order in which the person's memory, orientation, and other intellectual abilities are decreasing. Persons with organic dementia suffer not only the cognitive impairment but emotional and motivational impairment as well. There tends to be a general disorganization, desocialization, and regression of behavior. People functioning at a lower neurobiological level find it more difficult to control their emotions. Aggressive behavior may be marked in some people; clinging dependent behavior is evident in others.

Stages of dementia Three stages of this disease may be noted. In the first stage, mood swings, feelings of general inadequacy, and fatigue are felt by the individual. Failures are most conspicuous when the person is under pressure or faced with multiple tasks and he cannot fall back on the routine of performance. A decrease of interests, especially cultured interests, and a coarsening of interpersonal relationships are noted. In organic deficit states, in contrast to behavior disorders of old age in which the family is often overalerted for signs of impairment, this stage often goes unnoticed.

During the second stage the patient's inefficiency is obvious to everyone but himself. When confronted with his shortcomings, he tends to make excuses or else denies them. Gross impairment in social and intellectual functioning appears, for example, crude, tactless, and impulsive behavior. A decrease in reality testing, suspicious and paranoid attitudes, and misinterpretation of relationships are common. Memory, attention, and concentration may be impaired.

In the third stage of dementia the patient is very helpless and unable to care for himself. Intellectual deterioration is so affected that even the routine tasks of everyday living cannot be accomplished. The patient has great difficulty communicating and requires constant nursing care for prevention of infection, safety measures, and hygienic measures.

Community health nurses are excellent resource people in helping families to keep the person at home as long as possible. This will prevent the increase in dependency that institutions and nursing homes cannot help but foster. The nursing assessment of the various phases of dementia and teaching the family various psychological approaches that aim to maintain the person's level of functioning are most helpful.

Nursing procedures that the family cannot carry out can be performed by the Visiting Nurse Association, which will also facilitate keeping the person in his familiar environment.

[1]Thomas P. Detre and Henry G. Jarecki, *Modern Psychiatric Treatment* (Philadelphia: J. B. Lippincott Co., 1971), pp. 396–404.

Organic syndromes

Korsakoff's syndrome, a dysmnesic syndrome, usually follows an acute delirium, twilight state, or stupor. In its classical sense, the syndrome is associated with chronic alcoholism, polyneuritis due to thiamin (vitamin B_1) deficiency, and, occasionally, pellagralike skin lesions.[2]

Frequently, the person shows conspicuous memory loss. At the same time, the mechanism of *confabulation*—the making up of stories—is used to compensate for this memory loss. It has been hypothesized that this memory failure is not due to the defective storage of information but rather to a lack of access to information in storage and to the lack of new input.[3] A major defect is the person's inability to form new associations. The answers given in the mental status examination will usually show marked defects. In contrast, this condition may or may not be observed in patients with acute brain disorders due to surgery or immediately following electroconvulsive treatments.

This kind of progressive mental deterioration was described by Alois Alzheimer in 1906. Although this disease usually begins in persons in their early sixties, it occasionally begins in a person's fourth decade of life. This disease can be differentiated from Pick's disease. The person with Alzheimer's disease appears to be overactive, as compared with the loss of initiative seen in Pick's disease. Emotional distress and agitation are common, specifically a distressing awareness of impending disaster is described by the person. The usual duration of this disease is 2 to 5 years, although isolated cases have been reported for longer survival periods.[4]

This disease was first described by Arnold Pick in 1892. Pick's disease is much rarer than Alzheimer's disease and there is considerable evidence in the literature that this disease is a specific heredodegenerative process that is not associated with rapid progression in the normal aging process. In the early stages, the memory is not significantly involved, but the attention span is progressively affected, and this, in turn, is followed by a decline in memory. As deterioration continues, restlessness, aimless activity, and increased talkativeness can develop. Speech is difficult to understand. There is intellectual deterioration with early loss of abstract thinking. In the final stages of deterioration, paralysis, contractures, and epileptic seizures are often present.[5]

[2]Henry W. Brosin, "Brain Disorders, III: Associated with Trauma, Poisons, Drugs, Infections, and Neoplasm," in *Comprehensive Textbook of Psychiatry,* edited by Alfred M. Freedman and Harold I. Kaplan (Baltimore: The Williams & Wilkins Co., 1967), p. 752.

[3] Ibid., p. 752.

[4]Ewald W. Busse, "Brain Syndromes Associated with Disturbances in Metabolism, Growth and Nutrition," in *Comprehensive Textbook of Psychiatry,* edited by Alfred M. Freedman and Harold I. Kaplan (Baltimore: The Williams & Wilkins Co., 1967), pp. 730–31.

[5]Ibid., pp. 729–30.

Huntington's chorea is a genetically inherited disease and has a progressive degenerative process involving the cerebrum with onset usually in middle age. It is characterized by involuntary movements in the limbs and face and ultimately of the whole body. Dementia is the most notable psychiatric change, but personality variations can be noted one to two years prior to the overt signs. A person who has seemed fairly even-tempered may become unexplainably irritable and given to episodes of rage. A mild apathy with loss of interest in work, family, and friends comes on early. The patient complains that he is unable to concentrate. Judgment and insight gradually fail and the patient reaches a very regressed state. The suicide rate tends to be high with this group and the complication of alcoholism is common.

Nursing management of neurological conditions

Management of excitement and delirium: Calmness, firmness, and patience are essential nursing skills to being therapeutic with a person who is disoriented, excited, and frightened. Speaking and moving slowly, softly, and deliberately will help convey to the patient that the nurse is there to help him.

Constant observation and supervision of the patient are necessary to prevent his falling out of bed or wandering off the ward. The suicidal intent of many of these patients should not be ignored.

It is essential to leave a light on at night because the patient becomes more confused and frightened in the dark. The nurse can decrease the patient's agitation if she can be readily available to him or within sight.

Exposure to stressful procedures, such as X-rays and diagnostic tests, may precipitate delirious patients into a panic. Team consultation is most important in the planning and carrying out of procedures.

Medical control: Opinion on the use of medication in controlling excitement and delirium is divided. Sedation and/or tranquilizing drugs may be ordered. If they are, there is always a danger present of giving too much on top of an unknown cause for the delirium. The patient's vital signs must be carefully noted at least an hour before and an hour following administration of any medication. The possibility of helping the patient to ventilate is to be kept in mind in case of respiratory depression or cessation.

Drugs should not be given to the patient who is in shock or coma or who shows a decrease in vital signs. Patients who are in a stupor because of other drugs, narcotics, or alcohol should sleep off the effects before they are administered additional medication. And whenever possible, the oral route of administration is preferred.

Case illustration

The following case example illustrates behavioral disorders from surgical, psychological, and neurological situations. The referral form on Mrs. Round states that the husband has been told that nothing could be done for his wife and that the husband may be expected to be depressed for he had come to the psychiatrist "hoping for a miracle." The only other information is that the onset of her symptoms was 7 years ago and that a son was killed in an automobile accident 7 years ago.

Mrs. Round, age 59, was referred to the psychiatric clinic for a consultation and evaluation interview. Her problem dated back several years to when she became "depressed and slowed down." Four years prior to this interview the patient was operated on for a strangulated bowel and was quite ill. She was transferred postoperatively to the neurology service for evaluation of "dementia" that had become precipitously apparent after surgery. She was medically discharged home following her recovery.

Mrs. Round functioned fairly well at home, but there was a gradual decline in her ability to remember, make judgments, and solve problems. For example, she had a car accident four months after returning home because she mistook the accelerator for the brake and crashed into a tree.

Her progressive difficulties have worsened over the past 6 months to the point that she has become unintelligibly aphasic, confused, and disoriented. She must be asked simple requests several times. She cannot be left alone. She can feed and dress herself with directional assistance. She is not incontinent. A right hemiplegia, a leaning to the left while walking, and dropping objects from her right hand have been noted. She cries in apparent frustration every two–three days.

A diagnosis of pre-senile dementia caused by bilateral vascular disease was made. The results of the neurological examination showed that Mrs. Round was profoundly dysphasic with nearly unintelligible stammering, stuttering, and confusion. She could follow one-part commands but nothing more complex. An abnormal EEG with diffusely slow readings was confirmed.

SUMMARY
Nurses need to constantly think about the four conditions of pharmacological, medical, surgical, and neurological situations related to behavior disturbance when they evaluate a patient who has psychiatric concerns. For instance, when a nurse is seeing a patient out in the community who says she is feeling poorly, the nurse should ask about medications, illnesses, and recent hospitalizations. The nurse should include in the history taking of the patient any head injuries, seizures, or loss of memory. It is helpful to use the mental status examination with the patient. The areas of orientation, memory, intellect, judgment, insight, thought content, and mood can be useful in testing for either something organically wrong with the patient or something functionally wrong.

The nurse is in an evaluative position in her work both in the hospital and in the community. The information and judgments made by the nurse have direct input to the treatment or referral then decided.

REFERENCES
Detre, Thomas P., and Henry E. Jarecki (1971). *Modern Psychiatric Treatment.* Philadelphia: J. B. Lippincott Company.

Freedman, Alfred M., and Harold I. Kaplan (1967). *Comprehensive Textbook of Psychiatry.* Baltimore: The Williams & Wilkins Co.

Redlich, Frederick C., and Daniel X. Freedman (1966). *The Theory and Practice of Psychiatry.* New York: Basic Books, Inc.

PROBLEMS OF
CHILDREN AND ADOLESCENTS

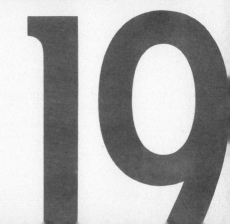

Marianne Tipmore Cannon

This chapter provides an introductory discussion of the nurse's role in the hospital and the community in working with children and adolescents. By using selected case examples of patients in a long-term residential treatment center, a short-term diagnostic hospital, and an out-patient clinic, a variety of interventions that the nurse can perform are illustrated.

CHILD PSYCHIATRIC NURSING

From two basic perspectives of educational preparation and life experiences, nurses provide an important role in the diagnosis and treatment of the emotionally disturbed child or adolescent. Students can examine and appreciate their own personal experiences as caretakers of children. Most students possess a natural background of experiences such as babysitting, camp counseling, and helping with younger brothers and sisters. Within the framework of these responsibilities, they function as caring, nurturing, protective authority figures for infants, children, and young adolescents. For example, when a child injures himself in play or when another child hurts him, he runs to his counselor or older sister for support, comfort, and attendance to his wounds. Infants and very young children show their sense of loss and fear of abandonment by their parents when they discover they have been left with a babysitter. The babysitter, in turn, approaches their cries of anger and sadness by giving them realistic expectations as to when their parents will return, empathizes with them, and then begins to redirect their attention. An older sister shows her younger sister that she loves and cares about her when she refuses to let the child play in the street. Each of the above examples demonstrates important principles of child psychiatric nursing.

The knowledge and skills acquired in nursing education provide another perspective from which the nurse can function in child psychiatric nursing. Nurses bring to this specialty an understanding of such basic concepts of sociology and psychology as the structure of the family; the cultural,

Marianne Tipmore Cannon, R.N., M.S., is child psychiatric nurse-clinician at the Newton-Wellesley Hospital Outpatient Department, Newton, Mass.

psychological, social, and biological dynamics of health and illness; the meaning of loss and separation through hospitalization, illness, death, divorce, or adoption; and, particularly important, an understanding of human growth and development. Not only should students realize the value of their theoretical knowledge, but they should also appreciate their clinical experiences which equip them with the skills to apply knowledge to patients and their families. To a large extent, nursing in child psychiatry requires that the nurse pool her experiences in pediatrics, adult psychiatry, maternity, medical–surgical, and community health nursing. The nurse's wide range of skills and broad educational background facilitate an essential position on the multidisciplinary diagnostic and treatment team common in many child psychiatric facilities.

Normal child development

In order to optimally apply concepts and skills, the nurse needs a theoretical framework for practice. Previous chapters included concepts of physical and psychological development. By observing the child at play, the team can assess the child's abilities to master normal developmental tasks. Using observational data in the assessment process is crucial in making an accurate diagnosis and planning an effective treatment plan.

The nurse uses perceptual senses in observing young patients because of the child's limited verbal abilities. The nurse should include the observations of the child's behavior such as how he physically cares for himself, his language skills, his play activities alone and with a group, his eating and sleeping habits. These data can then be compared with normal developmental patterns for his age and sex. It is important to observe the child when he is interacting with his parents as well as with other authority figures. For example, note how easy or stressful it is for the child to separate from his mother and father, especially after a visit.

Two guidelines for the nurse to follow when she observes a child's interactions are (1) the wide range of normal variations, e.g., the "spurts and lags" within the normal developmental pattern and (2) the normally very rapid growth rate, with many physical and emotional changes in children. The highest rate of growth takes place in infancy and continues until the third year of life. In latency, growth and developmental changes are less dramatic. In puberty and adolescence, the rate increases sharply and behavior becomes labile once again.

These two guidelines are important for the nurse when she is working with parents. Consider the young mother who calls her pediatrician because she is distressed about her extremely active 1-year-old who is not saying as many words as her neighbor's child of the same age or who has not learned to walk independently of her mother's hand. Even though most parents today intellectually understand that children develop at different rates, they frequently need to be reminded of this when they begin to rear their own children. Similarly, parents need support in accepting that their child is "normal" even though he may not have mastered all of the tasks or goals of a specific developmental phase at the same rate as another child. Of course, the nurse must be careful to observe extreme spurts or lags in a child's development because they may indicate physical and/or psychological disturbance. It is important to emphasize that even severely disturbed children have normal aspects to their behavior and personalities. Not only the deficiencies, but also the healthy parts of their psychodynamics should be recorded in nursing observations.

Therapeutic skills

All the therapeutic tasks identified in Chapter 8 apply to child psychiatric nursing. The specific skills of autodiagnosis, limit setting, and management of the milieu assume major emphasis in the nursing of disturbed children. The use of touch as a therapeutic task is also of great importance.

Autodiagnosis   Emotionally distressed children and adolescents evoke a gamut of feeling in the people who work with them closely. In most cases, parents themselves have been unable to cope effectively with their own feelings about their children, and, consequently, they have sought help from professionals in clinics and hospitals. Thus, it is of substantial importance that the nurse and the child care staff use the self-assessment process called *autodiagnosis*. This therapeutic task is especially important to the nurse who works with children whose strong dependency needs and low frustration tolerance place considerable stress on her own equilibrium. Often, these children are extremely deprived, to varying extents symbolically "hungry," and are seeking to be nurtured by a maternal figure. Therefore, the nurse and staff must set limits on how much they can give to their patients so that they may have sufficient energy to devote themselves to other areas outside their work.

Nurses who care for the troubled adolescent must acknowledge their own attitudes toward sex and sexual issues. It is normal for teenagers to be preoccupied or involved in some way with sexual issues. However, adolescents who are emotionally disturbed often have greater difficulty dealing with their sexual feelings and impulse control and are prone to act upon sexual conflicts. For example, adolescent patients may be found together engaged in sexual activity either in their hospital beds or on the hospital grounds; it may be homosexual or heterosexual behavior. Intervention in terms of disruption of the activity followed by careful discussion with the adolescents separately is very important. One partner may be more frightened or threatened by the sexual activity than the other or one may have become psychotic or more withdrawn as a result of the sexual encounter. For hospitalized patients, firm limits may need to be set on the amount of time adolescents spend together.

Staff need to autodiagnose their feelings because patients may be verbally seductive to staff members and attempt to touch or have physical contact with them. Adolescents may become angry and aggressive toward staff who set limits on their sexualized behavior and such situations need carefully negotiated treatment plans in order that an entire ward not be disrupted.

Touch The sense of touch is a frequently used observational medium in child psychiatric nursing. Children are often very clinging and want to touch, kiss, or hug the nurse in an effort to satisfy their tactile needs. Being physically close to the nurse during stressful times, for example, bedtime, can be anxiety reducing to children, including the latency age child.

Bedtime for hospitalized children is usually easier when the nursing staff is able to provide a period of physical closeness with the children. Staff spend time sitting beside the child's bed reading a story. Many times the children lean their heads back against the staff member or hold the staff member's hand during the storytelling. Gentle back rubs at bedtime are another form of contact the staff use to soothe an anxious child and help him counteract some of the fear he feels before going to sleep. The staff often notice that on nights when they are unable to provide physical contact to the patients, the amount of hyperactivity, usually oppositional and attention-getting behavior, increases.

Touch can be a useful therapeutic approach. The following example shows how the nurse helped a child say goodbye by using human contact in an appropriate and special way for this parting.

> Craig had been in several institutions during his 8 years of life. Now he was preparing to be transferred to a "long-term" residential center where he would spend 2 years. He was a very clingy child who was always eager to hold his nurse's arm, to try to hug her, and to "whisper a secret" in her ear.
>
> He constantly sought attention by touching the nurse on her hand, who observed after a few days that Craig derived sexual stimulation when he was allowed to touch female staff in the manner described. He became very anxious when this behavior was not redirected. Therefore, any attempts on Craig's part to touch female staff in such a way that he became anxious were stopped and he received attention in other ways from them.
>
> The one behavior that Craig had difficulty tolerating was when he was told he could not "whisper" in the nurse's ear. She had learned earlier that Craig did not want to "whisper," but that he wanted to kiss her. Then he started acting agitated because of the stimulation. Thus, he was told by the nurse that he could show he liked her by their doing other things together, for example, reading books or playing checkers.
>
> However, on his final afternoon on the ward, Craig approached the nurse, looked up at her and said, "I'm going now." The nurse said, "I'll miss you, Craig, but I hope you meet some nice friends at the new hospital." After a pause she told him good-bye. He said nothing for a moment and then softly asked, "Can I whisper a secret in your ear?" The nurse could sense the child's difficulty in verbalizing his good-bye but realized the importance of helping him resolve his conflicts at terminating. She knew he wanted to tell her good-bye in the only manner he could. She looked down at Craig and said, "You want to kiss me good-bye, don't you?" He shook his head affirmatively and the nurse smiled and bent down to let him kiss her on her cheek. He then walked toward the door.

In this example, the nurse helped to put the boy's request, which was nonverbal, into words. By observing when the boy's need to touch was too disturbing for the child to handle, the nurse set limits on the behavior. When touching the nurse was an appropriate way to deal with a situation, as in leaving the hospital, the nurse helped the boy state his request and then agreed to it.

Limit setting　　A third important therapeutic task is limit setting. The presence of limits, or external control, is vital to the healthy growth and development of the child. Limits can be divided into two conceptual categories: The first category includes limits that give direction; the second category includes limits that are disciplinary. Direction is provided by setting expectations, defining boundaries of acceptable behavior, and giving guidance and advice. Disciplinary limits are provided in the form of restrictions, restraints, and the use of physical intervention.

From early on, the infant and child need to experience both kinds of limits. If limit setting is consistent and effective, the infant learns to decrease impulsivity and to gain self-control on the one hand and to relinquish omnipotency and accept his own limitations and the limitations of others on the other.[1] Thus, limit setting is one of the most important functions of parenthood; it is a major process by which a child learns to adapt to the physical and social milieu in which he exists. In addition, the child's trust and affection for his parents are strengthened as he learns to distinguish between rejection (disfavor) and direction. Feeling cared for and protected, the child develops a sense of worth which means that his ego is strengthened and, consequently, anxiety is decreased.

A characteristic shared by many "hyperactive" children and adolescents is their exposure to destructive limit-setting practices in the family. This aggravates the hyperkinesis as well as the poor self-image; both disturbances leave the child feeling anxious and disorganized. Other consequences of pathological limit setting are temper tantrums, impulsivity, and a generalized sense of entitlement which the child imposes on his environment. Following are five kinds of destructive methods of setting limits on infants and young children:

1. Parental postponement of limit-setting procedures during the infant's expanding neuromotor development.
2. Inconsistencies in limit setting.
3. The use of harsh or abusive methods in the setting of limits.
4. Avoidance of setting limits.
5. Inadequate provision of opportunity for the infant's expression of frustration at the acceptance of limits.[2]

One of the most important therapeutic functions performed by the nurse is not only setting effective disciplinary limits on behavior, but also outlining safe, secure boundaries in which the child can live while he is in the

[1]Herman A. Meyersburg, Steven Ablon, and Joel Kotkin, "A Reverberating Psychic Mechanism in the Depressive Processes," *Psychiatry,* **37,** No. 4 (1974), 374.
[2]Ibid., p. 374.

hospital milieu. One means of accomplishing this limit setting is to establish rules and routine on the ward. Of course, in the ideal situation, parents establish rules and regulations at home so that their children know what the boundaries are. Another way is to establish realistic expectations of a child before he engages in a new activity or takes advantage of a brand new privilege he has earned for which there is no behavior precedent set.

Touch has previously been discussed as a mode of observation for nurses. However, the tactile modality can also be used as an effective means of communicating boundaries which provide concrete direction, especially therapeutic for anxious, disorganized children. The nurse's putting her hands on the child's body, such as on shoulders and arms, or by taking the child's hand can decrease some of the confusion perceived by the preoccupied child. In some situations, verbal communication may only further confuse the child.

> Ronnie was balking at having to make his bed before he went to breakfast. He was whining and playing with the sheets. A brain-damaged child from birth, routine tasks always took Ronnie longer than usual to accomplish. But this morning he was having a very difficult time. The nurse who was with him leaned down and put her hands on his shoulders in order to establish eye contact with him and hold his attention. She looked at him and said, "Ronnie, you must make your bed now. I will help you by staying here with you and watching. But I will have to leave when the hands on my watch get to here." When Ronnie did not look at her watch—even though he understood the meaning of telling time—she took one hand from his shoulder, gently moved his head in the direction of her watch, and explained again when she would leave.

> Although the nurse had to put the bed linen in his hand two or three times during the task, Ronnie was able to successfully complete the bedmaking in the desired time limit.

When using touch, it is always necessary for the nurse to assess whether or not the child's anxiety is increased by this physical contact. If he withdraws or becomes restless, the nurse should stop touching him and use alternative methods for setting limits.

In disciplining children on the ward, the nurse and staff will often be in the position of having to interrupt the hostile behavior of patients. Hostility can be self-directed as well as directed at others and in either case, the behavior needs to be limited. Ideally, the nurse should interrupt or respond at the first sign of hostility and aggression so that these forces are not allowed to escalate into an overwhelming or crisis situation.

A study was done of the effectiveness of a nursing staff in interrupting hostile behavior exhibited by latency-age boys in a residential treatment center. The children's hostile behavior was effectively interrupted 41% of the time when the staff responded "positively" by using the following behaviors: (1) verbal or physical limits; (2) interviewing techniques (explore, interpret, clarify); (3) restructures or regroups situation; (4) removes cause of hostility.[3] However, the study revealed that the children's hostile behavior was

---

[3]Elizabeth Boldizar and Marianne Cannon, "The Effects of a Nursing Staff's Responsive Acts on the Hostile Behavior Exhibited by Emotionally Disturbed Children in a Residential Treatment Center," Master's thesis, Boston University, 1970, p. 27.

uninterrupted 95% of the time by staff responses such as ignoring, threatening with loss of privileges, or laughing at the child.

This study points out the effective responses that the nurse can use to set limits on hostile behavior of latency-age children with emotional and behavioral disturbances.

Like the adult psychiatric patient, the youngster becomes more agitated when he is unable to control his behavior, and there is always a high risk of either self-abuse or abuse directed toward others. It is especially important for the nurse to remember this when she is treating adolescents. Also important is the fact that it is not therapeutic for the patient to suffer guilt feelings because of actions committed when he was angry and not in control of his impulses. It is best to use a system of progression in setting disciplinary or restrictive limits, for example, the following: (1) Verbally warn the child what will happen if you have to interrupt him again; (2) follow through on setting the limit; (3) if the child's oppositional behavior increases and if he refuses to abide by the limit set, with assistance, separate him from the group in order to cool him down (in the quiet room or his room if he can tolerate it); (4) if he resists physical isolation, you may have to give him medication, as well as keep him in the quiet room. Rarely with children, but frequently with adolescents, mechanical restraints, i.e., leather wrist and ankle bands, must be used, especially if the adolescent is in serious danger of hurting himself or others. If an adolescent patient is restrained in this way, he must be supported and protected by staff for the duration of the time he is confined.

Managing the milieu

The final therapeutic task to be stressed in this chapter is the nurse's functioning as the manager of the milieu. For reasons not entirely clear, children whose ego boundaries are impaired are extremely sensitive to nonverbal communication. They immediately sense anxiety, fear, and anger emanating from other patients or from staff; these feelings may be consciously or unconsciously conveyed to the patients. Therefore, the nurse should be able to detect an untherapeutic "feeling tone" on the ward, to assess the source of the feelings, and to intervene by problem-solving approaches.

Children and adolescents are particularly vulnerable to anger and fear.

During morning report the head nurse was hearing from one of the care workers who had worked the evening before what a difficult shift last night had been. He said the tone of the ward milieu was anxious and hostile but that the staff could not find a reason for these feelings in the patients. Then the nurse asked him how he had been feeling that evening. He said, "Well, I was really mad and upset over some of the changes that are going to take place around here. That new director talked to us in staff meeting yesterday and she is even going to change our schedules."

The staff were talking about how their ward was "turning into an adolescent ward." Many of the new admissions had been 13- and 14-year-old boys. One child care worker said, "I'm so used to working with little kids that these new boys look a lot bigger than I suppose they really are. I think I'm kind of afraid what they will do if I try to set limits on them. Last night Bobby picked up on my fear and hesitancy and got scared because he thought I couldn't control him. It ended by his getting himself in the quiet room."

Another important way a nurse manages the ward milieu in an effort to make it as therapeutic an atmosphere as possible is to establish a goal-oriented activity program for the young patients. It is impossible to elaborate on all aspects of this task; however, important considerations in planning activities include the child's developmental level, the age, high-energy vs. low-energy periods, and "wind-down" or transition times.

NURSING CARE OF CHILDREN AND ADOLESCENTS WITH EMOTIONAL DISORDERS

The fact that emotional disorders of children and adolescents usually have more than one etiologic factor cannot be stressed enough. In 1970 the Joint Commission on Mental Health of Children described an approach identifying the following five areas as at least some of the possible origins for such disorders:

> (1) Faulty training and faulty life experiences; (2) surface conflicts between children and parents which arise from such adjustment tasks as relations among siblings, school, social, and sexual development; (3) deeper conflicts within the child (these are the so-called neuroses); (4) a difficulty associated with physical handicaps and disorders; (5) difficulties associated with severe mental disorders, such as psychoses. It is estimated that 80% of emotional problems are related to the first two categories; 10% to the third category; and 10% to the fourth and fifth.[4]

The role of hereditary factors in the etiology of some of the above is a major research area.

Any combination of the above may contribute to a psychiatric disturbance that may arise in a child in any phase of his development. In this section we will identify some of the symptomatology of emotional distress associated with the oral, anal, oedipal, latency, and early adolescent phases of development. Implications for nursing care will be stressed.

Symptoms of the oral phase

Relatively few infants are seen in the child psychiatric clinic; they are far more frequently treated for emotional difficulties in the office of the pediatrician or general practitioner. Many, unfortunately, are not diagnosed or treated at all. Parents are often too frightened to admit that something may be wrong with their infant; often, real or potential emotional disorders are not easily identified in the infant. With such a strong emphasis on prevention in mental health, it is unfortunate that so many emotional disorders cannot be diagnosed in infancy when the problems are amenable to treatment.

Children who have emotional disorders during the first year usually show one or several of the following symptoms: listlessness, lethargy, disturbed feeding and sleeping habits, an abnormal amount of crying, failure to

[4]Joint Commission on Mental Health of Children, *Crisis in Child Mental Health: Challenge for the 1970's* (New York: Harper & Row, Publishers, Inc., 1970), p. 251.

gain weight, and social unresponsiveness, i.e., lack of smiling and cooing, and a general inability to form specific object relationships. A fundamental aspect of the relationship between the infant and the parent or parent substitute is characterized by the term *object specificity,* or the infant's ability to distinguish one human being from another and to interact with the person. The very first object the infant learns to relate to is his mother and/or his father for they are the ones who gratify his basic needs for safety, comfort, security, and attention. This early relationship of the infant is an egocentric one in which the infant receives immediate gratification of his needs. Trust between the parent and the infant is developed through the consistent and adequate satisfaction of mutual needs.

If, however, the infant is deprived of a consistent, nurturant parent because of death, illness, or some other kind of separation, the infant senses the loss and may develop physical and emotional symptoms. Anxiety increases as mistrust develops toward his environment. If the infant is deprived of a parent for too long a time, or if the substitute is not adequate to anticipate and meet his needs, serious behavioral reactions such as depression may be observed. The child's ability to form attachments in the future may be impaired.

Although they are rarely diagnosed at this age, two kinds of psychoses begin in the first year of life. These are the symbiotic and autistic psychoses. The child suffering from symbiotic psychosis does not separate his self-identity from a fused identity with his parent, usually the mother. "In failing to take this step, reality testing is impaired, since the child attempts to cope with the world by clinging solely to the symbiotic relationship.[5] The older the child becomes, the more he is faced with the overwhelming task of relating to others in his play and at school. His level of anxiety increases and he becomes very withdrawn and narcissistic—much like the young infant he psychologically actually is. Like autism, the symbiotic psychosis requires intensive, psychiatric treatment of both the child and his family, particularly the mother. This intervention usually happens long after infancy.

The nurse in the child guidance clinic felt strongly that 4-year-old Ruthie should be hospitalized for an intensive psychiatric and physical evaluation. The child's development seemed grossly impaired to the nurse, who had made a visit to the home of the child and her mother. Ruthie still wore diapers and exhibited very little verbal behavior. She looked pale and thin and she moved very lethargically.

Ruthie's mother spoke for her all the time, disregarding the fact that the nurse had asked Ruthie herself questions. Mother spoke of "we," not "she" and "I," and she used babyish language. She also talked of many fears which she defended against by overprotecting her daughter, who was not permitted to play on the floor for fear of getting dirty and sick. Nor could Ruthie go outside without her mother because of her mother's worry that she may be hurt by the other

[5]C. Glenn Clements, "Emotional Disorders of Childhood," in *Basic Psychiatric Concepts in Nursing,* 3rd ed., Joan J. Keyes and Charles K. Hofling, eds. (Philadelphia: J. B. Lippincott Co., 1974), p. 365.

children. The mother and child slept together in the same bed. Mother refused to allow Ruthie out of her sight and was extremely threatened to think of hospitalizing her daughter.

The nurse must have realistic, short-term goals when she plans an effective therapeutic intervention to a symbiotic mother–child relationship. Gaining alliance with the mother is a primary goal before the child can be helped. Usually, when the child is separated from the mother through hospitalization or school, the mother herself becomes very depressed or physically ill, and she may develop an overt psychotic reaction. The mother of a school-phobic child may be so overwhelmed at the thought of being separated from her child that she develops a physical illness, which, in turn, makes the child feel guilty and anxious. These feelings then lead to the child's developing a fear of school as a reaction.

The following example illustrates these feelings and reactions.

> A young boy diagnosed as school phobic is extremely withdrawn and fearful. He often isolates himself in his room by setting up a "barricade" with his bookshelf against the door. After many verbal and physical arguments, his parents gave in and allowed him to refuse to go to school.

> His mother had been overly protective of him all of his life; she never gave up helping him dress and wash his hair. He had no responsibilities around the house and put forth no effort to make or keep friends.

> After several months of individual and family psychotherapy, the mother revealed that when her son was 5 months old she learned she had cancer and thought she was going to die. She was separated from the baby for several weeks following surgery, but vowed after her recuperation that she would never leave her son again "as long as she lived." As the boy grew up, he associated his birth with his mother's illness and near death. He retained this magical thinking and feared that if he became independent of her, she would again become ill and die.

One of the most challenging experiences of the nurse in child psychiatry is that of caring for the autistic (atypical) child. The term *autistic* means governed by self; thus, the child lives in a totally subjective world. This patient is one in whom, some sources believe, a physical or emotional trauma distorts growth, particularly growth in the ability to communicate. Others feel that the atypical child suffers from a constitutional or functional defect which causes deviation in his development. To date, we can only speculate on the etiology of infantile autism.

Classic symptomatology of autism was described originally by Dr. Leo Kanner, a child psychiatrist. The most striking feature of this disorder is the child's lack of affect. The symptoms are as follows:

1. Socially withdrawn—child is unresponsive to parents and unrelated to other people.
2. Unaware of his physical environment.
3. Inexhaustible (hyperactive) energy—keeps families awake all night by screaming and uttering bizarre noises.
4. Tendency toward ritualization—child moves toward destination by alter-

nating two steps forward and one step backward; or, child fears even as slight a change as turning a street corner.

5. Infantile play—child examines objects by tapping, smelling, tasting and touching.
6. Verbal communication impaired—mutism to echolalia to limited vocabulary.
7. Attention span severely limited.
8. Intelligence average but scattered—child is not retarded in most cases of autism but intellectual capacity inconsistent; e.g., he may be unable to tie his shoes but can memorize long lists of facts.[6]

The atypical child may begin to manifest symptoms soon after birth or between the ages of 2 and 3 years. Prognosis for these patients is guarded and nursing management is complicated.

Four-year-old Peter was an autistic child who had been a patient in a long-term residential center for 2 years. His parents described him as never having been a "cuddly" baby, even when he was a young infant sucking from the bottle. Although he learned to walk at a normal age, he never developed speech nor the ability to be toilet trained. He was always an irritable, easily provoked child.

Although his parents and younger brother visited him regularly, Peter showed no signs of recognizing them and, in fact, seemed unaware of most of the nurses and care workers in the ward. He could not tolerate being touched, even slightly or by accident, and became enraged when this happened. He did not speak, but uttered unintelligible sounds as he roamed about the ward like a caged animal. He often made eerie whining sounds when he was frustrated. Peter was an overly active child who seemed to be in perpetual motion. He had well-developed rituals which he used to move from one place to another on the ward; he walked sideways or twirled himself along the wall in the corridor rather than walk normally.

His attention span in play was limited to a few seconds with a particular toy. He wanted to spend hours sitting on the floor rocking with his eyes closed. Occasionally, Peter sat in front of the television, but showed no facial response to what he was watching.

Peter needed assistance in getting dressed and in bathing. Because of his hyperactivity, bedtime was particularly difficult and he needed one of the staff members with him until he fell asleep, sometimes on the rug on the floor rather than his bed. He often soiled in the bathtub. He ate with his fingers and smeared food on the table or himself, as would an infant.

One of the basic goals of the nursing staff was socialization of Peter. He was expected to follow the ward rules like the other children. Thus, he was expected to get up, make his bed, and get dressed in time for breakfast with the other patients. He was expected to eat with a spoon rather than his fingers and was not allowed to play excessively with his food. He was encouraged to share toys rather than aggressively grab them from other patients. In order to help Peter meet the expectations staff had set, after warnings, limits, and restrictions were set, "rewards" were withheld or he was removed from a situation and placed in his room with the staff member outside the door. He required constant assistance and structuring of a task in order for him to even partially complete it. He was dealt with by staff similarly as with the other patients in an effort to encourage his adapting to the norms of the ward milieu.

[6]Leo Kanner, "Early Infantile Autism," *American Journal of Orthopsychiatry,* **19** (1949), 416–26.

In addition to the socialization goal, the second nursing objective was to limit his maladaptive activity. At specific intervals during the day, the nurse would require that Peter sit and play a game or look at a book with her on a one-to-one basis. He received candy and a great deal of social reinforcement from the nurse after each of these episodes. He received a "bonus" if he said a word or touched the nurse; in other words, if he made an effort to communicate with her, he was specifically rewarded for that behavior.

The nurse was also very active nonverbally as well as verbally during the times she administered his phenothiazine to him.

Peter will probably spend most of his life in a sheltered, but socializing atmosphere.

Although consistency among staff who work with an atypical child is beneficial in helping him learn to relate to another human being in a meaningful, socially acceptable way, responsibility for this child should be shared. Physical and emotional care is challenging and involving. Progress is extremely slow. A therapeutic milieu with medication (usually phenothiazine) is the most widely known treatment for this disorder.

Problems of the anal phase of development

Emotional disorders originating in this phase center around conflicts the child has with his parents regarding this phase specific training. As the child learns to use his rapidly developing neuromuscular system in his striving for autonomy, he often meets parental resistance, which can cause serious inhibitions, depression, and even psychosis. The attitudes parents have toward their child's walking, toilet training, and talking help determine the success or failure of the child's mastery of a sense of independence from his mother. For example, the seeking of autonomy by the child can cause retaliation by the mother which leads to a withdrawal of love. The mother may misperceive autonomy as the child's running away from her.[7] Parental characteristics, such as overpermissiveness, extreme rigidity, and inconsistency, should be assessed when a child is presenting any of the following difficulties: (1) *constipation*—symptomatic of withholding from the parents due to anger, opposition; (2) *diarrhea*—anxiety, particularly from the angry child who feels rejected—may lead to severe paristalsis and ulcerative colitis; (3) *excessive soiling or encopresis;* and (4) *enuresis.*

Although 7-year-old Billy had been hospitalized several times during his lifetime for a variety of surgical and medical problems, he was now being admitted for his first psychiatric evaluation. He appeared to the nurse who was helping with the admission to be very frightened. When the doctor was interviewing Billy's parents, he frequently interrupted by saying, "I'm not going to stay here." He got up and walked around the room, always stopping in front of the door.

Because Billy had been adopted when he was a year old and had lived through

[7]Rachel M. Rosenberg, and Barbara C. Mueller, "Preschool Antisocial Children; Psychodynamic Considerations and Implications for Treatment," *Journal of Child Psychiatry,* **7** (1968), 422.

many separations from foster mothers, his adoptive parents tried for a long time not to submit him to another separation. However, because of Billy's severe soiling problem which interrupted his relationships at school and at home, they had to have help.

Billy was also refusing to eat, sleep, or talk to his parents. His opposition and negativism subsided when he wanted something.

Billy's oppositional behavior was inhibiting him from making friends. He appeared to the nurse to be an intelligent but lonely, angry little boy. During Billy's first few weeks on the ward, his behavior continued to be hostile and provocative toward staff and the other patients. He continued to soil as much as two and three times a day. An added difficulty was that he seemed to be hiding his soiled clothing, for articles were missing.

One Friday afternoon when the nurse was helping Billy prepare to go home for a visit, she discovered several pairs of soiled underpants and trousers stuffed into his suitcase. Two of the other patients laughed and teased Billy, who looked ashamed. Suddenly, he struck out at one of the boys. The nurse and a care worker separated the boys, but Billy's rage was out of control and the nurse stayed with him in the quiet room in order to help him regain control as quickly as possible and also to communicate to him that she was not going to reject him because of the soiled clothing or his anger. The isolation also protected Billy from further scapegoating by the other children.

In the next team meeting the nurse outlined an approach to Billy's soiling problem. "It is important that Billy learn to assume responsibility for cleaning up after he soils. We can tell him that if he does continue with this behavior, he will be the one who cleans up. We will keep a chart which identifies what the situation was when he soiled and what Billy's outward reaction was. Someone should be also assigned each day to count Billy's underwear along with him so that we can help him control his soiling that way, too."

In the meeting the team also learned of the family dynamics that contributed to Billy's oppositional behavior, especially the soiling. Disagreements among family members were numerous but, more important, they never were talked about openly, and, therefore, anger was never dealt with directly in the family. Billy's only alternative was to express anger and frustration by soiling and refusing to eat and sleep. The cycle was completed because the family focused on Billy's soiling rather than on talking about and resolving their own conflicts. Therefore, the team decided that before the parents could hear about their own issues, the staff would have to help Billy resolve the soiling problem.

During the first month in which the nurse's plan was implemented, the records showed that as Billy began to assume responsibility for his soiling, the frequency decreased. However, it remained consistent whenever he got into an argument with another child or a staff member; it also remained frequent during the visits home. But the parents were also involved in the underwear count and in helping Billy assume responsibility for himself. Over the period of 2 months, the problem was no longer a problem and Billy was succeeding much better in his school work and in his peer relationships. After he was discharged from the hospital, he and his parents continued in the out-patient clinic in family therapy.

Encopresis is an expression of hostility by the child toward an authority figure with whom he is experiencing conflict. Soiling is a complex developmental problem because of the resistance and negative attitude on the part of most adults toward acknowledging and becoming involved in treating the problem. Nurses must be comfortable with their own attitudes toward fecal soiling before they can become invested in a therapeutic intervention.

Enuresis, or bed-wetting, is most commonly a problem occurring at night when a child is sleeping. Studies indicate that etiologically this problem may have physiological, psychological, and hereditary roots. Because the etiology is still unclear, staff can help to counteract the feelings of shame and guilt that very often have been instilled in the child from projected attitudes of parents. A variety of treatment interventions may be tried. The biologic model of prescribing and administering Tofranil, as a mood elevator, is being tried with varying degrees of success. This medication works on the basis of raising the child's deep sleep level so that he is able to awake at the time he feels the urge to urinate. Fluids may also be restricted prior to bedtime. Sometimes the behavioral model of intervention is used; here buzzers are attached to the child's bed linens before he retires. Urine causes a bell to buzz and the child awakens. The goal is to interrupt by negatively reinforcing the enuretic behavior. The child is positively rewarded by staff when he successfully goes through the night without wetting. Psycho-social methods of intervention include encouraging dialogue with the child about the problem, allowing him the freedom to express his feelings of inadequacy about his failure to perform this developmental task. Whatever model of intervention is used, the child needs considerable support, within the framework of firm expectations, in order to achieve mastery of nocturnal bladder control.

Two personality disturbances that begin in the anal phase are excessive rebelliousness and excessive conformity. These behavior extremes should not be confused with the normal 2-year-old's expression of negativism and opposition, which causes parent–child conflicts. When a child says, "No" to seemingly all parental requests, it is difficult for parents not to overreact by using harsh punishment or, even more distressing for the child, by abandoning any attempts to set limits.

In contrast, there may be cause for alarm when a parent boasts of his or her "perfect" child. Excessive conformity may be the basis of severe obsessive, compulsive, or ritualistic behavior in later stages of development.

Disturbances in the oedipal phase

The emotional problems of this phase of the child's development reflect the increasing complexity of the child's personality. His intellectual curiosity is growing. He is also becoming aware of not only his now less egocentric relationship with his mother, but also his relationship with his father. A child vies for the attention of the parent of the opposite sex and feels a sense of rivalry with the parent of the same sex.

The child's expanding awareness includes heightened interest in his own body, particularly the pleasure he derives from exploration and stimulation of his genital area. Fondling and touching his genitals are natural behaviors in the child from 4 to 6 years of age. However, excessive masturbation and erotic preoccupation are two of the most frequent symptoms of emotional turmoil in the oedipal child.

Frank, 4-years old, asked numerous questions about "how, why, who, and where?" He had many questions about not only his own body but also the bodies of the members of his family. His mother told the nurse in the pediatrician's office that she was very upset one day when Frank asked her why her breasts were bigger than his were.

She said that she now is very careful he doesn't see her without being fully clothed. She seemed to the nurse to be feeling very guilty about this reaction. She went on to say that her husband thinks Frank is "too young" to be talking about "sex" and, consequently, sends him to his room every time he asks "provocative" questions. Frank's mother says that since this pattern began, he has started spending more and more time in his room, especially when his father is at home. Mother is particularly concerned because she has found Frank lying on top of his toy dog and rocking back and forth. She feels that he feels rejected by his parents and seeks comfort in the security of his room and the pleasure of masturbatory activity. He appears to the nurse to be a very anxious, frightened child who may become increasingly disturbed if there is not psychiatric treatment for the child and his parents.

The parents and the nurses must examine their own attitudes toward sexuality, specifically, self-exploration and masturbation. The young child should not be dealt with in a rigid, punitive manner when he is engaged in the above behavior, because this approach will only increase his anxiety and fears.

A careful assessment of a child's masturbatory behavior needs to be made. Is there a pattern to the behavior such as an upsetting event just prior to the masturbating? How frequently does the child masturbate? Is the behavior done privately or where many people can observe? One method of intervention is to redirect the child's interest to show an alternative method of dealing with anxiety. In the hospital setting, the child who masturbates excessively also needs to be protected from becoming a scapegoat by the child's peers. The nurse can talk with the child to find out if something specific is troubling him or her and should answer any questions the child has about sexuality in an open manner that does not overwhelm the child.

Another symptom of the oedipal phase is excessive fears in a child. Again, excessive must be accurately determined, since normal children express many fears, or phobias, such as of animals, the dark, noises, machines, etc. The following case example demonstrates how a 5-year-old child converted excessive fear and anxiety into action; a discussion of nursing interventions follows:

John, age 5 years, came to the hospital because his mother was having difficulty with his management, particularly in controlling his extremely active behavior. In fact, she described John as "hyperactive"; he had great difficulty going to bed at night and frequently was awakened with nightmares. In addition, he had lately begun to wet the bed and also to express his fears of shadows and "people" in his room. He continued to have difficulty at bedtime when he came to the hospital. He was also very curious, yet frightened by mechanical devices around the ward, such as the janitor's vacuum cleaner and the flush of the toilet. At times, John appeared very regressed; he often talked in an infantile manner, grabbed other children's toys, and destroyed books. When he seemed especially worried and upset, he sucked his thumb.

John lived with his mother and grandmother; he was an only child whose father was in the military and was gone 6 months out of the year.

The child who is overly active because of excessive fear and anxiety needs considerable support from the nurse at transition times, such as bedtime, upon awakening, before and after a doctor's appointment, and around a visit time from parents. Although it is unrealistic to expect him to verbalize his concerns, he will gain a sense of security from the physical presence of the nurse during periods when he is moving from one experience to another and where expectations are unclear.

The nurse must also remember that the young child has not fully developed the ability to verbalize his thoughts and feelings. Introspection and the development of insight are often difficult, even for the adolescent. Therefore, the nurse must be sensitive to all possibilities in assessing the cause of the child's fear and then dealing with the problem. Interpreting the cause of the child's fear and anxiety to him should only be done when one can predict the child's ability to use such information.

Other problems of this phase are psychoneurotic and psychotic disturbances and psychophysiologic disorders. Children in the oedipal phase more frequently come to the attention of the professional in the child psychiatric setting than do children in the earlier stages.

Expressions of emotional disturbance in latency

In the normal latency period (between 6 and 11 years of age) intrapsychically the three following major dynamics occur:

1. Repression of oedipal wishes and libidinal drives
2. Strengthening of the ego and defense mechanisms
3. Socialization and the development of morality[8]

Naturally, the emotional difficulties of the child in latency reflect the tasks of this phase. It is common for the disturbed child of this age to have difficulty socializing with peers and achieving in school. In fact, the clinical picture typically shows a child who shrinks from any competition to the extent that he excludes himself totally from interaction with others. Thus, the tasks of developing competency and confidence are thwarted. In contrast, the disturbed latency-age child may be so overly competitive that he cannot tolerate compromise in his interactions with his peer group.[9]

The child in this phase of development is normally very industrious; the troubled child may be seriously inhibited and withdrawn so that his basic, everyday habits of daily living are impaired.

Ten-year-old Ann was admitted to the hospital because she had begun withdrawing from her friends and family. She talked about hearing "strange" noises and mentioned things her mother could not understand. Ann grew increasingly

8Dean L. Critchley, "Nursing Intervention with the Disturbed Latency-aged Child," in *Nursing in Child Psychiatry,* ed. Claire M. Fagin (St. Louis: The C. V. Mosby Co., 1972), p. 29.
9Ibid., p. 31.

more fearful and suspicious of a close girlfriend and, except for attending school, she refused to go out of the house.

At home, she either watched television with such a fixed stare that her mother wondered if she was paying any attention to the programs. She often took an unusually long time to respond to her mother's questions; she appeared very preoccupied with her own thoughts. Ann's mother was very anxious because she was responsible for her daughter since her divorce from her husband 6 years ago.

When Ann arrived on the ward, the team nurse quickly introduced herself and noticed her frightened appearance as well as her reluctance to be introduced to the other patients. Later in the day, when the nurse went to talk with Ann in her room, the patient said, "Who are you?" The nurse told the child, who seemed very confused, "I am Miss Jones, I am a nurse on this ward." The nurse stayed with Ann for 10 minutes and while she was there, she answered the patient's questions in simple concrete statements.

During Ann's early period on the ward, she was permitted to alternate times in her room with times out on the ward. The latter gradually increased. The staff realized her need for a place where there would be little stimulation and a minimum of opportunities for her to become overwhelmed and frightened. At the same time, however, they had learned in a clinical conference of a goal for the disorganized, withdrawn child, namely to decrease her isolation by participating in the activities of the milieu. When Ann was out in the stimulation of the ward, she performed brief, simple tasks, such as sweeping, helping the ward secretary fold letters, or sewing.

One problem was Ann's disturbed behavior, which posed a threat to the other children. Needless to say, she had poor relationships with her peers on the ward. She was teased, or scapegoated, and became the target for abusive behavior. One day the nurse, who was doing routine checks on all the patients on the ward, found Ann standing on top of her chest of drawers surrounded by some of the other girls who were threatening to throw water on her. The girls were restricted to their rooms and Ann was placed on 10-minute checks for her protection. She acknowledged to the nurse that she had been scared.

The severely withdrawn, disorganized child has a very poor psychological defensive system and is easily overwhelmed with anxiety and fear in even a minimally threatening situation. An important nursing function is to help this child defend herself by providing external controls and protection for her. Medication, especially phenothiazines such as Thorazine or Stelazine, is one way of providing these controls. Another approach is through frequent, direct staff observation of the child. A third control is provided by the correct amount of activities. At first, stimulation such as noise, conversation, lights, play should be limited and gradually increased. Encouraging the child to participate in activities, especially concrete pastimes like simple games and chores, conveys to her that the nurse believes she is capable and competent to begin to master her environment.

Similarly, nursing interviews should be structured around a concrete activity with the child. Early in the child's illness the focus should not be on discussing her thoughts and feelings, because they are too anxiety provoking. Listening to the child, providing reality orientation, and talking in simple language are important tasks in caring for the latency-age child who is withdrawn and disorganized.

In sharp contrast to the inhibited child is the overtly hostile child. Most emotionally disturbed latency-aged patients manifest hostile emotional disorder and are often characterized as "hyperactive." Children whose behavior falls into this aggressive, tension ridden category are more likely to be boys. They characteristically display the following problems: learning difficulty in school, poor peer relationships, aggressive or assaultive behavior toward parents and other authority figures, impulsivity, and short attention span. In addition, these patients appear to have low self-esteem which contributes to their hyperactivity. By the time a child reaches latency, the disruptive behavior patterns are difficult to treat and the child usually requires intensive, long-term treatment. The use of medications, psychotherapy, and special education has been successful in the treatment of some cases of the tension discharge disorder among latency-age children.

Disturbances in early adolescence

For children who have not successfully achieved the goals of earlier developmental stages, the adolescent phase poses a serious threat. The ego which is already deficient is likely to become even further impaired. Even the adolescent who has a comparatively healthy psyche finds the years between 12 and the early 20s a crisis period full of conflict as he struggles to attain adulthood.

During adolescence, the individual's physical and emotional energy is so great that much of it must be sublimated or channeled into socially acceptable activity, i.e., sports, dancing, shopping, work, so that the ego may maintain equilibrium. Adolescents are normally very active.

However, the disturbed adolescent is active to the extent that he or she is unable to function adequately in school, at home, or in the community. Problems arise, for example, rebelliousness, in the form of antisocial behavior, i.e., lying, stealing, promiscuity, and running away. Running away from home is one of the most frequent manifestations of emotional disturbance in the adolescent, particularly in the early adolescent girl.

> "I can't stand this place. I'm used to being on the road whenever I want—you don't understand what it is like for me to have to stay in this ward all the time. On the road you can do whatever you want to. Here, the staff never let us do what we want to—just what they want us to do."

> "Talk, talk, talk. Talking doesn't help. What are you going to *do* about my problems?"

> "If I could be anywhere, where would I want to be? On the streets with just boys and dope."

The above dialogue took place during interviews between the nurse and her patient, a 13-year-old girl who had been admitted to the hospital by her parents for evaluation of multiple run-away episodes. One of the first observations of this girl is that she becomes hostile and easily threatened when the nurse limits her to talking about her feelings instead of allowing her to act her feelings out. One of the important interventions that the nurse is using is setting a limit on her patient's activity, namely, running away and compulsivity. Limit setting is an extremely important therapeutic task when working with adolescents. It is necessary, however, to use appropriate limits and restrictions—and privileges—in order to avoid infantilizing and sexual acting out.

Interviews with adolescents should always be goal oriented and should minimize the patient's attempt to manipulate. Another important task of the nurse is to build self-esteem. Usually, the acting-out adolescent has a low self-esteem, and the anxiety caused by this feeling encourages him to defend against the pain by running, drugs, etc. Ideally, parents should be involved in treatment; they need a great deal of support and guidance in order to provide limits, a sense of reality, and support for their adolescent. Adolescents with severe personality disorders may continue in antisocial behavior and further complicate their lives by breaking the laws of society and by becoming involved with law enforcement people and agencies.

CHILD PSYCHIATRIC NURSING IN THE COMMUNITY

The focus of this chapter has been primarily on the nurse's responsibilities in the caretaking of young patients who are hospitalized with emotional and behavior problems. Children and adolescents with less serious disturbances are seen by the nurse in the out-patient clinic, child guidance center, and in other types of community settings. Nursing in these situations is oriented toward diagnosis and treatment of the young patient.

Community mental health services

Mental health services for children are often rare and fragmented in many communities. Such facilities as preschool, kindergarten, after-school, holiday and summer programs, weekend and overnight recreation, day care, foster care, adoption plans, institutional care, and health-psychological programs may not even be available in some communities.

As a result of a national survey on mental health services, many states have placed priorities on developing comprehensive services for children. Concerted efforts are directed toward this focus in the following ways:[10]

1. Community mental health centers providing direct services to troubled children and their families.
2. Improvement of the quality of institutional care provided severely disturbed children.
3. Emphasis on the prevention of child behavior disorders through interdisciplinary collaboration at the centers.
4. Continued research on the dynamics of child development.
5. Identifying new treatments for childhood emotional disorders from problem behavior to childhood schizophrenia.

Regardless of the setting, nurses are in a strategic position to help in the prevention of mental and emotional stress in families with children. For example, practitioners of public health and maternal/child nursing are case finding and/or preventing physical and mental illness through daily inter-

[10]Julius Segal, ed., *The Mental Health of the Child* (Rockville, Md.: Program Reports of the National Institute of Mental Health, 1971), p. vi.

vention in home visits, well baby clinics, school programs, child day-care centers, and in local groups of children of alcoholic or divorced parents. As the nurse listens and guides the parent who is worried about training a stubborn two-year-old, feeding a finicky three-year-old, or limiting an overweight adolescent, she helps alleviate anxiety in the parent-child relationship which could become a serious obstacle if not identified and treated in the early stage.

In some states, nurses have recently been included, along with other professionals, in the evaluation of a child or adolescent who is showing signs of learning difficulties in school. Learning disability, as it is known, usually has an emotional and/or physiological component. The nurse in the school evaluation is involved in early case-finding, an integral process of prevention in medicine and nursing. Potentially serious psychiatric disorders of children and youth, such as depression and psychosis, are detected very early and are more accessible to treatment. Sometimes these disorders are prevented from ever occurring.

Nursing's increasing involvement in education and research has strong implications for the role of the profession in the prevention of mental illness in children. There is a need for a greater emphasis to be placed on the promotion of the health and well-being of children and adolescents in this society.

The problem of child abuse

The problem of child abuse through emotional neglect, nutritional neglect, medical neglect, or physical abusive handling is increasing. Pediatricians are reporting that the problem of the battered and abused child is growing worse. Children are being scalded, burned with cigarettes and lighters, flung against walls, beaten with fists or clubs, and poisoned by hard drugs, as well as being abused sexually by adults.

At one time parents "owned" their children and any behavior of the parents toward the child was accepted and unchallenged. Today the rights of children have been identified, and parents are held responsible for the well-being of their children.

Diagnosis It is essential to be able to distinguish the normal injuries of childhood from those caused by abusive treatment. Superficial injuries above the elbows, the shins, and the knees should be examined in order to determine if they are caused by rough handling, human bites, or cigarette burns or if they are only normal dermatologic conditions.

Although malnutrition is a key indication of abuse and neglect, it is difficult to identify as such. Community health nurses can often assess physical injury and malnutrition in the family assessment process.

Legal issues Every state has a law that child abuse must be reported. Medical personnel, as well as other community health professionals, are required to report these cases to the Child Welfare Agency.

However, the problem of complying with this request is complex. Physicians and mental health professionals fail to do this for a variety of reasons such as: the possibility of inappropriate accusation and perhaps a law suit; inadequate diagnostic guidelines; inadequate training of professionals for social-family assessment; the time-consuming aspect of the procedure; confidentiality; the social class factor whereby private physicians protect the family rather than the child; lack of community placements for the endangered child; the question of involving the police in this issue; the method of dealing with the parents and family of the abused child.

Mental health professionals and law enforcement personnel must work together much more closely so that they can understand the similarities and differences in each other's work, and in each other's goals. Concerted efforts might rechannel energies to help the child rather than to continue to ignore the pressing problem.

Prevention The goal in solving the problem of child abuse is to protect the child. As with other preventive issues, the most effective vehicle is education.

Nurses are key health professionals who are in touch with the potential problem and can be instrumental in dealing with the issue. Being aware of such situations as frequent pregnancies with little or no relief in between, marital strain, poverty, isolation, and overwhelmed mothers should be the concern of the community health nurse. Nurses should talk with families so that they (the nurses) can understand the families' problems and their perception of their difficulties in order to assess whether or not there may be potential danger for the children in the environment.

Understanding child-development and child-rearing practices should start early in the school system. Junior-high and high-school students who are babysitters should have this knowledge for their current work as well as for the time when they themselves become parents. The developmental tasks of children, discipline methods, and the human dimension of the child are essential for all to know.

Education in family planning continues to be a major issue. Nurses are currently dealing with this in clinics and the school systems. Unwanted children are in serious danger, as is seen by the rise in the number of child abuse cases. Parents need counseling in this area.

The rights of parents continue to be a major resistance to the prevention programs. Emphasis must be placed in better perspective on the rights of children for protection from noxious family conditions.

Community support is essential. Such techniques as crisis intervention and hotline service are possibilities. A troubled mother or father on the verge of losing control could call these centers for help.

Education in the school systems is one method for helping people to learn healthy ways of interacting with people. Other forms of communication, especially auditory-visual methods, need to be explored by nurses. Television is another possibility.

The actual treatment of the child victim needs redefining. A network of coordinating diagnostic and treatment centers to help the responsible agency with this problem would provide considerable back-up support for the Child Welfare Services. In too many cases the child is allowed to return to the same environment and is later found dead.[11]

Rehabilitation and treatment centers are needed where the battering parent can receive help with his or her aggressive and abusive behavior. This is an important area for continued research and study by nurses.

Case illustration

Mrs. Green, a 26-year-old white female, separated mother of three (boys aged 3 years and 3 months; a girl aged 2 years), was admitted to a psychiatric unit on a 10-day observation commitment from the court for assault and battery on her 2-year-old daughter.

Upon admission Mrs. Green was teary eyed, quiet, cooperative, answering questions with a yes or no, giving information factually as requested and appeared frightened and depressed. She related the following story:

Her 2-year-old daughter fell down the front stairway when she and her brother were playing. The 3-year-old opened the front door, which Mrs. Green had prohibited, and the two children continued to play on the front staircase. Mrs. Green checked her daughter after the fall, knew she felt hurt, but did not think it was serious. That evening the side of the girl's face and head became swollen but the swelling went down the next morning. For the next two days her daughter vomited. On the evening of the second day Mrs. Green went grocery shopping and left the children with her boyfriend. While the boyfriend was there, the little girl fell again, started shaking, and stopped breathing twice. The boyfriend used mouth-to-mouth resuscitation to start her breathing again, then called the police emergency station, and awaited their help.

When Mrs. Green returned from shopping, she found the police rushing her daughter out of the house on a stretcher, and her boyfriend very frightened and attempting to relate what had happened. Mrs. Green was taken by the police with her daughter in the ambulance to the emergency room of the local hospital. Her daughter was quickly examined by the doctor and taken immediately to neurosurgery. Mrs. Green was questioned briefly by the doctor who said her child had bruises on her ribs that she had sustained not from a fall but from being struck.

Mrs. Green was taken by the police to the women's retention center and held for court the next morning. In court she cried during the hearing, answered the judge's questions continually with the question, "How is my daughter?" She was then sent to the psychiatric unit for a 10-day observation to await a continuance of the hearing.

The condition of the child deteriorated and after the 10-day observation period was over, she went into a coma. The mother was then returned to the women's reformatory. The trial was delayed until it could be determined if the mother would be charged with child abuse or manslaughter.

Priorities become a major concern in a case such as this in which there are legal concerns. The legal issue must be settled first. Then, treatment or roles may then be defined. The issue for the psychiatric team is to determine if the mother is competent to stand trial and not if she is guilty or not guilty of the charge of child abuse.

[11]Segal, *The Mental Health of the Child,* pp. 343–69.

SUMMARY This chapter presented one specialty area of psychiatric nursing, the care of the emotionally disturbed child and adolescent. Case examples illustrated the therapeutic work of patient and nurse. The role of the psychiatric nurse in the hospital and the community in preventing mental disorders in children was also discussed specifically as it relates to child abuse.

REFERENCES AND SUGGESTED READINGS

Bentz, Willard K., and Ann Davis (1975). "Perceptions of Emotional Disorders Among Children as Viewed by Leaders, Teachers, and the General Public," *American Journal of Public Health*, **65,** No. 2, 129–32.

Bettelheim, Bruno (1962). "To Nurse and Nurture." *Nursing Forum*, **1,** No. 3, 60–72.

Brodie, Barbara (1974). "Views of Healthy Children Toward Illness," *American Journal of Public Health*, **64,** No. 12, 1156–59.

Byassee, James E., and Stanley A. Murrell (1975). "Interaction Patterns in Families of Autistic, Disturbed and Normal Children," *American Journal of Orthopsychiatry*, **45,** No. 3, 473–78.

Coles, Robert (1964). *Children of Crisis*. Boston: Little, Brown & Co.

Fagin, Claire M., ed. (1972). *Nursing in Child Psychiatry*. St. Louis, Mo.: The C.V. Mosby Co.

Freud, Anna (1971). *The Psychoanalytic Treatment of Children*, 4th ed. New York: Schocken Books.

Gelles, Richard J. (1975). "The Social Construction of Child Abuse," *American Journal of Orthopsychiatry*, **45,** No. 3, 363–71.

Gil, David G. (1975). "Unraveling Child Abuse," *American Journal of Orthopsychiatry*, **45,** No. 3, 346–56.

Gregg, Grace S. (1968). "Physician, Child Abuse Reporting Laws, and the Injured Child," *Clinical Pediatrics*, **7,** No. 12, 720–25.

Helfer, Ray E., and C. Henry Kempe, eds. (1968). *The Battered Child*. Chicago: The University of Chicago Press.

Hopkins, Joan (1970). "The Nurse and the Abused Child," *Nursing Clinics of North America,* **5,** No. 4, 589–98.

Inman, Merilee (1974). "What Teenagers Want in Sex Education," *American Journal of Nursing*, **74,** No. 10, 1866–67.

Kalisch, Barbara J. (1973). "Nursing Actions in Behalf of the Battered Child," *Nursing Forum*, **12,** No. 4, 365–77.

Krieger, Dolores (1975). "Therapeutic Touch: The Imprimatur of Nursing," *American Journal of Nursing*, **75,** No. 5, 784–87.

Mindex, Laurie (1974). "Sex Education on a Psychiatric Unit," *American Journal of Nursing*, **74,** No. 10, 1865–66.

Mitchell, Betsy (1973). "Working with Abusive Parents," *American Journal of Nurssing*, **73,** No. 3, 480–81.

Parker, Buella (1962). *My Langauge Is Me*. New York: Basic Books.

Polier, Justine Wise (1975). "Professional Abuse of Children: Responsibility for the Delivery of Services," *American Journal of Orthopsychiatry,* **45,** No. 3, 357–62.

Savino, Anne B., and R. Wyman Sanders (1973). "Group Therapy and Home Visits," *American Journal of Nursing*, **73,** No. 3, 482–84.

LIAISON
PSYCHIATRIC NURSING

20

T he following illustrates a reaction of patients that is of great concern to practitioners of liaison psychiatric nursing, that is, the psychological reaction of the medically ill patient.

> The intern and nurse stared, wide-eyed as Mr. R., who had just been hospitalized for a massive coronary occlusion, ran down the corridor. Mr. R's aberrant behavior did not cease after he was chastised for his defiance of his doctor's orders to stay in bed. When the staff explained that bed rest was essential for recovery, Mr. R. proceeded to demonstrate his strength by lifting his bed. He did push-ups in front of the nurse's station. Angry warnings that he might kill himself were to no avail.[1]

Dr. James Strain emphasizes that one half of ambulatory and at least one-third of hospitalized patients have significant psychological reactions that accompany their medical illness or physical condition.[2] Liaison psychiatric services have emerged to affect the ward environment of the patient, to develop the team approach to psychological care, to impart psychological dynamics to nonpsychiatric care takers, and to participate in studies to expand the understanding of the psychology of the medically and surgically ill.[3]

The introduction of the psychiatric nurse as a clinical specialist in the liaison psychiatric services is well documented by Dr. Lisa Robinson.[4] The liaison model in the hospital is intended to (1) practice the three levels of prevention (primary, secondary, and tertiary); (2) focus on the consultant and milieu in addition to the patient; (3) participate in case detection instead of awaiting referral; (4) clarify the care taker's status as well as the patient's (using the chart, the doctor, nurse, family, and patient as data sources); and

[1]James J. Strain, "Liaison Psychiatry: Treating Psychological Reactions of the Medically Ill," *Medical World News Review*, **1**, No. 2 (1974), 42.

[2]Ibid.

[3]Ibid.

[4]Lisa Robinson, *Liaison Nursing: Psychological Approach to Patient Care* (Philadelphia: F. A. Davis Co., 1974).

(5) provide an ongoing educational program that promotes more autonomous functioning by medical, surgical, and nursing personnel with regard
to handling their patients' psychological needs.[5]

**CONCEPTUAL
FRAMEWORK**

Liaison psychiatric services include various concepts that are basic to its
practice. Three concepts identified by Lisa Robinson are the concept of
adaptation, the concept of physical service component, and the concept of
anxiety.[6] Other concepts to be discussed are those of reactions to illness and
patient status.

Concept of adaptation

This concept identifies humans as an integral part of a dynamic system that
is constantly acting and reacting to incoming stimuli. Coping skills and adaptation strategies are key factors to be assessed. Illness, disability, hospitalization, medical treatment are all stimuli that generally create discomfort.
Patient status may threaten one's identity and self-concept. The person, in
turn, must use coping mechanisms to deal with the discomfort. If these
efforts fail, maladaptive behaviors frequently result, and in hospitals that
have liaison services, a liaison nurse may be called to help with the maladaptive behavior of the patient.

In the case cited, Mr. R. had experienced a severe myocardial
infarction. His subsequent behavior of running down the corridor, doing
push-ups, and lifting the bed disturbed and annoyed the staff. Their attempts
to set limits by reprimanding the patient made him more volatile. By working
with the staff, the patient, and his wife, the liaison nurse was able to demonstrate that the hyperactivity was a defensive reaction to worries about being
passive and feeling less masculine. The patient was told that the most difficult and manly job he would ever have was to stay in bed. He was asked to
chart his vital signs and progress and to offer suggestions to the staff on his
care. This plan helped the patient to put his thoughts into words instead of
actions.[7]

Concept of physical-health illness

Since the practice setting for liaison nursing is the general hospital, a knowledge of the patient's physical illness is essential. For this reason, a liaison
service has nurses with various subspeciality areas. For example, a nurse
who has medical–surgical expertise may not be effective in a gynecological
situation in which a patient has had a miscarriage. A liaison nurse who has a
background in gynecological and obstetrical nursing would be very helpful
to this patient because she could provide physical services and also deal with
the psychological component. Since the liaison nurses usually give direct

---

[5] Strain, "Liaison Psychiatry," pp. 42–43.

[6] Robinson, *Liaison Nursing*.

[7] Strain, "Liaison Psychiatry," p. 43.

services to the patient, they must be competent in the clinical area, especially in intensive and acute care settings.

Concept of anxiety

Anxiety—a feeling state of discomfort—is internally experienced as a threat to one's self or to one's sense of integrity. This feeling is a result of perceiving incoming stimuli in terms of previously experienced threatening events. For example, if a nurse prefaces her comments to a patient with the words, "I'm afraid I have bad news for you," the person will probably be flooded with anxiety because it relates to a previous experience in which there was distressing news. The person will simultaneously react physically and mentally to the words. Additionally, the person will attempt to maintain a steady balance in the face of the stressful stimuli.

A primary goal in liaison nursing is to support the person so that disequilibrium does not occur. Support means helping the person identify and better cope with feelings being expressed. As long as the person can cope with the incoming stimuli, the anxiety level is manageable. If coping mechanisms fail, the ego functions are affected, anxiety increases, and the person is in crisis. Uncontrolled anxiety precipitates an extremely vulnerable state. Liaison nurses must be especially knowledgeable in assessing anxiety and determining nursing intervention.

The patient's reaction to his illness

A person hospitalized for a physical condition has to deal with many feelings and reactions. Some reactions are the result of his feelings of helplessness at being confined in the hospital, his feelings of dependency at having to rely on other people for care, his feelings of inadequacy at not being able to do what he normally could and would do for himself, his feelings of anger at what has caused his present predicament, his feelings of anxiety over the uncertainty of the situation, or his feelings of sadness over the loss of his previous state of well-being and independence. Some factors contributing to his illness may be based on situations relevant to his family or community, his economic status, his religious needs, or his employment situation.

When patients are overwhelmed by these reactions, they respond in a variety of ways: Some may deny the seriousness of the illness; some may be excessively demanding; others may simply be outwardly depressed.

How a person copes with the reactions his illness provokes usually is dependent on his personality or character style, the nature of the illness, and how he perceives it. The impact of hearing about his illness and the environment in which he finds himself may compound the reaction.

Everyone brings his own unique way of coping into a situation. In other words, the patient who has an ulcer does not react in a "typical ulcer personality way." If the person has previously used rationalization when he was under stress, he will bring rationalization into this situation. To a large extent, the impact of the illness determines his method of coping.

When a patient perceives his situation as being a life–death one, he is then more likely to use denial. One person with a broken finger may find the inconvenience of a cast annoying, but a broken finger to a baseball pitcher may be catastrophic. When any illness achieves major psychological significance, an adequate coping defense is needed.

The environment in which the patient finds himself will also affect his coping abilities. If he finds himself in an intensive care unit with many electrical devices attached to him, his defensive reaction will be much stronger than if he finds himself in a six-bed ward for convalescents.

Coping mechanisms are used as protective devices by individuals who are overwhelmed by anxiety. The defenses may become pathological and ultimately interfere with the patient's treatment.

BEHAVIORAL PATTERNS IN ADJUSTING TO THE ILLNESS

We find it useful to view the patient's reactions to his illness within four patterns of behavior: (1) shock and disbelief, (2) awareness, (3) reorganization, and (4) readjustment.

When first confronted with the news of serious illness, the person generally reacts with *shock and disbelief.* This behavioral response brings defense mechanisms into play. The nurse's ability to assess the defenses will help to identify the therapeutic route to take with the patient in formulating a patient care plan.

The patient needs to use his defenses in this phase because he is overwhelmed. The nurse must recognize this as an appropriate reaction. The patient may say, "I don't believe I have a serious illness" or "I could not have diabetes. The tests must be wrong."

The nurse does not encourage denial or any defense any more than a patient is encouraged to talk about his delusion in the psychiatric setting. It is more therapeutic to ignore the defense and instead try to encourage the patient to talk and express his feelings about his illness.

A therapeutic response to someone who says that he cannot believe that he has a certain illness should be supportive: "It is hard to believe" or "What makes it so hard to believe?" The nurse supports and stands by him in the hopes that he eventually can come to terms with the illness and give up the defense by himself.

Some of the verbal responses and behaviors that demonstrate the common defense of denial are:

"I don't have it."

"I had it, but not now."

"It's not serious."

"It isn't what they think it is. My heart isn't the problem; it is my stomach."

Patient verbally agrees but acts in a way that the nurse knows is denial, e.g., he keeps smoking or overeating or drinking which are contra-indications to the illness.

Patient changes the subject.

Patient is evasive and does not talk about the issue.

Patient tries to get the nurse to talk about herself.

Patient is excessively cheerful and jokes about what is going on.

Patient goes from a specific topic to a general topic

Denial may interfere with the prescribed treatment. For example, the patient may refuse to take radiation therapy for a tumor because he insists that it really is not there. Or the patient who has an enlarged liver may continue to drink alcoholic beverages even though he has been warned of the possible consequences. The patient's denial may be so great that he wishes to sign himself out against medical advice. The therapeutic task is either to try to reduce the patient's anxiety and defense mechanism of denial so that they do not interfere with the treatment or to encourage him to express his feelings in order to gain some awareness of his illness.

The nurse should autodiagnose her own reactions in helping the patient during this behavioral phase because they may stall the therapeutic process in several ways. First, the nurse may become anxious while she is listening to the patient talk and therefore change the subject or deny that the patient should feel as he does. For example, the patient says, "I am afraid of the radiation treatments. I won't take them." The nurse who says, "Don't be afraid of them" or "You should do what the doctor says because he knows best" or "You should be thinking of going home" or "I am here to record the amount of fluids you have had today" is stalling the process of encouraging the expression of feelings.

Another stall may occur when the nurse upon entering the room and finding the patient perspiring freely, asks, "Are you too warm?" If he asks, "Doesn't everyone perspire after taking the tests that I have just taken?" his response may be interpreted as going from the specific to the general. The nurse may unintentionally support this by continuing to talk in generalities. This keeps the subject of the patient's distress from being discussed. The difficulty the nurse is having is her inability to relate to and to help the patient bear the painful feelings that he has. A more helpful statement to the patient would be, "How did you feel about the tests you took this morning?"

The second behavioral area in dealing with the news of a serious illness is when the patient develops *awareness* of the illness. Included in developing awareness are the feelings of anger, sadness, anxiety, and/or dependence. The patient still is not dealing directly with the reality issue of his illness.

The sign that a patient is moving into an awareness of his illness is seen when he makes such statements as "If I have had this" or "If this has really happened, then what about. . . ." There is neither complete acceptance nor acknowledgement yet, but there is a conscious attempt to deal with the reality that others see. This kind of verbal statement by the patient indicates that he is beginning to incorporate the news. This behavior is to be encouraged by the nurse.

It is in this phase that the patient often shows the feeling of anger. This may be because of the patient's feelings of helplessness, of having to depend on others, of not being independent and strong as he once was. The patient may be angry at having to give up his self-image as an independent person or he may be wishing to be cared for but feels uncomfortable about directly expressing this wish.

The anger is often displaced onto anything that is available, for example, the water in the pitcher is not the right temperature, the waste basket is not emptied, the food is cold, someone isn't coming to visit, or the nurse walks into the room.

For example, a surgical patient who appeared very angry and displeased at just about everything was a puzzle to the staff who tried in many ways to cheer her up. All efforts ended in failure until the day she had the gastric tube going to her stomach removed from her nose. After this the patient changed to a delightful person. When the staff asked her what had made the big change in her mood, she said that she was not aware of how dreadful she felt until the tube was removed and she realized how well she then felt.

It is important not to overlook the fact that people become quite angry and irritable when they are in pain or are hurt. And unquestionably many physical nursing procedures can and do hurt. Some people get angry with the person who hurts them. For example, when the dentist hurts his patient while he is drilling a tooth, the patient may react adversely by saying that the dentist is too insensitive and that he wishes to select another dentist.

Some people react unfavorably to nurses because they hurt them by making them get out of bed when it is painful to them, by making them walk when they feel very dizzy, or by pulling the adhesive tape off a dressing that covers a very sore spot.

The stall in this situation occurs when the nurse takes the anger personally and withdraws from the patient. In order to prevent the stall, the nurse needs to identify the issue about which the patient is really upset. The therapeutic task is to help bear the feeling the patient is experiencing. Even if she cannot identify what the patient is angry about, she cannot take the anger personally unless she knows that she has specifically provoked the patient. Otherwise, she has to realize that the anger is not because of her and that she has to bear the feeling.

When the nurse can openly bear the content of the patient's complaint and not become angry, this acceptance will be therapeutic. For example, if the patient is complaining that the food is cold or that the nurses seem busy and do not answer his bell when he rings, the nurse may be helpful by listening and thereby acknowledge and accept the feelings of the patient.

There may be a clue in the patient's behavior that can help the nurse understand the patient. If the nurse does find a clue, then she should not feel annoyed because the patient is so demanding or complaining; she can then begin to try to solve the puzzle. Dealing with the needs of the patient rather than with her own judgmental reactions is the goal for the nurse.

This phase of developing an awareness of one's illness blends progressively into the third phase, *reorganization*. It is at this time that the patient begins to ask questions. These questions may be masked or direct.

The question may be compared to an iceberg in that the manifest question may have little to do with what is really there and submerged beneath the surface.

The manifest question usually does not begin to tell the nurse precisely what is on the patient's mind. As a rule, she is usually unaware of exactly what precipitated the question because she does not have access to all the thoughts that have prompted the patient to ask the question.

Sometimes the nurse deals directly and openly with the question because she thinks that a "yes or "no" answer is indicated. Generally, it is more useful to reply to the patient, "You seem quite concerned about what is happening to you. I wonder what you have been thinking about or what your doctor has talked about." Or "You are asking if you have emphysema. What makes you think that?"

To respond to the patient's question with statements such as: "Don't worry about that" or "You should ask your doctor about that" or by changing the subject are all potential stall situations to the therapeutic process. In order to correct the stall, the technique of asking and answering questions might be reviewed (see Chapter 10).

The fourth behavior phase, the *readjustment* or *change* phase follows the reorganization of the patient's thinking that allows him to ask questions about his illness. This phase is necessary for him because it helps him to continue with his personal life goals. The acceptance of the changes that must be made implies that the person has dealt with the pain of the news of his illness and that he has come to terms within himself by accepting the demands or modifications that will be involved in his life.

Coming to grips with the loss that is inherent in the illness situation may mean indulging in some fantasy or substitution, but ultimately the patient must give up what has to be given up. For example, if the patient's leg must be amputated and the patient lies in bed fantasizing that he still can be a great runner, he is going to trip and fall when he gets up because he hasn't come to terms with the reality of the lost leg.

Or if the patient is facing the possibility of the removal of an organ, contingent upon unfavorable biopsy reports, and persists in fantasizing that surgery will not be necessary, he is not facing reality. The patient needs to face what it would be like if surgery is required. If he doesn't, the reactions, for example, depression, will likely occur during the recovery period. In this phase the patient has to be prepared to create a new self-image to fit into and to feel comfortable with.

The problem for the patient in this phase is in learning how to heal the pains received when he heard the news of the illness and how then to move on into the world of living.

Mastery is a critical part of this behavior phase. As the patient becomes skillful in his situation and realizes his control, he regains a feeling of adequacy and security. It is at this point that nurses need to evaluate the amount and degree of nursing care needed in helping the patient to master his situation.

Stalls in the therapeutic process may occur in several ways. A stall may occur when routine, impersonal care is given to the patient. This phenomenon may be seen in overcrowded institutional settings in which staff members are overworked and patients are neither motivated nor encouraged to change their situation.

A stall will also occur when nursing care is excessive and infantilizes the patient. Dependence is encouraged and the patient's efforts at mastery are inhibited.

Another stall situation may occur when the patient maintains the fantasy that prevents him from dealing with reality. For example, a 35-year-old man develops arthritis, takes to a wheelchair, and stays there because he cannot meet the demands of physical therapy or his reactions to his illness.

Patient status

When a patient is admitted to the general hospital for medical or surgical reasons, he brings with him many apprehensive thoughts, feelings, and reactions to the hospital setting. These thoughts, feelings, and reactions are usually present regardless of the severity of the physical condition.

How the patient comes to the hospital is important, especially the mode of transportation to the hospital. For example, if the patient began to hemorrhage at home and a relative called an ambulance, the memory of the trip to the hospital may still be uppermost in the patient's mind. To sit and listen to this recount would reveal how the patient reacted to the experience, how anxious and frightened she might be at suddenly being placed in a strange environment. If the patient has been scheduled for a series of diagnostic tests regarding vague, perplexing symptoms, the feelings she has between the time the physician tells her she should have the tests and the time a hospital bed is available will be important. Having to anticipate what is going to happen creates anxiety. If the patient has been scheduled for elective surgery, for example, a tubal ligation, the stress of waiting may have influenced the woman's feelings about this procedure and the ultimate meaning it will have on her life.

Assessing the significance of how the patient came to the hospital will give the nurse information on the patient's fears, anxiety, and level of adjustment to these reactions.

Patients are temporary occupants in a hospital; they are merely "passing through." They are at a distinct disadvantage in an established, highly organized, bureaucratic institution. Patients are anxious in their new setting and they are separated from people who normally support their identity. Their being ill and hospitalized compounds the anxiety. It is to be expected that they will use defense mechanisms to suppress anxiety. The pressures of running an institution often foster staff to encourage a patient to regress to a dependent position which then allows the professional to make the decisions for the patient as to needs and nursing care. Social isolation may develop quickly. Staff relationships are usually superficial and patients are attended to on a priority of care basis.

Referral

On in-patient units, the liaison nurse often receives a referral to see a patient. The referral may be made by a physician, nurse, or other staff member. Using the data on the referral, the nurse must identify *who* needs help, *who* is seeking it, *what* is the real problem, and *how* the intervention must be structured.[8]

When the nurse is employed by the hospital, there are four considerations: the hospital, the attending physician, the liaison nurse, and the patient. All four must agree on the purpose of the liaison service.

Assessment

The nurse has a variety of data available: the patient's record which includes age, sex, occupation, diagnosis, and orders. The order sheet may be analyzed in order to evaluate medications and to see if behavior reactions may be a result of drugs. Temperature rise may indicate delerium. The ways in which orders are written may alert the nurse that patient behavior is not matching the frequent change in orders.

The manner in which physicians write orders may indicate poor communication between the physician and nurse. Progress notes may indicate that nursing and medical observations are either similar or different and they should be followed up by an observation of subsequent patient behavior.

Talking with staff provides useful background data. Asking strategic questions about subtle or obvious changes in patient behavior under varying circumstances may provide helpful clues to understanding the patient.

Interviewing the patient

The entry to the patient is a very important step. Liaison staff make it a special point to be direct and open as to who they are and why they are called to see the patient. For example, the liaison nurse may say, "I was asked to see you because the nurses knew you must have been upset last night when you slapped Mr. Jones." Or, "The nurses are concerned about you. They saw you were worried about your surgery."

The remaining part of the interview, following the introduction, then deals with the concerns of the patient.

Patient's perception of his illness

The question, "What do you think is wrong with you?" will evoke a variety of responses from the patient. How the patient describes his illness in his own words is a significant point to record. As with the psychiatric patient, these words may tell you more than the several paragraphs that follow.

For example, if the patient says that he is in the hospital because of an ulcer, in what terms does he describe this? Does he use medical terminology, for example, "I have a duodenal ulcer." Or does he say that his stom-

[8]Robinson, *Liaison Nursing,* p. 67.

ach burns after he eats, or does he say that the doctor told him he had an
ulcer?

The patient might say he is in the hospital because of high blood pressure or that his wife thought he should come to have some tests in order to find out why he was tired all the time. These words help determine the patient's perception of his illness.

The family's perception of the illness

During the assessment process the nurse can ask the patient how he thinks his family perceives his illness. If the patient's family does visit, it will be useful to ask each member directly what his or her own interpretation of the illness is, what impact this news has on each of their lives, and whether the family will be able to continue to function as a family unit.

Does the family want the patient in the hospital? Does the family feel that he should be in the hospital? Would the family rather have him home? Does the illness frighten and keep the family from visiting the patient?

The patient's goals for treatment

How does the patient see the hospital helping with the illness? What does he expect from the hospital? What previous experiences has he had with hospitals, medical treatment, and nursing care?

If the patient is having diagnostic tests, what does he plan to do when the results of the tests are known? Will he continue to do what medical judgment advises and does he feel the need to be a part of the treatment process?

From a comprehensive health care standpoint, does the patient indicate any need for follow-up visits by a community health nurse to assess his readjustment back into the home and community setting? Does he see hospitalization as an isolated experience? The in-patient nursing staff should include posthospitalization health care plans in every nursing assessment.

The family's goals in the treatment process

How does the family see its role in the treatment process? Do the members feel involved with the treatment the patient is receiving and how may they be of support to the patient both in the hospital and at home? Do they see any need for comprehensive health care follow-up?

For example, if the patient has had a myocardial infarction, does the family see this as a frightening experience that may happen again? Are the family's feelings and reactions considered? Is the community health nurse or the home care coordinating service of the hospital of help to meet the family's needs?

Psychological assessment

What is the dynamic issue for the patient in relation to his illness? Are his needs to be cared for uppermost in this hospitalization or is his need to be in control of the situation more the issue? Does the patient feel he has "lost" because of the forced dependence and does he become defensive because of this lowered self-concept?

What coping mechanisms is the patient using to deal with the stress of the news of the illness? What defenses should be strengthened and supported?

What is the meaning of the illness to the patient? What does this illness do or not do for the patient? Does he respond positively to family and visitors and enjoy cards he receives or does he leave his mail unopened? Does he get secondary gain from the illness?

Are there any unrealistic fears in connection with the illness? For example, does the patient's anxiety about having an intravenous pyelogram seem out of proportion to the procedure? Or does the patient who is facing cardiac catheterization seem cheerful and totally unconcerned?

Social assessment of the patient

What has the patient heard about the illness from friends or relatives? Does she know anyone who has had this illness? What experiences has she heard about? For example, if she is having a surgical procedure, what other women does she know who have had a similar operation and how does she relate this to herself?

Does the illness help the patient identify with an important person who has had the illness? For example, does the patient who has had a heart attack say, "Look at all the presidents who have had what I had."

When the family visits, what visiting style does it have? Do the members talk with the patient about the illness or do they avoid it?

Is the patient worried about finances?

What are his religious needs?

Behavioral assessment

What behavior does the patient present? Is the patient aware that his behavior is different or changed because of the stress of hospitalization? How does the staff describe and react to the patient's behavior?

Medical assessment

What symptoms has the patient been having? How clearly can the patient describe her symptoms? Does she say she has pain in her stomach or does she point to the area and describe it as either sharp or dull pain? Does she gloss over the symptoms or go into great detail during the interview?

Strengths of the patient

What was the patient doing before he became a patient? Does he talk of his work, his family, his community involvement? Does he seem anxious to be back in that role again or is he concerned only with the illness?

What questions is the patient able to ask the nurse? This can be an area of strength. It means that the patient wants to be involved in his illness and the treatment and it is essential that the nurse support this strength.

Does the patient want to know what will be happening during the hospital course? What has been his reaction to the hospitalization so far?

How does the patient feel he will be able to deal with the illness? Does he say, "I know I can get through this; I have made it through other surgical experiences." "This illness isn't going to get me down." Or does he say, "I don't know whether I can fight this time. I am so tired." Statements of either nature may be therapeutic.

CLINICAL SITUATIONS There are various clinical situations in which a liaison nurse may be called. They will be described briefly in the following pages.

Newly admitted patient

The crisis of hospitalization begins the moment the person learns that he must be hospitalized and it becomes most apparent as he sits before the admissions clerk. Being subjected to the impersonality of admission forms, questions, and the ritual of receiving the wrist band (the badge of patienthood) and observing an array of uniformed people with their professional aloofness are only the beginning. Vital signs, urine sample, weight, and history may be immediately taken and followed by the order to remove one's clothing and to put on the uniform of patienthood, the gown. The medical examination, serology, and chemistry testing follow.

The basis of the patient's anxieties is the threat of loss of identity. All procedures are done routinely by the staff, but the patient is alone and is often ignorant of the procedure. A primary nursing intervention to be provided by nurses is patient teaching. Presenting the facts prepares the patient to better handle his anxiety.

Patient with undiagnosed illness

The person who enters the hospital to find out the etiology of symptoms will undoubtedly experience many unsettling feelings and thoughts. Uppermost in the patient's mind is that something very serious might be found. The symptoms are a nagging reminder and may be overwhelming if the person thinks about them constantly. The stress of uncertainty weighs heavily on the mind of the patient.

The pre-operative patient

The person facing surgery is usually preoccupied with the immediate aspects of surgery: the reason for the surgery, and the unknown element or the loss of consciousness during the surgical procedure.

Reason for surgery The seriousness of the surgery or the potential for seriousness is important. For example, a person scheduled for a hemorrhoidectomy may be less preoccupied with the surgery itself than with what he has heard about the pain he will experience after the operation. A woman scheduled for a breast nodule biopsy will undoubtedly be under great anxiety regarding the outcome of surgery.

Element of the unknown

Surgery allows one's internal organs and body system to be examined while one is unconscious. The element of the unknown in terms of what might be discovered, or if one will recover from the surgery, registers with the patient. When people are faced with possible danger, an alternative to the surgery might be selected. It is not surprising that people do not always accept the physician's advice for surgery.

The pre-operative patient is generally preoccupied with safety and survival issues; thus he has minimal energy to respond to outside pressures. Learning is difficult because it requires cognitive input and the person is only thinking of the surgery. If the patient is in conflict about the surgery, emotional energy is doubly invested in worry and debate.

Pre-operative tests may be viewed as legitimate assaults to the body. Gynecological exams, proctoscopy, cystoscopy, cardiac catheterizations are all done while the patient is awake. These procedures are painful and the patient has to cope with his feelings and anxieties.

Methods to decrease anxiety regarding the unknown are patient teaching, for example, showing the patient the room in which the examination will take place or explaining the X-ray equipment. In cases of extreme stress, the liaison nurse may go to surgery with the patient. The goal is to condense the anxiety producing experience and focus the patient's attention on one area so that he is not overwhelmed by many stressors at once.[9]

Patient in pain

Pain is a defensive reaction to alert the body that there has been injury or damage to the body. Pain may register psychologically, physiologically, or both. The sensory experience of pain is complex and varying theories have been proposed regarding the etiology of pain.

The assessment of people experiencing pain may be made through the following areas: motor responses (movement of body, clenching of teeth, writhing, twisting); vocal responses (crying, screaming, groaning); verbal responses (asking for relief, complaining, cursing); social responses (withdrawal, changes in social manners or communication style); or the absence of overt behavior (hiding pain).[10]

Factors that influence a person's response to pain are personality style, race, culture, intellect, family, environment, occupation, and life-style.

Patients in pain are usually referred to the liaison nurse for one of two reasons.[11] The patient's pain is causing him to feel intense anxiety which heightens the actual pain and hinders the action of routine analgesia. Or the

[9]Ibid., p. 117.

[10]Laurel Archer Copp, "The Spectrum of Suffering," *American Journal of Nursing,* **74,** No. 3 (1974), 492–93.

[11]Robinson, *Liaison Nursing,* p. 138.

patient feels very anxious and simultaneously he experiences uncontrollable pain. The staff can neither control the patient's pain nor identify its unremitting intensity and thus they feel helpless and frustrated. The liaison nurse then deals with staff's reaction to the patient as well as with the patient's reaction to staff and to his pain.

Pediatric patient

The liaison nurse is called to work with children who are presenting serious problems to the pediatric staff. For example, infants who have a diagnosis of failure to thrive and shriek at human contact, children who have been rejected by parents, children who experience stress severe enough to threaten personality structure.

The developing psyche in the child does not have the repertoire of defenses that the adult has to protect against overwhelming stress, such as long periods of hospitalization, painful treatments, isolation from family.

Childhood is a period of life characterized by helplessness, powerlessness, and authority figures. This situation may be intensified in the pediatric setting if the staff is rewarded in terms of getting the job done (a procedural orientation) rather than in terms of having a positive relationship with a patient (humanistic orientation). Nursing of children perhaps tests this dichotomy most intensely; that is, how much to protect the rights of children and how much to take a stand against procedural and nonhumanistic treatment of patients.

The seriously ill patient

In helping the patient deal with his feelings and reaction to the news of serious illness the nurse's therapeutic task is to provide those human elements essential in interaction with patients—being supportive and helping to bear painful feelings.

The emergence of depression is always a consideration to be observed. For example, in the first phase (shock and disbelief) upon hearing the news the patient says, "I don't have a lump in my breast. That is just a gland swelling." In the second phase (awareness) the patient says, "It really provokes me to have to go without breakfast for these tests. Are you sure you know what you are doing? Nurse, could you please comb my hair? Nobody cares if I get breakfast or not (crying)." In this phase the feelings of anxiety, anger, dependence, and sadness are all expressed.

In the third phase (reorganization) the patient says, "What does it mean to have a lump in my breast? Do I have cancer? What will happen to my breast?" The patient is asking questions and expressing anxiety, fear, and concern.

In the fourth phase (readjustment) the patient says, "I hear I have to have surgery on my breast. The doctor may have to remove it." The patient is crying during this conversation.

It might be helpful to know that some patients pass very quickly through these stages but others take a long time, even months. Some never go through the entire cycle. Although patients cannot be pushed into expressing their feelings, the nurse should be aware of the ways in which she can facilitate or stall these processes.

Adaptation to illness generally includes hope as well as a variety of defense mechanisms. Although he relinquishes control of his body to staff, he still clings to hope which generally means returning to one's former lifestyle.

If the situation is deteriorating, the alternative must be addressed. To many, chronicity is a hopeless state. Robinson describes this state:[12]

> Patients crossing the boundary from acute illness to chronicity must realign their body image with the limitations of a chronic condition . . . they must redefine their social roles and functions. . . .

During this period of redefinition, the person must define a new concept of self and a new concept of the environment as he will experience it. Personality integrity is a main goal in working with the chronically ill.

Patients in intensive care unit

An intensive care unit is very different from other areas of the general hospital. It is usually a small area set aside to care for acutely ill people. Units may be called ICU, coronary care, special nursing care, critical care, or trauma units. The pace of the unit is tense and fast. Economy of movement by staff is observed.

Life supporting equipment is readily available. Many units are completely open so that all may be seen and heard. Artificial light is used so that patients are prevented from perceiving time changes.

Time loses all meaning. There is no way to orient a person to time. The unit is isolated from the rest of the hospital. Very often staff is involved with nursing, monitoring, and hospital equipment instead of with the patient. The liaison nurse has to be able to provide direct care if she works in these units.

The dying patient

One of the most difficult situations for staff is caring for the dying patient. The nursing process involved in caring for the person who is dying provokes a variety of reactions in the nurse. Very often, a liaison nurse may be called to help in this situation.

The person who is dying struggles with many thoughts and feelings. There are two specific feelings that the nurse may be able to help the person bear: these are the feelings of loss and sadness.

Bearing the feelings of loss and sadness   One of the essential therapeutic tasks in the general hospital setting for the nurse is to help patients bear their painful feelings, especially the feeling of sadness. Since sadness is a healthy emotion and since its avoidance leads to medical and psychiatric pathology including depression, it is important to

[12]Ibid., p. 178.

look at some of the ways in which the nurse may be therapeutic to the patient in dealing with loss and the subsequent feeling of sadness.

In the hospital setting the patient is reaching out. He may be searching for the slightest cue from the nurse to confirm that what he feels is acceptable to talk about. He begins to discuss his personal life or his feelings about his illness. It is at this point that the nurse may easily stall the process of the patient's expressing his feelings. An example is when the patient cries. The nurse may cut the patient off in several ways: She may directly state that the patient should not cry and that he be brave; she may quickly reassure the patient that everything will be fine; she may change the subject or busy herself with straightening the patient's room; she may refer the patient to a psychiatric nurse clinician; or she may dismiss the patient in her own mind as "feeling sorry for himself."

There are many understandable reasons why nurses stall this process and wish to avoid the patient's sadness.

1. It is painful to listen to someone's psychological distress.
2. The nurse, as she sees the outflow of tears and affect-laden thoughts, is afraid of opening Pandora's box. Can she handle what she fears will come next?
3. The nurse's own discomfort may be further exaggerated because some unresolved sadness in her own life is reawakened by the patient's experience.
4. When loss is related to a medical procedure (surgery, for example), the patient's sense of loss and sadness is often accompanied by feelings of anger toward the hospital and staff. It is very difficult for the nurse to be understanding toward someone who is angry with her.
5. The nurse feels helpless as she listens. She wants to do something and has not yet had the experience of knowing that listening is doing something.

In order to prevent the stall from occurring, the nurse must realize that there is a great deal that she can do to help to bear the patient's feeling of sadness. The nurse should assume that the patient who experiences serious illness has feelings of sadness over the loss of function and/or change in body image. For example, the patient with a myocardial infarction may have to give up otherwise normal activities. The patient needs understanding and encouragement to talk with someone about these feelings. If she appears upset, tense, sad, or tearful, the nurse should call her attention to these feelings by saying: "You seem troubled today" (pause). The patient may correctly perceive the statement and the expectant pause as a show of interest and a willingness to listen on the part of the nurse. When the patient does not appear to be upset or strained, the nurse might then be more direct: "What does having a hysterectomy mean to you?" "How do you feel about your child having surgery?" The patient then thinks: "The nurse is perceptive enough to know I am suffering and she can bear to hear me talk about how I feel." Sometimes expressions such as "your heart is heavy," "your heart is aching," "your heart is full of tears," or "you hurt inside" may seem appropriate for a particular patient and situation. These phrases, sincerely expressed, may elicit a great outpouring of feeling.[13] The patient needs to know that it is natural to have these feelings. And the nurse needs to learn how to cope and bear with the intensity of the emotion.

In summary, the nurse can be most effective in helping the patient to deal with the news and implications of a serious illness. Aiding in the healing process involves helping the patient to become involved in mastering his illness and accepting his feelings. As he is able to make peace with that which must be, he then finds the strength to move on, which may include the process of dying.

People also need to talk about the "letting go" of life. As one elderly patient said;

> I don't want to die. I am old and in one sense I am old enough to die. But I don't want to. It is hard to go. . . . The letting go of life. I just don't want to let go.

The liaison nurse may also be asked to talk with the family after there has been a death. The nurse helps the family members begin the grieving process by letting them know that it is all right to feel and express sadness. Her presence communicates that what was done for the patient was done with respect. The nurse can bear to face and talk with the family. The reality of what has happened is present. People will be grateful to be acknowledged in such a respectful manner.

If nurses are able to minimize their feelings of helplessness, deal with their own reactions to death, and find the active as well as the passive ways to be therapeutic with the dying patient, they have achieved a high degree of competence. Being physically present and attending to the physical comfort of the patient are essential. Whether or not nurses are able to increase their sensitivity in helping the dying person depends on how they autodiagnose their own feelings about dying and on how therapeutic they are to the patient.

It is not necessary to have a liaison nurse care for the patient in his dying process, but it may be helpful for staff to be able to call upon the liaison services in difficult situations. We believe that caring for the dying person is a vital part of every nurse's credo.

The liaison nurse may help staff with their feelings about caring for the dying patient and thus help the staff avoid potential stalls.

Stalls in helping the person to die are common and occur for specific reasons. The stalls occur because of nurses' feelings about caring for the dying patient.

1. One stall situation develops from the feeling of helplessness experienced by the nurses. They say, "I can't help the patient to live; therefore I am helpless." What has to be understood is that the nurse need not feel helpless to the point that the patient is abandoned as he is dying. Nurses cannot

---

[13]Aaron Lazare, "The Difference between Sadness and Depression," *Medical Insight,* **2,** No. 23 (1970), 26.

stop the actual dying process and to that extent they are helpless, but they can be most therapeutic in helping the person be comfortable as he dies. The presence and caring of another person during this very difficult and lonely life experience is one of the most human aspects of all nursing.

2. A second common stall situation in the patient's dying process is staff identification with the illness. Staff members who are close in age with terminally ill patients may experience feelings of identification with them. These patients are difficult to care for if staff members are unable to express their own feelings of anxiety and fear over the possibility of this illness in themselves.

Other factors heighten the identification process of staff with patients. Sometimes the occupation or the socio-economic factor affects this reaction. The similarities between patient and staff all contribute. The staff person thinks, "This could be me and I wonder how I would react if it were me? What would I do?" These feelings can be explored in staff meetings in order to help sift out the feelings and thus enable the staff to care appropriately for the patient and not to withdraw because of conflict of feelings.

3. A third stall occurs over the issue of whether or not the patient knows his diagnosis. The nurse may use this issue as the reason not to get involved in a therapeutic way in caring for him. The nurse will say, "How can I talk to the patient? I don't know what the doctor has told him." This is not a valid reason for not talking with the patient.

Although it is helpful to know what the doctor has told the patient and what the family has told the patient, it gives no information on what the patient really knows or has heard. He is the only one who can supply that information.

Whether or not the patient knows his diagnosis should not interfere with the nurse's listening and trying to understand what the patient is experiencing. She can learn from the patient what his illness means to him.

Once the patient has told the nurse what he feels and worries about, he then knows someone else knows about it. This in itself is therapeutic. He knows the nurse is not afraid to hear whatever else he may want to tell of his fears. The nurse does not have to avoid the patient anymore because now there are no secrets between nurse and patient.

4. A fourth stall situation may occur when the patient asks something the nurse feels cannot be answered. Nurses also say they fear that the patient will request something they would not know how to handle. Or they say, "I might give something away or tell something the doctor should tell." All that these excuses do is keep the nurse from the patient. Other evasive methods used by the nurse in dealing with the patient are to send other staff in, to keep busy with the records or reports, or to be in staff meetings. The nurse has to work through her feelings of discomfort and insecurity when talking with patients about troublesome subjects.

The stall warning should sound when the nurse feels herself withdrawing from the dying patient or when she finds herself reacting personally to the patient's expressed feeling. For example, the patient will often feel angry and sad when he realizes he is dying. He may tell the nurse to leave him alone or to go away. He may turn his back on staff or turn the radio up loudly when staff members enter the room.

The therapeutic task is to help him bear the painful feelings he is having: those feelings of having to let go and leave this world alone.

5. Hospital rituals may enhance the stall process and interfere with people's being able to express their feelings. Single rooms are often assigned to the dying patient so that he does feel isolated, different, segregated, and abandoned.

Following the death of the patient (if in a ward setting) the curtains are drawn around the other patients, the body is whisked away, the corridors are cleared, and a special elevator is used. The mystique of the ritual increases people's fantasies as well as their own fear of death. Who then sits down to talk with other patients in the ward or with the family?

SUMMARY This chapter discussed liaison psychiatric nursing services within the hospital setting to help nurses integrate psychiatric–mental health concepts into nursing care. The theoretical framework for liaison nursing included the concepts of adaptation, direct physical care, anxiety, patient reaction to illness, behavioral patterns in adjusting to illness, and patient status. The clinical situation often determines which patients are to be referred to the liaison nurse; they are identified as the newly admitted patient, patient with undiagnosed illness, pre-operative patient, the patient in pain, pediatric patient, seriously ill patient, the patient in the intensive care unit, and the dying patient. We included some management aspects of patient care, although we realize that not all hospitals have liaison services.

REFERENCES
AND SUGGESTED
READINGS

Bergerson, Janet H. (1971). "A Patient Plea: Tell Me, I Need to Know," *American Journal of Nursing,* **71,** No. 8, 1572–73.

Burch, Judy W., and Joan L. Meredith (1974). "Nurses as the Core of a Psychiatric Team," *American Journal of Nursing,* **74,** No. 11, 2037–38.

Cassem, Ned H., Thomas P. Hackett, Carolyn J. Bascom, and Howard A. Wishnie (1970). "Reactions of Coronary Patients to the CCU Nurse," *American Journal of Nursing,* **70,** No. 2, 319–25.

Grace, Mary Jo (1974). "The Psychiatric Nurse Specialist and Medical-Surgical Patients," *American Journal of Nursing,* **74,** No. 3, 481–83.

Hall, Benita L. (1968). "Human Relations in the Hospital Setting," *Nursing Outlook,* **16,** No. 3, 43–45.

Hoffman, Esther E. (1971) "Don't Give Up on Me," *American Journal of Nursing,* **71,** No. 1, 60–62.

Holstein, Shirley, and John Schwab (1965). "A Coordinated Consultation Program for Nurses and Psychiatrists," *Journal of the American Medical Association* **194,** No. 3, 103–5.

Jackson, Harriet H. (1969). "The Psychiatric Nurse as a Mental Health Consultant in a General Hospital," *Nursing Clinics of North America,* **4,** No. 3, 527–40.

Johnson, Betty Sue (1963). "Psychiatric Nurse Consultant in a General Hospital," *Nursing Outlook,* **11,** No. 10, 728–29.

Klagsbrun, Samuel C. (1971). "Communications in the Treatment of Cancer," *American Journal of Nursing,* **71,** No. 5, 944–48.

Kligerman, Martin, and F. Patrick McKegney (1971). "Patterns of Psychiatric Consultation in Two General Hospitals," *Psychiatry in Medicine,* **2,** No.2, 126–32.

Mervin, Frances (1971). "The Plight of the Dying Patients in Hospitals," *American Journal of Nursing,* **71,** No. 10, 1988–90.

Mendelson, Myer, and Eugene Leyer (1961). "Countertransference Problems of the Liaison Psychiatrist," *Psychosomatic Medicine,* **23,** No. 2, 115–22.

Meyer, Eugene, and Myer Mendelson (1960). "Psychiatric Consultations with Patients in Post-Graduate Medical Training," *Journal of Nervous and Mental Diseases,* **130,** No. 1, 78–81.

Robinson, Lisa (1968). "Liaison Psychiatric Nursing," *Perspectives in Psychiatric Care,* **6,** No. 2, 87–93.

Steen, Joyce (1973). "Liaison Nurse: Ombudsman for the Chronically Ill," *Americal Journal of Nursing,* **73,** No. 12, 2102–4.

Zahourek, Rothlyn, and Katherine Morrison (1974). "Help with Problem Patients," *American Journal of Nursing,* **74,** No. 11, 2037–38.

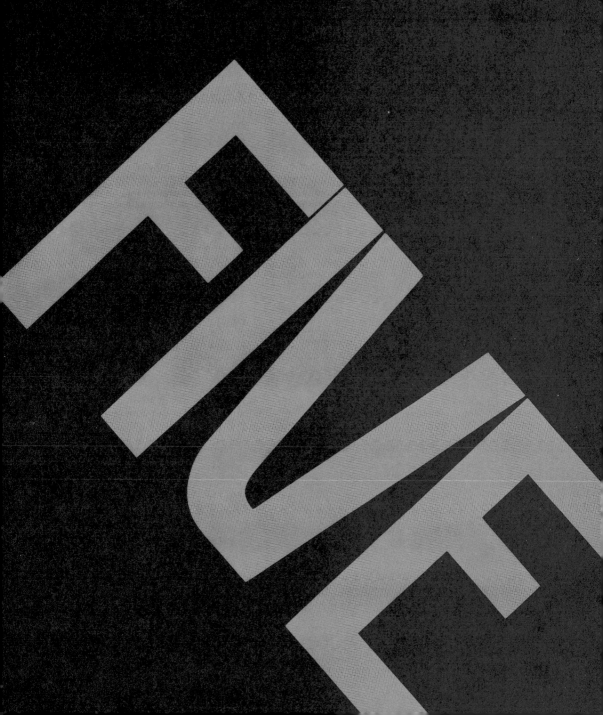

THE COMMUNITY

FIVE

To successfully achieve the goals of understanding the diversities and similarities of human behavior, there is the need to develop insights to see patients in their own reality and in their own community. By doing so we avoid the pitfall of merely projecting our theories about the person and his behavior in a judgmental and nontherapeutic way.

The changing quality and values in our society present a mandate that nurses be socially conscious in their practice. The issues described in this part really test the nurse's humaneness. Of the many elements of individual–family–community interaction in the framework of psychic distress, the following have been portrayed in this section:

Chapter 21 **Social Forces in Mental Health Practice**

> *Social and psychological factors strongly influence human behavior. Social forces that involve political and economic policy have had an important effect on mental health practice: the community mental health movement, the feminist movement, and patients' rights.*

Chapter 22 **Patients' Requests and Clinical Negotiations:**
The Customer Approach

> *The concept of the customer approach to patienthood shows how the health seeker can help the provider. This concept ensures that the rights of health seekers are taken seriously by recognizing that patients' requests for health care are usually reasonable and are always negotiable.*

Chapter 23 **Diagnosis and Intervention in Crises**

> *Crisis theory and intervention is discussed specific to developmental, situational, and victim crises.*

Chapter 24 **Unresolved Grief**

> *The crisis dimensions of grief are discussed in terms of the normal bereavement and grief process and the unresolved process.*

Chapter 25 **The Elderly in the Community**

> *The elderly in the community are a contemporary concern of all health professionals.*

Chapter 26 **Alcoholism as a Community Problem**
by John A. Renner, Jr.

> *Clinical examples and the historical aspects of the community problems of alcoholism are presented.*

Chapter 27 **Treating the Drug Abuser**
by John A. Renner, Jr.

> *Current treatment modalities are described for this topical problem.*

SOCIAL FORCES IN MENTAL HEALTH PRACTICE

21

Significant sociopolitical developments in American society during the past two decades have directly affected the mental health field. This chapter examines the social context of mental illness and contemporary social forces in community mental health, including the community mental health movement, the feminist movement, and the patients' rights movement.

SOCIAL FACTORS IN MENTAL ILLNESS

Social factors that strongly influence mental illness are family and social network relationships, child-rearing practices, peer groups, race, migration, socioeconomic status, unemployment, war, and social crises. It should be noted that different population groups in the society differ in frequency and kind of mental disorders. Social scientists have tried to discover the reason why some population groups have a higher incidence of mental illness than do other population groups.

To view mental illness as a social issue means to understand the following:

1. Mental illness may handicap a person over a long period of time.
2. Mental illness is expensive, not only in terms of family disruption and personal suffering, but also in social and economic terms.
3. Current treatment methods, facilities, and personnel are inadequate to cope with the problem.
4. There is an uneven distribution of mental illness in the society. This observation has implications for the social and political structures of the society.
5. Psychiatric symptomatology is affected by such social forces as population growth, automation, industrialization, poverty, racial conflict, and international relations.

The individual and his group

The individual has a role expectation as he relates to his family and to his community. These cultural expectations of individuals may be potential stress factors that, in turn, may lead to the breakdown of the individual.

Individuals first learn expected role and attitude behavior in the family group. The socialization process then progresses through schooling and interactions with other groups, for example, peer group, religious group, neighbors, and colleagues. How each group views health and illness and the behavior that it allows teaches the individual his attitudes.

The mentally ill in society

Cultural factors in a society refer to those aspects or ways of life for a given population that distinguish it from other populations.

The definition of the mentally ill differs from culture to culture. In some cultures, women who are mentally ill are thought to be possessed by demons. In one culture, the mentally ill are thought to be possessed by magic and other special powers. In other cultures, the mentally ill person is the outcast or scapegoat for the community. What happens to the mentally ill person is also determined culturally.

Psychiatric hospitalization as a social process

As previously stated, the multitude of social factors influences to a large degree the diagnosis and incidence of mental illness. Nevertheless, psychiatric institutions that have been designed to deal with the disturbances of behavior have evolved with a certain degree of uniformity.

To view patienthood as a social process means to understand the following factors:

1. The reaction to being labeled mentally ill.
2. The decline of intimate, socio–emotional family relationships (family betrayal).
3. Social isolation.
4. The loss of social identity and role responsibility.
5. The status of unemployment.
6. Social deterioration.

Several historic trends are evident when viewing the function of the psychiatric institution as a social system responding to society's need to care for its mentally ill. At the start of the twentieth century the main concern of mental institutions was the safe and economic custody of patients. This meant locked windows and doors, a warning system when someone tried to escape, and a poorly paid and untrained staff to manage large patient populations. By midcentury (1950) it was not unusual to have 1 registered nurse for 50 patients or 1 physician for 200–1000 patients in the large state hospitals of 1500–2000 patient population.

In 1958 Goffman presented the view that mental illness is a social process rather than a disease process.[1] He vividly described what it felt and looked like to be a mental patient. He believed that the arbitrary power of the mental hospital staff bred a coercive and corrupting political system that

[1]Erving Goffman, *Asylums* (New York: Doubleday & Company, Inc., 1961).

was degrading and disrespectful to the patient. He pointed up the fact that institutions required all patients be treated alike and that they adhere to schedules designed for the efficient management of the institution rather than for the needs of the patients.

The system of nursing care at this time was primarily oriented toward controlling patient behavior (custodial care) rather than toward care that was creatively therapeutic. For example, "bad" patient behavior was dealt with by loss of privileges, transfer to a different ward, or social isolation from staff.

The concept of the therapeutic community, originally developed by Maxwell Jones, follows:

1. The current social behavior of the patient is the focus.
2. The patient is an active participant in his own treatment and that of his fellow patient.
3. Increased communication between staff and patients is a goal designed to decrease social distance.
4. Psychodynamic insights of personality and the psychopathology of the patient are de-emphasized.

The concept of "token economy," a form of behavior modification, was subsequently developed to deal with the problem of socially deprived, "hard core," backward, untreated, and older chronic patients. The desired, healthy, and approved behavior, as defined by the hospital staff, was rewarded (positively reinforced) through a token reward system of increased privileges or in some cases money. Studies indicated that therapeutic change is possible if the social environment in the hospital setting is restructured.

Contemporary concepts of psychiatric hospitalization that have been developed from the comprehensive mental centers are discussed later in this chapter.

Social class and mental illness

A study by August Hollingshead and Frederick Redlich reported that adult deprivation resulting from lower class position was a determinant in severely disordered psychological functioning. This study further indicated that the lowest status groups show the highest rates of hospitalized psychiatric disorders. Relevant to this is the fact that cultural patterns associated with social class status influence diagnostic judgments. That is, the lower the status, the more severe the psychiatric diagnoses are.

Biosocial variables influencing mental illness

Age is a biological factor of mankind. Studies indicate that psychiatric disturbances increase with age. For example, the Midtown Manhattan Study reported an estimate of the mental health of a metropolitan community. Eighty percent of the population studied were found to have some psychiatric symptoms. One striking relationship was age. There was an increase in poor mental health with age by decades, the 50–59 year group indicated 15%

well and 31% impaired as compared to the 24% well and 15% impaired in the 20–29 age group.

It is difficult to assess the significance of sex in psychiatric disorders from mental hospital statistics. Usually, there are as many beds for male patients as there are for female patients. However, there are studies in progress to determine which institutions have what percentage of males and females. For example, are there more women or men in long-term continued care psychiatric institutions and nursing homes?

In out-patient settings there are usually more females than males. The sex difference may be seen when certain features of a culture tend to place men or women in advantaged or disadvantaged positions. This position may protect or contribute to stress situations that lead to symptom formation. For example, the organization of groups to influence the exercise of individual rights is a contemporary force in the society.

Marital status is a blending of biocultural factors. Many cultures specify marriage rules, for example, who may marry whom, and how the change from single to married to unmarried status shall be formalized, and what are the obligations of the married pair to family and community. From this standpoint, many varying cultural patterns exist.

The reports on marital status and psychiatric hospitalization are uniform and state that first admission rates for hospitalization are consistently higher for divorced people than for any other group. The descending order for psychiatric admissions is divorced, single, widowed, married.

The disenfranchised and minority groups

There is evidence that undue social and economic pressures on any particular minority group lead to social disintegration. The high rate of alcoholism, the high rate of suicide among its youth, and the low morale of the American Indian are examples from one culture group.

The concept of blaming the victim[2] is a psychological mechanism of society that can be applied to many American problems. Ryan gives the example of why majority groups hate minority groups. The majority group is really blaming the minority group for that which the majority group has caused.

At every social class level, the minority groups often suffer a greater and more intensive range of overt deprivation than do the majority groups. For example, blacks in the American culture are more prone to mental illness, crime, and other maladaptive behaviors. Undoubtedly, this is a result of social and economic situations, which are a consequence of group prejudices.

Psychiatric hospital statistics show that the rates of first admissions for blacks are consistently and overwhelmingly higher than the rates for whites in every age range and for both sexes. The suicide rate among blacks reaches its peak in the youthful years. Suicide rates among whites increase in direct relationship to advancing chronological years.

[2]William Ryan, *Blaming the Victim* (New York: Pantheon Books, Inc, 1970).

Etiological explanations offered for these statistics are urban stresses, poverty, inadequate schools, unemployment, and father-separated households. Social deprivation is so widely experienced among blacks that it is considered a major cause of psychological impairment.

Sociocultural integration

When morale in a society is high and when the economics are good, there is a healthy society in which there are few psychiatric symptoms. When morale is low and where the economics are poor, there is social disintegration, depression, and a high rate of mental illness. A sociocultural view is that the mental illness of any given person is attributed to a maladjusted social system rather than to a singular fact of individual pathology.

It has been hypothesized that communities as units of culture can be assessed on a range of integration from near zero at one end (disintegration) to a well-functioning societal system that provides for its sociocultural needs at the other end. Indicators to determine where a community ranks are as follows:

1. Stability of families.
2. The poverty-affluence dimension.
3. The viability of its religious system.
4. The overall coherence of its cultural values.
5. Leadership and followership.
6. Communication networks.
7. Supportiveness of interpersonal relationships in the community.

SOCIAL FORCES Three significant social forces have occurred within the last two decades which have made an impact on the society. They are the community mental health movement, the feminist movement, and the movement for individual (patients') rights.

The community mental health movement

In 1963, under President John F. Kennedy, federal legislation was passed toward developing new methods to treat the adult mentally ill in terms of decreasing the physical size of state mental hospitals, improving their resources, and extending services into the community.

The new model developed was the community mental health center. The center required a consolidation of services, change in operational and fiscal policy, incorporation of the lay public into its structure, and an increased focus on comprehensive care. The Community Mental Health Centers Act of 1963 authorized $150 million in federal aid to the states for the construction of comprehensive centers over a period of 3 years, 1965–1967. These centers were to provide a program of mental health services to the community, not just a new or separate building. In order to qualify for federal funds, the program had to provide at least the five following essential services:

1. *In-patient Care:* This unit offers treatment to patients who require 24-hour care.
2. *Out-patient Care.* This unit offers treatment programs for adults, children, and families on an out-patient basis.
3. *Partial Hospitalization.* This unit offers day care or night care for patients who are able to return home evenings and weekends or who are able to work during the day. The night care provides temporary arrangements for the person until more suitable arrangements can be made.
4. *Emergency Care.* Twenty-four hour emergency service is available in one of the three units named above.
5. *Consultation and Education.* The center's staff offers consultation and education to community agencies and professional personnel.

Full comprehensive service includes five more services that complete the comprehensive community mental health program. If these additional services are also included, special consideration is given to the application requesting federal support.

6. *Diagnostic Service.* This service provides diagnostic evaluation and may include recommendations for appropriate care.
7. *Rehabilitative Service.* This service includes both social and vocational rehabilitation. It offers such services as prevocational testing, guidance, counseling, and job placement.
8. *Precare and Aftercare.* This service provides screening patients prior to hospital admission and home visiting before and after hospitalization. Follow-up services for patients are available in out-patient clinics or in foster homes or halfway houses.
9. *Training.* This program provides training for all kinds of mental health personnel.
10. *Research and Evaluation.* The center may establish methods for evaluating the effectiveness of its program. It may also carry out research into mental illness or cooperate with other agencies in research.

In this program a patient may move easily from one kind of treatment to another as his needs change. This is called "continuity of care" and represents a key concept of the mental health program.

A variety of treatment methods become especially important in implementing this concept: group therapy, family therapy, crisis intervention, multiple impact therapy, and therapeutic community. Emphasis is placed on short-term treatment and on follow-up care.

Operating concepts for community mental health centers

Catchment area. The catchment area concept divides a population into small enough segments so that collaborative working relationships may be established between community agencies and the mental health center. Optimally, the geographical boundaries and functional relationships define the area as a community. The catchment area concept helps to reallocate responsibility between hospital and a designated community. This expanded responsibility allows the professional to practice in the community as well as in the hospital.

Community participation. Citizen participation and community control are contemporary issues in all of society today. Currently, these issues tend to be directed toward minority groups, for example, the poor, the medically indigent, specific ethnic groups, and women.

Today's increasing demands for citizen participation in community programs are a result of the failure of health programs previously prescribed by professionals and politicians, a growing awareness by minority groups that they are relatively powerless, and a growing desire by the groups to gain real power by taking an active role in shaping their destinies.

The population in a technological age, whether a minority group or not, tends to feel disenfranchised, and with good reason. As a result, everyone wants more control over his destiny. This occurs in mental health as well as anywhere else. It includes all men, women, students, teachers, and patients. People want their rights. Any group that feels that it does not have a say in its destiny is part of this current movement. People who pay federal, state, and local taxes want to know where their money goes. They want to know that their money is being spent wisely and in their best interest.

The powerlessness that people in this society feel comes from rising taxes, increased technology, reaction to federal and state government, urbanization, mobility of the population, disillusionment with the political process, and many other reasons.

Therefore, it is essential for the success of any community mental health program that citizen involvement be assured.

Many communities are able to participate in the administration of health care by means of area boards. These boards are formed by the community and the board members are local residents. All members of the board—be they members of the medical profession or laymen—join together to work on the problems of health care.

Interdisciplinary collaboration. The interdisciplinary collaboration of the mental health team is an important concept in the effectiveness of the community program. For optimal collaboration, questions of role, authority, and territory must be carefully resolved by the members of the team. Inevitably, the rigid role boundaries of the past must be made more flexible. At the same time, it is important that each member of the team maintain his area of expertise. The team will stall when either too much separatism exists as a result of role and authority issues or when the whole team becomes so homogenized that there is no differentiation of expertise.

The overall areas of expertise include skills in community organization, research, in-patient and out-patient services, and emergency treatment.

With the high cost of mental health services and the uneven health care delivery system, the mental health profession can ill afford not to maximize its efficiency by interdisciplinary collaboration.

Concepts of intervention   Community mental health is often referred to as preventive with an emphasis on health rather than on care services. Caplan states:

... the topic of prevention can be considered under three main headings .... Primary Prevention ... the processes involved in reducing the risk that people in the community will fall ill with mental disorders. ... Secondary Prevention ... the activities involved in reducing the duration of established cases of mental disorder and thus reducing their prevalence in the community. Involved here is the prevention of disability by case-finding and early diagnosis and by effective treatment .... Tertiary Prevention ... the prevention of defect and crippling among the members of a community. Involved here are rehabilitation services which aim at returning sick people as soon as possible to a maximum degree of effectiveness.[3]

Primary prevention. Primary prevention programs try to lower the rate of emotional disorders in two ways: The first approach is to try to counteract the potentially noxious social conditions in the community. The second approach is to directly intervene when such a condition does exist. These programs depend on the community participation of social agencies, schools, churches, health care workers, local political leaders, and families for their implementation.

Secondary prevention. Secondary prevention is the early identification of emotional disorders that require prompt treatment. Work in this area requires knowledge of the signs and symptoms of the disturbances in infancy, early childhood, the school-age child, the adolescent, the young adult, the adult, and the elderly adult.

Treating the acute phases of the major psychoses of schizophrenia, depression, and manic–depressive illness is part of secondary prevention. The clinical syndromes described previously represent almost all the emotional difficulties requiring in-patient and out-patient care. Much of psychiatric nursing deals with problems in secondary prevention.

The community mental health services aim to treat the acute phase of illness as early and as quickly as possible. In-patient care is only used when it is apparent that out-patient treatment or partial hospitalization will not suffice. In general, it is best to treat the patient without removing him from the community. When the patient must be hospitalized, the health team should try to return him to the community as quickly as possible.

Tertiary prevention. Tertiary prevention is the attempt to reduce the residual effects of mental illness. This is accomplished by planning the rehabilitation program as soon as the illness is identified. Rehabilitation efforts may involve partial hospitalization, home care programs, foster home care, halfway houses, and organizations for former patients. Nurses have traditionally played an important role in the processes of rehabilitation.

The feminist movement

A second social movement has occurred within our society in the past dec-

---

[3]Gerald Caplan, *An Approach to Community Mental Health* (New York: Grune & Stratton, Inc., 1961), pp. vii–viii.

ade. The feminist movement is and promises to be a significantly influential social force in the last quarter of the twentieth century. Jesse Bernard writes:[4]

> How was it possible for small bands of women . . . to change our thinking so radically in so short a period of time? . . . Yet less than a decade after their inception, with no foundation funds, no formal structure, no mass support, no consensus, no access to the media, and against strong opposition, they changed our minds (if not our hearts) with respect to sex roles to an incredible extent.

The beginning: A purpose

A series of protest movements—peace, civil rights, the New Left, antipoverty—were in full swing in the late 1960s when the feminist movement began. This movement—the revival of feminism—was more often than not the object of many jokes and sarcastic remarks. For example, "women libbers" were accused of being sexually deprived, man haters, or sexually promiscuous. They were portrayed as rejecting marriage and motherhood and unwilling to sacrifice any personal whim for the sake of their children; they were described as physically unattractive, hostile, hysterical, maladjusted, and they were feared as "wanting to take over the world," to subordinate men. As Maren Lockwood Carden said, "The press and other mass media had a field day making fun of the women."[5]

However, the dust cleared and despite this initially strong opposition, the goals of the movement have held firm and purposeful. The feminist movement is a serious reform movement, one that identifies itself with the person's right to find out the kind of individual she or he is and to be free to pursue and become that person.

The new feminist ideology

Today's feminists argue that too much emphasis has been placed on the biological differences between men and women. Their belief is that the socialization process instead of biological differences accounts for the larger part of the observed differences in male and female behavior. Feminists protest the degree to which social institutions have channeled women into narrowly defined sex roles. They bring into awareness how tightly society has defined the role of wife and mother, for example, society uses the term housewife, as though a woman could be married to a house. Feminists argue that if roles were not so rigidly defined, women could combine career roles with that of wife and mother if they so elected. A recent study[6] reveals that the two-career family is an increasingly workable reality. In fact, both husband and wife may be deeply committed to serious professions without sacrificing a full and complete family life. In that case, the career wife will then feel less pressure placed upon her to justify her working not solely for financial reasons. At the same time, she will not necessarily be the one censured if one of their children develops "problems." As one woman stated, "It is a tremen-

[4]Jessie Bernard in *The New Feminist Movement* by Maren Lockwood Carden (New York: Russell Sage Foundation, 1974), p. x.

[5]Maren Lockwood Carden, *The New Feminist Movement* (New York: Russell Sage Foundation, 1974), pp. 1–3.

[6]Lynda Lytle Holmstrom, *The Two-Career Family* (Cambridge, Mass.: Schenkman, 1972).

dous relief to be able to pursue my career as I want to and not to have to reassure people by adding, 'And yes, my children are not juvenile delinquents.' "[7]

Feminists remind us of how oppressive conditioning or the social process is practiced both consciously and unconsciously. For example, girls are encouraged to be pretty and charming. Boys are encouraged to be strong and manly. Young women are taught to be concerned with their appearance and not their intellect. They are encouraged to dress to please men instead of dressing for comfort. Mass media contribute heavily to fostering the socialization process by portraying women as sex objects and by stereotyping women as dependent, nonintellectual, and passive. Studies indicate the difficulty women have experienced in climbing beyond the middle management rung of the "career ladder" in business.

Children's toys and grammar-school textbooks have been criticized by feminists for focusing on this sex role stereotype. Both historical and contemporary writing use the terms "man" and "mankind" instead of humans and human history. Adult women are reminded of their secondary role when they are asked to perform community services. For example, in community organizations, the woman solicits for campaigns, bakes cakes, types or telephones, or engages in secondary roles instead of organizing, managing, and developing the purposes of the organization. In employment, her job very often involves complementing others--usually men—and carrying out orders under male supervision. The predominate female careers (teaching, social work, nursing, and secretarial or administrative assistants) validate this.

The concept of sisterhood is a central force in the feminist movement. The premise is that if women cease living their lives through men, they will be freer to establish relationships with other women instead of avoiding and competing with other women.

Participation in the movement

There are two primary vehicles in which women participate in the feminist movement: consciousness-raising sessions and women's rights groups.

Consciousness-raising sessions. In consciousness-raising sessions women gather in small groups to talk, to question, to rethink, and to revise their old concepts of womanhood. The focus is on their own unique position as women. Personal experiences form the basis for the discussion; members contribute equally, for there is no designated "group" leader. The women examine a wide range of topics, including their sex roles in a family. In these sessions many questions are asked, for example, the following: Should a woman devote herself solely to her husband? Do women have to sacrifice more than men for the sake of companionship and the intimacy of marriage? Should a mother be in sole charge of her children and how involved should the father be? Why is the whole family uprooted if the husband decides on a job in another city?[8]

[7]Consciousness-raising session.
[8]Maren Lockwood Carden *The New Feminist Movement,* pp. 33–37.

Many feelings about stereotyped sex roles are expressed and discussed. Women describe the resentment they feel about having to wait on family members or the anguish and frustration they feel about having to wait for a man to call to ask for a date or the discomfort they feel when men whistle or stare at them when they walk down the street. Many women are beginning to realize that they have too little control over their lives, that, in fact, life revolves around men, and that the way men treat women in this society is disturbing. After discussing these conditions, conditions they have taken for granted most of their lives, women begin to consider changing their behavior. They cease to support only the male ego, and they expand to support both the women and men whom they respect. They begin to identify and to subsequently ignore male devaluing comments. They avoid relationships in which men see them primarily as sex partners. They seek relationships in which they are viewed as human beings. They discuss and negotiate housekeeping responsibilities with their husbands and they insist on their personal rights in terms of having equal time to themselves in order to pursue educational courses.[9]

Sexual partnership is an important topic in consciousness-raising sessions. Women readily talk with one another about apprehensions, feelings, and values that have concerned them since they were children. They were usually too embarrassed or fearful to talk about them and consequently, they became suppressed. Single women, younger and older married women, divorced women, and widowed women all help to provide various perspectives and guidelines. A valuable component of these sessions is the sense of communal interest these women share within our large impersonal society. Women learn to talk freely, meet people, and understand the emphasis finally placed on sisterhood.

Consciousness-raising groups strengthen self-confidence among their members. Women discuss their lives frankly and with dignity. They begin to listen and to understand the common problems that they have as women. They receive true and accurate information about their real potential, they explore new roles for social behavior, and they support women who wish to depart from the traditional female roles.

Women's rights. A second kind of group for women who participate in the feminist movement are formally organized groups. The oldest and largest of the women's rights group is the National Organization for Women (NOW), which was organized in 1966. This organization includes both men and women. The original officers were 1 man and 4 women. The 24-member board of directors included 4 men. The organization's primary goal is to take social action in order to bring women into full participation in the mainstream of American society.

Consciousness-raising sessions are also an integral part of many of the groups' overall programs. Task forces form an important component of NOW.

Members of NOW work through legal methods and employ other

[9]Ibid., p. 35.

strategies in order to place social pressure on political groups. They have taken action in a variety of ways, for example, filing proceedings against sexist organizations, pressuring companies and banks to grant women credit, and promoting child care on a national scale.

Feminists generally agree that the objectives of feminism will be difficult to achieve within the current American social structure. Hopefully, a structural change will facilitate a redefinition of male and female roles. For example, feminists believe that child care facilities might socialize American children and help them to become more sensitive to interpersonal relations. Thus, if men and women work together as colleagues, they may abandon stereotyped definitions of each other. Many feminists believe that such goals will provide a general improvement in the quality of human life.

Implications of the feminist movement in mental health

There are serious considerations for mental health professionals to review as they encounter the impact of the feminist movement. Feminists, who reject the idea of male superiority, point out that for decades males have been interpreting female behavior within male parameters. Women strongly reject such psychoanalytic thinking as Freud's theory of penis envy, Erikson's modification of Freud's argument that, for women, anatomy is destiny,[10] and Bruno Bettelheim's assertion that women want "first and foremost to be womanly companions of men and to be mothers."[11]

Feminists point out that scholarly discussions during the first 60 years of this century aided in sustaining the traditional role of women and that they will no longer accept these interpretations from psychologists and psychiatrists. This rejection of contemporary psychiatric thinking has greatly increased the need for feminist therapists. In many cities, feminist therapists and feminist physicians are listed in women's journals.[12]

The impact of the feminist movement on mental health professionals is evidencing itself in the continuing educational programs that are being offered to mental health clinicians. Male and female mental health professionals have become increasingly aware of sex-role differentiation and of sex stereotyping, and conferences are being arranged to deal with these issues. One conference states its purpose as follows:[13]

> Conference participants will explore the ways that sex-role differentiation and sex stereotyping influence psychological evaluation, establishment of mental health goals, and choice and use of preventive and remedial techniques with men and women clients. The implications of sex stereotyping for those receiving mental health services as well as for those providing them, and the implica-

[10]Erik H. Erikson, "Inner and Outerspace: Reflections on Womanhood," in *The Woman in America,* ed. Robert Jay Lifton (Boston: Beacon, 1965), pp. 1–26.

[11]Bruno Bettelheim, "The Commitment Required of a Woman," in *Women and the Scientific Professions: The M.I.T. Symposium on American Women in Science and Engineering,* eds., Jacqueline A. Mattfeld and Carol G. Van Aken (Cambridge, Mass.: The M.I.T. Press, 1965), p. 15.

[12]Carden, *The New Feminist Movement.*

[13]Conference on Sex Stereotyping and Mental Health, sponsored by the Mental Health Continuing Education Consortium of Boston University School of Social Work, McLean Hospital, Tufts-New England Medical Center, Department of Psychiatry, December 6–7, 1974, in Waltham, Mass.

tions for policy and service issues, will be presented by keynote speakers and discussed by conference participants.

There are many who believe that the impact of the feminist movement has just begun and that future developments are promising. It certainly needs to be fully understood by professionals who will be dealing with female and male clients of all ages.

Patients' rights

A third important movement in the past decade is that of patients' rights. This movement is different from those previously mentioned in that people other than those directly involved are being instrumental in protesting and pressuring for social action. Jonas Robitscher describes it as follows:[14]

> The mentally disabled do not have minority pride like blacks, do not organize like grape pickers, do not agitate like students, and do not rebel like prisoners. They passively wait for action to be taken on their behalf.

General hospitals have been responding to this issue of patients' rights since the early 1970s. They formally published a patients' bill of rights. These rights, implicit in human history, are based on civil rights as defined in the constitution. Publishing this bill of rights has been one giant step toward accountability by the administration of the hospital. It remains to be seen how responsible, individual professionals will integrate this humanistic focus into their clinical practice.

Psychiatric hospitals have additional concerns about the civil rights of an individual. The conditions prevailing, under which many people are hospitalized for psychiatric reasons, have encouraged the denial of a person's inalienable rights. Litigation procedures are currently being instituted to test the individual's rights vs. the institutions' rights. We will discuss some of the rights that have been ruled on in the courts.

Right to education   The mentally ill and the mentally retarded person's right to education is being considered a constitutional right in more and more states. Using the courts as a means of testing the legal aspects of cases is increasing. For example, in one state, the mother of a perceptually handicapped child with a learning disability was awarded damages when the school program in her town failed to offer her child a special education program.[15]

Right to vote   One concern regarding the rights of institutionalized patients is the right to vote. What is the election procedure for people who are hospitalized? A recent study[16] reported that the state division of mental health in St. Louis intervened and encouraged in-patients to exercise their right to vote. Each

[14]Jonas Robitscher, "Medical, Moral, and Legal Issues in Mental Health Care," *Hospital and Community Psychiatry,* **25,** No. 7 (1974), 466.

[15]Milton Greenblatt, "Class Action and the Right to Treatment," *Hospital and Community Psychiatry,* **25,** No. 7 (1974), 449.

[16]Bernice Thompson and Julian Hall, "Helping Psychiatric Inpatients Exercise their Right to Vote," *Hospital and Community Psychiatry,* **25,** No. 7 (1974), 441.

patient in the state institution was asked to complete a questionnaire in which he was asked if he were registered to vote, if he planned to vote, and if he had obtained an absentee ballot? Ward staff met with groups of patients to further discuss plans and to arrange transportation and escorts for the patients who wished to vote in their own precincts on election day.

Patient's advocate office Some state hospitals have established a patient's advocate office. One study at Fergus Falls, Minnesota, reports the implementation of such a program. The office is staffed with social workers, social work students, and a law intern who investigate in-patients' complaints and have access to all treatment areas, plans, programs, and records. The channels and procedures have been identified in a document agreed upon by the advocate and the hospital administrator.[17]

New patients are informed of their legal rights and their welfare benefits and they are given a pamphlet which explains the function of the office. The advocate also reviews the chart of new admissions to see that a treatment plan has been formulated and implemented within one week of admission. The study reports that the largest category of complaints about legal rights comes under the state's hospitalization and commitment law. Other complaints involve treatment issues, staff relations, and ward living conditions.

Right to treatment The issue of the patient's right to adequate treatment is a complex one. The development of this issue concerning mental hospital patients began with the case of mentally ill John Baxstrom who, in 1961, was incarcerated in a New York prison and was held long after any sentence for his crime would have terminated. Although it had not been established that Baxstrom was dangerous, he was detained in prison on the basis of his mental illness and the belief that the community should be protected.

In 1966 the Supreme Court of the United States held that Baxstrom had been denied equal protection by the law and he was transferred to a civil mental hospital. This precedent allowed 900 other psychiatric offenders, who were believed to have been illegally detained, to be transferred to civil mental hospitals. In due time approximately 200 of these patients were released. Subsequent follow-up indicated that relatively few of them had to be returned to institutions.[18] This New York precedent prompted other states to review cases involving psychiatric offenders, and subsequently many of them were transferred to civil institutions.

A second legal case made history in 1966 in Washington, D.C. Charles Rouse was charged with carrying a dangerous weapon and was found not guilty by reason of insanity. He was committed to a state mental institution. The offense was legally defined as a misdemeanor and punishable by a maximum sentence of 1 year. Four years later Rouse's lawyer filed a habeas cor-

[17]Bill Johnson and David Aanes, "Patients' Use of a Full-Time Patient Advocate Office in a State Hospital," *Hospital and Community Psychiatry* **25,** No. 7 (1974), 445.

[18]R. C. Hunt and E. David Wiley, "Operation Baxstrom After One Year," *American Journal of Psychiatry,* **124,** No. 7 (1968), 974–78.

pus petition stating that Rouse was not getting adequate treatment. The district court denied the petition on the grounds that it refused to consider quality of treatment as a cause.

The case was appealed. The historic value of the case was in the appeal decision. The judge decided that adequate treatment is an inalienable right of anyone who is mentally ill and involuntarily committed. The judge stated that the purpose of involuntary hospitalization is treatment, not punishment. The judge's decision turned the case back to the district level for a determination of adequacy of treatment. The court did find that the patient was being provided adequate care.

Class action suit　Another legal action aimed at making states responsible for the treatment process involves class action suits.

In one case an in-patient at a state mental hospital alleged that he was not getting adequate treatment, and he sought transfer to another institution. The results of a hearing showed that the patient had been receiving only custodial care. Further investigation revealed that the staffing at the institution was grossly inadequate and that the patient was indeed not receiving suitable treatment. The court then allowed the state reasonable time to improve its treatment program.

As a result of the increasing number of legal cases over this issue of patients' rights, there have been released several publications in which the rights of the mentally handicapped have been outlined. Among the publications are *Basic Rights of the Mentally Handicapped* and *Legal Rights of the Mentally Handicapped,* both prepared by the Mental Health Law Project.[19] The American Civil Liberties Union has published *Handbook on Mental Patients' Rights.*[20]

Reaction to patients' rights　The other side of the coin regarding patients' rights includes the rights of the patient's family, the community, and the professionals who say that they are there to help the mentally handicapped. Milton Greenblatt, in discussing the issue of class action and the right to treatment, raises serious questions from the standpoint of the institution. He asks:

> Is it a constitutional right? Does it apply to involuntarily committed patients alone, or also to voluntary admissions who are dependent on the state? Where will the states find the trained personnel and billions of dollars necessary to meet the standards of adequate treatment? What should those standards be? Will the federal government provide funds to help the states accomplish this upgrading? Will the whole effort result in the rapid phasing-out and ultimate disappearance of the state institutions? If so, what will take their place?[21]

States vary on commitment laws and on their criteria for involuntary commitment. Follow-up reports of released psychiatric patients reveal a

[19]Mental Health Law Project, *Basic Rights of the Mentally Handicapped* and *Legal Rights of the Mentally Handicapped* (Washington D.C.: U.S. Government Printing Office, 1973).

[20]Bruce Ennis, *Handbook on Mental Patients' Rights* (New York: American Civil Liberties Union, 1973).

[21]Greenblatt, "Class Action," pp. 449-521.

need for a very careful review of all patients who sign 3-day papers and leave against medical advice. The major concern involves possible and probable dangerous behavior. Because of the liberalized hospital rules and the emergence of the 3-day papers, there has been a marked increase in dangerous behavior either to self or to others.

If a patient is allowed to sign himself out, there has to be someone who is to be concerned with family and community reaction. It may be that the family is not ready to have the patient home and there may be fears and concern about the behavior of the patient.

The concept of aggressive behavior and dangerousness has been seriously neglected by clinicians. How much is known about the nature of aggressive impulses, the stimuli of aggressive behavior, and the discharge of such behavior? One group working with sexually dangerous men has been researching these questions for over 14 years at Massachusetts Treatment Center in Bridgewater, Massachusetts. They have defined a dangerous person as "one who has a high probability of inflicting serious bodily injury on another."[22] They are currently working on the problem of predicting such behavior in a person.

There is a conflict between the safety of the community and the restrictions upon a person's liberty, and serious consideration must be given to this conflict. It is the duty of society to protect its members from unwarranted violence and to protect the rights of the individual.

The following chapters in this book deal with some of these community problems. These discussions point up the need for sociological, political, legal, and psychological input.

Implications for psychiatric nursing

SOCIAL FACTORS FOR NURSING Conditions are changing so quickly that when nurses see new problems emerging, they have to think of what kind of new social factors are occurring. If nurses do not consider these social influences, they will develop a narrow, myopic view of mental illness.

The implication of these general data is that they should broaden the perspective of the nurse in understanding mental illness. Mental illness is not limited to something biochemically going on in a person's head; it is a function of the group involvement of the individual, the economic conditions, or even of the individual's current housing situation.

Nursing management

The nurse may have to join efforts with larger groups to deal with broader issues. For example, if a public health nurse tries to help someone who continually has colds and she finds that the temperature in the patient's house is 30 degrees, she is, in a sense, wasting her time treating the cold. The factor to deal with is the temperature in the house. Here the nurse has to join forces

[22]A. Nicholas Groth and Murray L. Cohen, "The Diagnosis and Treatment of Aggressive Sexual Offenders," in *Community Mental Health: Target Populations,* by A. W. Burgess and A. Lazare (Englewood Cliffs, N.J.: Prentice Hall, Inc., 1976).

with other groups, for example, the social service or local housing authorities, to help exert the proper pressure on the landlord.

If the children are eating paint, the public health nurse cannot just advise the mother not to let her child eat paint. She will have to be involved with other groups in helping to remove lead paint from the market, as well as in working with screening detection centers.

The public health nurse has to learn to deal with the many variables contributing to the larger problem. Since she is not in a hospital setting, where variables are more easily controlled, she should work with other groups who can help bring pressure to bear on the problem at hand.

SUMMARY   Beginning steps have been taken toward understanding the interrelationship of psychiatric disorder and the biosociocultural components of a person's experiences. The sociocultural implications are inherent in such activities as urban planning, community development, status integration, social relationships, social improvement, relief from poverty conditions, and increased health care delivery systems.

The social factors inherent in viewing mental illness were identified as family and social relationships, child-rearing practices, peer group influence, race, migration, relocation, socioeconomic status, unemployement, war, and social crises.

Discussed in this chapter were the effects of socialization upon individuals and their groups, the mentally ill in society, psychiatric hospitalization as a social process, social class and mental illness, the disenfranchised and minority groups, and sociocultural integration. Three social movements that originated in the 1960's were identified as strong influences on mental health practice: the community mental health movement, the feminist movement, and the movement for patients' rights.

REFERENCES   Baker, Frank (1974). "From Community Mental Health to Human Service Ideol-
AND SUGGESTED   ogy," *American Journal of Public Health*, **64,** No. 6, 576–81.
READINGS   Bradner, Patty (1974). "Women in Groups," *American Journal of Nursing*, **74,** No.
                9, 1661–63.
            Brown, Frances G. (1970). "Social Linkability," *American Journal of Nursing,* **71,**
                No. 3, 516–20.
            Clark, Kenneth B. (1965). *Dark Ghetto*. New York: Harper and Row.
            Dumas, Rhetaugh (1969). "This I Believe . . . About Nursing and the Poor," *Nurs-
                ing Outlook*, **19,** No. 9, 47–50.
            Goffman, Erving (1961). *Asylums*. New York: Doubleday and Company, Inc.
            Goffman, Erving (1965). *Stigma*. Englewood Cliffs, N.J.: Prentice-Hall, Inc.
            Heide, Wilma Scott (1973). "Nursing and Women's Liberation — A Parallel," *Amer-
                ican Journal of Nursing*, **73,** No. 5, 824–26.
            Hollingshead, August, and Frederick Redlich (1958). *Social Class and Mental Ill-
                ness*. New York: John Wiley & Sons, Inc.
            Holmstrom, Lynda Lytle (1972). *The Two-Career Family*. Cambridge, Mass.: Schenk-
                man Publishing Company.

Janzen, Sharon Ann (1974). "Psychiatric Day Care in a Rural Area," *American Journal of Nursing,* **74,** No. 9, 1632–35.

Jones, Maxwell (1968). *Beyond the Therapeutic Community.* New Haven: Yale University Press.

Klerman, Gerald (1969). "Mental Health and the Urban Crisis," *American Journal of Orthopsychiatry,* **39,** No. 5, 818–26.

Lamb, Karen Thompson (1973). "Freedom for Our Sisters, Freedom for Ourselves: Nursing Confronts Social Change," *Nursing Forum,* **12,** No. 4, 328–52.

Madden, Barbara P. (1975). "Raising the Consciousness of Nursing Students," *Nursing Outlook,* **23,** No. 5, 292–96.

Quinn, Nancy K., and Anne R. Somers (1974). "The Patient's Bill of Rights: A Significant Aspect of the Consumer Revolution," *Nursing Outlook,* **22,** No. 4, 240–44.

Regester, David C. (1974). "Community Mental Health – For Whose Community?" *American Journal of Public Health,* **64,** No. 9, 886–93.

Roberts, Joan T., and Thetis M. Group (1973). "The Women's Movement and Nursing," *Nursing Forum,* **12,** No. 3, 303–22.

PATIENTS' REQUESTS AND CLINICAL NEGOTIATIONS: THE CUSTOMER APPROACH

22

ssues of patients' rights, malpractice insurance, and consumer advocates are making headlines daily. The implications of these issues have served to heighten nursing's consciousness about the problems inherent in the delivery and financing of health services. One obvious yet frequently omitted step both in practice and in the professional literature that could counteract this wave of consumer rebellion is to include the patient in the therapeutic process. This chapter will discuss the use of patient requests in the process of clinical negotiations.

THE CUSTOMER APPROACH TO PATIENTHOOD For many years such mental health professionals as Sigmund Freud, Kurt Lewin, and Herbert Maslow studied the concept of human need. Although these men were scientists investigating specific human problems, they did not necessarily attempt to meet the needs they were studying.

For several decades meeting patients' needs has been a major goal in planning nursing care. The nurses, as therapeutic implements of care, have been putting the concepts and theories into practice. Ida Orlando Pellitier,[1] a nurse-clinician, describes the development of treatment methods based on the hypothesis that satisfaction of needs leads to mental stability and that dissatisfaction of needs leads to mental instability. For the most part, however, what the patient has "needed" has been determined by the professionals' clinical judgment rather than by direct verbal response from the patient.

In our attempts to describe a customer approach to the psychiatric patient, we shall share some of our clinical observations and research findings.

The patient, in most situations, knows how he would like to feel and how he hopes the professional can help him to achieve this end. However, because the patient may be afraid of being disappointed or being made to feel

[1]Ida J. Orlando, *The Dynamic Nurse-Patient Relationship* (New York: G. P. Putnam's Sons, 1961).

ridiculous, he seldom relates his expectations to the professional. Consequently, the professional often assumes that the patient doesn't know what he wants. For this reason it is important for nurses to demonstrate their concern for their patients and to continually ask questions to find out what the patients really want.

Based on the assumptions that the patient knows how he would like the nurse to help and that the nurse can be more effective by learning the patient's requests, the authors attempted to explore the range of requests.

The patient request

It is important to distinguish between patient request, patient complaint, and patient goal. Sometimes nurses think they know the request after hearing or reading in the chart the patient's chief complaint.

The complaint is the patient's initial statement as to what is bothering him; for instance, "I am in pain." The goal is what the patient would like to accomplish or how he would like to feel; for instance, "I would like to feel well enough to be able to work." The request is how the patient would like the nurse to respond to help him achieve the desired goal. He might request *medical* intervention: "Give me some medicine for the pain." He might request *clarification:* "Help me understand why I am having this pain." He might make an *administrative* request: "Would you write a letter to my employer that I am ill?" In the studies of how well clinicians elicit these three data points, it has been found that the complaint is invariably elicited, the goal is usually elicited, but the request is often not elicited.[2] In such situations, the negotiation process will be seriously impaired if the nurse does not know the patient request.

Research on patient requests has been conceptualized from various population groups. The original research project was led by author A. L.[3] The clinical research team set out to learn from patients at the Massachusetts General Walk-In Psychiatric Clinic what they wanted from the professionals who were there to serve them. From the analysis of several hundred interviews, patients' requests were classified into fourteen categories as follows.[4]

Administrative request   The patient is seeking administrative or legal assistance from the clinic to help him with his current dilemma. The specific request may be to provide a disability evaluation, a draft deferment, a medical excuse to leave work, medical permission to return to work, permission to drive, admission to a hospital, or testimony in court. The power to grant or deny these requests is delegated by society to particular professionals or institutions. The power

[2]Aaron Lazare, Sherman Eisenthal, and Linda Wasserman, "The Customer Approach to Patienthood," *Archives of General Psychiatry* **32**, No. 32 (1975), 553–58.
[3]Aaron Lazare, et al., "The Walk-In Patient as a Customer," *American Journal of Orthopsychiatry,* **42**, No. 5, 872–83.
[4]Lazare, Eisenthal, and Wasserman, "The Walk-In Patient as a Customer."

may be subsequently rescinded, or, as in the case of therapeutic abortions, may no longer be necessary.

Advice   The patient wants guidance about what to do in personal or social matters. He may already have formed an opinion, but he now wants professional advice. He wants to know the "right" thing, the "best" thing, or the "wisest" thing to do. He may want the advice in order to have the clinician share the responsibility for a decision he is about to make.

Clarification   The patient wants help to put his feelings, thoughts, or behavior in perspective. He does not want to be told what to do but would rather take an active role in the therapeutic process. Often, the patient wants the help to be able to make a decision. He wants to understand; he wants to see his choices. The patient usually sees his problem as being acute and not a part of an ongoing neurotic pattern.

Community triage   The patient is requesting information on where in his community he can get the help he needs. He sees the clinic as an available resource which has the necessary information.

Confession   The patient feels guilty about what he has said, thought, or done. He hopes that by talking to the therapist he will feel better. Specifically, the patient wants to be forgiven. He hopes the clinician (authority figure) will see the misdeed as medical or psychological in origin and therefore not bad.

Control   The patient is feeling overwhelmed and out of control. He may fear hurting himself or someone else, or going crazy. He is saying, "Please take over. I can no longer manage."

Medical   The patient sees his problem as being physical in origin, like any other medical condition, as opposed to psychological or situational in origin. He often refers to his problem as "nerves" or as a "nervous condition." The patient, accordingly, hopes for medical treatment, for example, pills, ECT, hospitalization, or medical advice. He expects to take a passive role in the treatment.

Psychological expertise   The patient believes that the source of his problem is psychological rather than physical or situational. He is asking the professional to explain to him why he thinks, feels, or acts the way he does. The patient anticipates playing a passive role in the interaction, contributing only that information which the expert requires.

Psychodynamic insight   The patient perceives his problem as psychological in origin, as evolving from his early development, and as having a repetitive quality. As a result, he is left feeling unhappy, unfulfilled, but not overwhelmed or out of control. He expects to take an active, collaborative role in talking about the roots of his problem and hopes that a better understanding of his problem will enable him to change.

Reality contact   The patient feels that he is losing hold of reality. He wants to talk to someone who is psychologically stable and "safe." He is requesting the clinician to help him "check out" or "keep in touch with" reality so that he will feel that he is thinking straight and not losing his mind.

Social intervention   The patient sees the problem as residing primarily in the people or situations around him. Because he feels that he does not possess the resources to effect the necessary change, he is asking the clinic to intervene on his behalf. He is asking not for the legal powers of the clinic but for its social influence.

Succorance   The patient is feeling empty, alone, not cared for, deprived, or drained. He wants the clinician to care, to be involved, to be comforting, to be warm and giving so that he can feel replenished and warm inside. It is not so much the content of the interchange that is requested as its affective quality of warmth and caring.

Ventilation   The patient would like to tell the clinician about various feelings and affect-laden experiences. The patient anticipates that "getting it out" or "getting it off his chest" will be therapeutic. He feels that he is carrying around a burden which he would like to leave with the clinician. In contrast to confession, the patient does not feel guilty and does not need or want forgiveness.

Nothing   Patients who make no request are a heterogeneous group. They may have been referred without proper preparation; they may be psychotic; they may have problems, but they are not seeking help at this time; they may want help, but they are reluctant to state the problem; they may not need help; they may be in the wrong clinic.

Eliciting the request

CLINICAL TECHNIQUES   An important clinical technique is how to elicit the patient's request. Sometimes the patient will state the request spontaneously at the beginning of the interview. If this does not happen, the patient's request is best elicited after the nurse learns the patient's complaint and some background of the present concern. This early interaction establishes the rapport and alliance necessary for elicitation of the request.

Eliciting the request too early in the interview and before the patient states his problem increases the probability of placing the patient in the position of adversary rather than collaborator in the assessment process. "You asked me what I want. You do not even know what is wrong with me." Eliciting the request at the end of the interview deprives the nurse of the opportunity to negotiate or work with the patient.

The most successful way of eliciting the request is by asking: "How do you hope (or wish) I (or the hospital or clinic) can help?" Try to avoid questions such as "What do you want?" or "What do you expect?" because they are apt to be perceived as a confrontation. The words "wish" or "hope," in contrast, give the patient permission to state requests he does not necessarily expect will be granted.

Sometimes the patient's response to the question will be, "I don't know. You are the nurse." Or, "I just want to feel better." In this case, the patient may have a rather specific request in mind that he is reluctant to state. Thus, eliciting the request then requires persistence, persuasion, and compassion. "You must have some idea when you decided to come to the clinic," or "It is important for me to know what your wishes are even if I may not be able to fulfil them."

It is not easy for patients to tell nurses what they want. Patients often perceive that it is their role to state their problem but not to evaluate how the help should be provided. The patient, however, does have the right to take his business elsewhere if he is not satisfied. Patients often perceive a health care person or agency as having the power to say "no." As a result, the patient must hint at his request rather than boldly state it. Or patients may find it difficult for a variety of personality reasons, for example: "A caring nurse would know what I wanted without my saying," or "Who am I to ask for anything?" Others feel a loss of pride in having to ask for something. The difficulty in stating what one wants, wishes, or hopes for is not limited to the nurse-patient relationship. It is deeply rooted in our culture. In seeking certain employment positions, one does not always believe his best chances are when he asks for the job but rather if someone else submits his name for the position. The childhood ritual of blowing candles out after a wish or breaking a wishbone carries with it the pressure to keep the wish to oneself in order to have the best chance of its coming true. In academic settings, students are often reluctant to express their wishes regarding either lectures or clinical experiences for fear of influencing a grade.

The initial statement of the request may be incomplete or stated in such general terms that it requires elaboration to achieve more detail for clinical utility. "You said you want me to help you to understand this situation better. What in particular did you want me to understand?" Or, "You thought you would feel better if I talked with your family. How do you hope I can talk to them?"

When the request has been finally stated and elaborated, it is important that the nurse acknowledge that she has heard and understood the request. Otherwise, the patient may wonder whether the nurse heard the request, was offended by it, or didn't believe it worthy of a response.

The elicitation of the request undoubtedly depends on more than timing and phraseology. Certainly the nurse's attitude of interest and receptivity is crucial. One frequently observes a patient hinting or alluding to the request, apparently waiting for some response from the nurse that will indicate that it is acceptable to continue to be more specific.

As the interview progresses, the nurse should listen for elaborations of or changes in the request resulting from the developing relationship between the nurse and patient. The patient thinks to himself: "Now that I have more trust in you, let me tell you what I really want," or "Now that you have responded to my initial request, it occurs to me that there is something more important that I need."

Negotiating the patient's request

The negotiation is the heart of the clinical nursing process. It is the coming together, the interaction, the dialogue between the patient who is formulating what he thinks he needs and the nurse who is formulating what she hopefully thinks is clinically appropriate.

In an ideal negotiation, the patient exerts his influence in several ways. First, since the request has considerable diagnostic value, the patient is providing the nurse with valuable information. Second, the statement of the request itself obliges the nurse to consider the legitimacy of the perceived need and to explain why an alternative formulation might be more valid. Third, the patient has the right to evaluate and ultimately accept or reject any treatment proposal. In the process, he may expect to receive from the nurse a further explanation, an alternative treatment plan, or a statement that the staff cannot meet the request.

The nurse is simultaneously exerting influence by the clarification and evaluation of each request in regard to whether it is clinically appropriate, clinically sufficient, and clinically feasible. If a request is clinically inappropriate, such as a request for medication where there is little chance that the medication will be effective, the nurse attempts to educate the patient so that he will change the request.

It is not uncommon for the request to be appropriate, but not sufficient. For example, the patient who wants to talk out his fears and concerns about a chronic medical illness may also need referral for diagnostic tests. Or there are situations where the request is clinically appropriate but not clinically feasible because of the treatment facility. This dilemma should be stated directly and honestly to the patient. At least the patient has received clinical confirmation of what he wishes and can be referred elsewhere if necessary.

Impasses in negotiations are common, and remedial strategies are varied. It may be helpful to understand the patient's perception as to the nature of his health concern and to inquire what he has tried before. It may be helpful to know the patient's fears about his health and what he specifically does not want to happen. It may be helpful for the nurse to restate the formulation in the patient's words in order to facilitate communication.

Stalls in the negotiation process

There is apt to be a great deal of wasted time and energy during an interview in which the patient request is verbalized either late in the interview or not at all. Instead of speaking freely about the problem, the patient may be preoccupied, wondering whether the nurse is kind enough, respectful enough, wise enough, understanding enough, and flexible enough to hear the request. "When will the nurse be ready to hear? When will I have the guts to come right out with it?" The nurse, meanwhile, often unaware of these concerns, goes about the business of establishing nursing care plans not understanding why the patient participates only reluctantly during the interview. On the other hand, when the patient has stated the request early in the interview and feels it has been supportively heard, he is apt to participate more freely and feel more satisfied at the end of the interview.

There are several situations in which the nurse may stall the process of eliciting the request.

1. The nurse may unwittingly discourage the patient from stating his request by changing the subject after the patient has hinted at the request.

2. The request elicited too late in the interview. The patient may feel there is no opening till the end of the interview: "By the way, would you . . .?" Or the patient comes to a medical clinic for a general exam, and, as he is ready to leave the office, states the real request: "Please tell me if I have cancer." Had the patient made the request earlier and had the nurse perceived the request as legitimate and important, the nurse might have explored the reasons for the patient's concern and learned what kind of explanation would be most appropriate.

3. Progressive aspect of requests. In many clinical situations, acknowledging the request or giving the patient what he asks for satisfies needs that must be met before a second request can be made. In cases of sexual assault, victims very often have a medical request upon entry to the emergency ward. Once reassured of their medical condition in terms of treatment of physical trauma, wounds and prevention of venereal disease and/or pregnancy, the victim then makes a request for psychological assistance. "I keep thinking about the attack. Help me get rid of these thoughts."

Implications of clinical negotiations

The customer approach is an attempt to conceptualize the initial interview as a process of negotiation between the nurse and the patient, taking the patient's request as a starting point. A basic assumption is that a patient's request for care is usually reasonable and always negotiable. This customer approach makes the patient more understandable and diminishes the nurse's sense of helplessness. It is the nurse's task to elicit the patient's request, collect the relevant clinical data, and enter into a negotiation. As a result, it is hoped that the patient will feel his perceived needs have been heard and responded to while the nurse will feel that she has not only been comprehensive but responsive to the patient. The negotiation should facilitate a relationship of mutual influence between nurse and patient to the benefit of both parties.

There are many clinical situations in which the patient's statement of what he wants is exactly what he needs. "I don't want to be woken up at midnight for my medication. I wish to sleep." Using the customer approach, the nurse has the chance to learn important information early in the interview and profit from the patient's ideas, a commonly ignored source of diagnostic data.

When the patient's request is clinically appropriate, making a careful diagnosis of the request can be very important in determining the precise clinical intervention. For example, the patient who needs "ventilation"—

talking over fears and concerns about his mental health—requires the nurse to take the role of an interested listener. If the nurse breaks in to make interpretive comments and provides advice or some other intervention the patient has not requested, the clinical plan can fail.

Some nurses may find the word *customer* difficult to integrate in their concept of patient care. We believe it is a useful metaphor to describe a relationship in which the patient has the right to ask for what he wants, to negotiate, and to take his business elsewhere if he so desires, while the nurse has the obligation to listen, to negotiate, and to offer interventions that meet professional nursing standards. This customer relationship, we believe, is in the interest of both parties. On the other hand, a relationship characterized either by the patient taking whatever he wants or can pay for (as in the supermarket) or by the nurse acting independently of the patient's wishes runs the risk of being ineffective or even destructive to both parties.

SUMMARY Technical and social changes are presenting new clinical demands for nurses. Increased pressure on nurses and physicians results not only from limitations of the diagnostic system and clinical formulations but also from our approach to patients. In this chapter, we have attempted to conceptualize a clinical approach to patienthood based on the mutual influence between nurse and patient.[5] Such an approach results in improved patient care, patient satisfaction, and better staff morale.

SUGGESTED READINGS

Levinson, Dan, John Merrifield, and Ken Berg (1967). "Becoming a Patient," *Archives of General Psychiatry,* **17,** 385–406.

Borghi, John (1968). "Premature Termination of Psychotherapy and Patient-therapist Expectations," *American Journal of Psychotherapy,* **22,** 460–73.

Coleman, Jules V., and Rhetaugh Dumas (1962). "Contributions of a Nurse in an Adult Psychiatric Clinic: An Exploratory Project," *Mental Hygiene,* **46,** No. 3, 448–53.

Saper, Beatrice (1974). "Patients as Partners in a Team Approach," *American Journal of Nursing,* **74,** No. 10, 1844–47.

[5]Sections of this chapter are reprinted with permission from Aaron Lazare, Sherman Eisenthal, and Linda Wasserman, "The Customer Approach to Patienthood," *Archives of General Psychiatry* **32,** (1975), 553–58. Copyright 1975, American Medical Association.

Sections of this chapter are reprinted with permission from Aaron Lazare, Sherman Eisenthal, Linda Wasserman, Thomas C. Harford, "Patient Requests in a Walk-In Clinic," *Comprehensive Psychiatry,* **16** (5), 467–477.

DIAGNOSIS AND INTERVENTION IN CRISES

23

C ommunity mental health staff are in daily contact with people who are in crisis. The patient who is hospitalized is in a situational crisis because his normal life-style is disrupted. A family member dealing with the news of the death of a loved one is facing a crisis situation. The stress of hospitalization and of the subsequent financial costs predisposes a person to possible economic crisis. Crisis is a time when a person can either gain strength psychologically or regress to a mental ill-health level. Gerald Caplan, a crisis theorist, has defined crisis as follows:

> Crisis . . . a psychological disequilibrium in a person who confronts a hazardous circumstance that for him constitutes an important problem which he can for the time being neither escape nor solve with his customary problem-solving resources.[1]

Psychiatric nurses have the opportunity to practice primary prevention of mental illness specifically by intervening in crisis situations to aid or strengthen the coping process of the client. It thus becomes essential that nurses be able to diagnose crisis situations and to plan the appropriate interventions.

CRISIS THEORY Over the past several years, social scientists and mental health clinicians have been studying the effects of crises on individuals, families, and communities. Crisis theory has begun to attempt to define systematically differences in the many kinds of crises. However, crisis theorists and practitioners point to the difficulty in making precise distinctions because there are gaps in the current state of knowledge of the elements of crisis patterns, for example, stress, response, and settlement of the crisis. There is no general theory of crisis behavior. Hopefully, as research in crisis situations continues, publications or results will develop such a theory.

[1]Gerald Caplan, *Principles of Preventive Psychiatry* (New York: Basic Books, Inc., 1964), p. 53.

TYPOLOGY OF CRISES

People in crisis feel helpless and unable to deal with their problem by themselves. They are in a state of emotional disequilibrium. Their normal ways of coping with stress are not available to them. As a result, they are in an extremely vulnerable position psychologically.

Currently, clinicians talk of two main forms of crises: the internal or maturational crises of the life cycle and the external or situational crises.

Internal crises

Sigmund Freud's theory of psychosexual development and Erik Erikson's formulation of the eight stages of development in the human life cycle provide the theoretical basis for analyzing developmental or maturational crises. Erikson conceptualizes personality development as a succession of differentiated phases, such as infancy, childhood, adolescence, and adulthood, each being qualitatively different from its predecessor. Between one phase and the next, periods of transition are characterized by disorganized behavior. The person may be aware of minor mood swings as well as fluctuating emotions and thoughts experienced during the phase. The solution arrived at from the previous phase is then applied to the next phase. Erikson emphasizes the relationship between the person's social development and his social environment. He also emphasizes the normal aspect of the stages of development. For example, he goes into considerable detail in describing the normal "identity crisis" in the adolescent developmental crisis phase, stating that the phase includes increased conflicts with which the person must deal concurrently. Erikson identifies these eight major developmental crises in terms of the tasks that must be resolved in each phase (see Chapter 5).

Developmental or internal crises are expected life events which normally occur in most individuals' life spans. Because these crises are expected, an individual has the opportunity during his development to prepare for these events. This approach is designed and encouraged by clinicians in order to decrease the crisis experience and increase the person's internal control over the normal event. However, in discussing motherhood as a stage in the life cycle, Lopata[2] emphasizes that this developmental task permits little preparation and arrives with shocking suddenness.

Mastering these internal crises plays a large part in determining the ego strength of the individual. Coping skills are learned in order to deal with the various maturational tasks. For example, Lynda Lytle Holmstrom identifies three coping skills of two-career parents in dealing with the developmental task of child rearing as husband participation, modified work schedules, and hired help.[3]

Negative settlement of a developmental crisis may be termed a *fixation* which may lead to a characterological defect. The defect may interfere with the person's interpersonal relationships, and correction of the defect may

[2]H. Lopata, "The Life Cycle of the Social Role of the Housewife," *Sociology and Social Research,* **51,** No. 2 (1966), 2–22.
[3]Lynda Lytle Holmstrom, *Two-Career Family* (Cambridge, Mass.: Schenkman, 1972), pp. 73–75.

require psychotherapy. Grunebaum, Weiss, Cohler, Hartman, and Gallant
write of motherhood as being almost a classic example of a developmental
role crisis. They say:

> During pregnancy, a woman, her husband, and their extended families can pre-
> pare for the new role, but no preparation can anticipate the full reality of the
> event itself. With the baby's birth, the mother must have the welfare of another
> uppermost in her thoughts: at least in our culture, concern for self is explicitly
> secondary to concern for another for the first time in a woman's life. Time,
> energy, and emotional resources must be shared, and even sleep is sacrificed
> for the baby's welfare.[4]

Carol Hartman, the nurse-therapist who provided the nursing intervention
to the mothers and their babies during the joint admission project, states:

> Successful working through of the conflicts encountered in becoming a mother
> holds significant potential for improved mental health. Failure to deal with the
> maturational tasks of motherhood may bring a woman to the hospital, but the
> accomplishment of those tasks will facilitate her more mature development.[5]

External crises

Anticipated life events

Anticipated life events may be nontraumatic, growth promoting, or hazardous. In a study by Heisel and his associates[6] specific life events were identified in the life cycle of the child, adolescent, and young adult. These life
events are important to understand because all events involve stress which
implies a need for coping as well as possible adaptive measures if the event is
seen as hazardous. These anticipated life events may be identified as follows
and always involve a certain degree of participation by the person. That is,
the situation is usually agreed upon by the person; the hazardous event may
be superimposed.

> SCHOOL-RELATED: beginning nursery school, first grade, seventh grade or high
> school; change to a different school; failure of a year in school; being accepted
> into a college of one's choice.

> FAMILY-RELATED: birth or adoption of a brother or sister; change of father's
> occupation requiring increased absence from the home; marital separation of a
> parent; divorce of a parent; marriage of a parent to a stepparent; addition
> of a third adult to the family (e.g., grandparent, aunt, uncle); change in parents'
> financial status; increase or decrease in number of arguments between parents
> as well as with parents.

> SELF-RELATED: having a visible congenital deformity; change in acceptance
> by peers; outstanding personal achievement; becoming involved with drugs or
> alcohol; failing to be involved in an extracurricular activity one wished to join
> such as band or athletic team; breaking up with boy friend or girl friend; begin-
> ning to date; fathering an unwanted pregnancy; unwed pregnancy.

[4]Henry Grunebaum, Justin Weiss, Bert Cohler, Carol Hartman, and David Gallant, *Mentally
Ill Mothers and Their Children* (Chicago: University of Chicago Press, 1975), p. 319.

[5]Ibid., p. 86.

[6]J. Steven Heisel, Scott Ream, Raymond Raitz, Michael Rappaport, and R. D. Coddington,
"The Significance of Life Events as Contributing Factors in the Diseases of Children, III: A
Study of Pediatric Patients," *Journal of Pediatrics*, **83**, No. 1 (1973), 119–23.

Unanticipated life events The unanticipated life events are generally distinguished from the anticipated life events by the variable of prediction. Caplan defines these situational crises as chance events that are viewed by the person as unpredictable.[7] These are often considered to be hazardous. The element of unpreparedness increases the disruption in life style that an individual will experience. This factor, in turn, reduces the person's control over the situation.

These hazardous events may be related to a failure, for example, in school, in work, or with an individual person; a death of an important person; imprisonment of a family member or friend; hospitalization of a family member or oneself.

Research studies are looking at such events as the birth of a handicapped child, the birth of a premature infant, and widowhood. These problems often demand solutions that are new for the individual. These external situations are in addition to the internal or developmental task confronting the person.

Erik Lindemann's classic work on grief[8] provides the main focus for understanding the symptomatology of the bereavement crisis. From his experience with bereaved individuals, Lindemann continued his research around the concept of emotional crisis. He identified certain inevitable events in human life that were potentially hazardous. Each situation contains emotional strain in which stress would be expanded and would necessarily call for additional resources or adaptive behavior. In turn, adaptive behavior would lead to either mastery or failure.

Victim crises There are life situations in which an individual faces an overwhelmingly hazardous situation and in which the individual may be physically or psychologically injured, traumatized, destroyed, or sacrificed. Such an event involves physically aggressive and forced action by another person, by a group of persons, or by an environment.

Examples of victim crises are national disasters (war), civilian disasters (riots and racial persecutions), and violent crimes (murder, rape, and assaults).

Not only crisis theorists, but other disciplines as well are taking an increased interest in the victim. For example, people interested in law and criminology are beginning to look more and more at the victim. Attorney B. Mendelsohn has proposed the term "victimology"—the study of the victim—in order to develop an independent field of investigation. And a major study on the criminal and his victim was made by Hans von Hentig. Over a 25-year period, the number of publications on the study and understanding of the victim in various situations has increased considerably.[9]

[7]Caplan, *Principles of Preventive Psychiatry.*
[8]Eric Lindemann, "Symptomatology and Management of Acute Grief," *American Journal of Psychiatry,* **101,** No. 1 (1944), 141–48.
[9]Ann Wolbert Burgess and Lynda Lytle Holmstrom, *Rape: Victims of Crisis* (Bowie, Md.: Robert J. Brady Co., 1974).

Speculating whether or not a crisis will develop is an important clinical concern. We believe that the question is not whether or not a crisis will develop, but rather, what is the ripple effect or the severity of disruption and disorganization during the acute phase of the crisis and what is the length of time needed for the reorganization back to a normal life-style.

We believe that all life events are stressors and have the capacity to disrupt the homeostatic status of one's life-style. The life event has the potential to disrupt multiple areas of a life-style, and it is these areas which have a cumulative or ripple effect.

For example, a 32-year-old woman moved into an urban city after ending a 3-year marriage and leaving a job that she had had for 10 years. She moved into a new area and apartment and was job hunting when she was seriously injured in a car accident. The subsequent hospitalization disrupted her life physically and emotionally. The situation also created a personal and financial crisis. Her recovery physically will be only one part of her return to her normal life-style. She has other areas of her life to put back into order, all at a time when she is settling her feelings about dissolving a marriage, a job, and moving to a new environment.

ASSESSMENT People in a noncrisis state are in a homeodynamic state, that is, they have an even balance of stress and coping mechanisms to deal with the hazardous event. In contrast, the person in the crisis state is not able to use usual coping mechanisms to deal with the stressful situation. This lack of balance of stress and coping skills and the event prove disruptive to their normal life-style, and subsequently the normal anxiety increases. As Lorna Mill Barrell states, ". . . with the increase in anxiety, the coping powers further decrease. The resulting crisis is clearly the person's reaction and inability to cope, not the event or obstacle."[10]

According to Aguilera, Messick, and Farrell, the three important factors to study when assessing a crisis are perception of the life event, situational supports, and coping mechanisms.[11]

Perception of the crisis event

How does the person view the life event? Where in the life cycle is this person and how does this factor affect the perception of the event? How does the person view the positive and negative factors of the event? Are they evenly balanced or are they balanced too heavily on the negative side? To what degree will this alter the life-style of the person? What kind of crisis is the person describing?

---

[10]Lorna Mill Barrell, "Crisis Intervention: Partnership in Problem-Solving," *Nursing Clinics of North America*, **9**, No. 1 (1974), 5–17.

[11]Donna C. Aguilera, Janice M. Messick and Marlene S. Farrell, *Crisis Intervention. Theory and Methodology*, 2nd ed. (St. Louis: C. V. Mosby Co., 1974).

Situational supports

Who are the significant people to the person? How does the person plan to discuss this situation with them? How has the social network responded to the person thus far? How secure is the person in his relationship with the social network? How does the person perceive himself in relation to the social network and how accurate a perception is this? With whom is the person readily able to share thoughts and feelings about the situation?

Personality structure and coping mechanisms

How has the person handled stressful situations before? What coping mechanisms have been useful previously? What is the person's dynamic issue and how does the stressful situation relate to the dynamic issue? Does the person use coping mechanisms that have worked previously? Why is this situation different from others that he has dealt with?

DIAGNOSIS The clinician gathers all available data relevant to the crisis situation. The data are gathered from the individual, the social network, and other sources, for example, previous contact with professionals and agencies.

Crisis formulation includes a description of the precipitating events leading to the crisis, the perception of the stressful situation by the individual and the social network, the support the individual has available, and the individual's strengths and weaknesses with specific focus on coping skills. It must be determined if the crisis is an anticipated life event, an unanticipated life event, or a victim experience.

The crisis the person faces can then be analyzed by looking at the interaction between the developmental phase the person is in, that is, the internal crisis and the external imposed life event. The clinician must look at the developmental point of the individual and try to understand what the situational crisis means to the person at that age or position in the life cycle.

INTERVENTION The crisis state, as viewed by the helping person or agency, may be viewed as a therapeutic opportunity for the following reasons: The person, because his coping skills are not adequate, is now ready to learn new coping skills. He also may be in a better position to restrengthen ties with people in his social network with whom he may previously have been alienated. For example, the teen-ager who withdrew from parents for various reasons may be now inclined to talk with parents because of the crisis situation. If the teen-ager is on drugs and has become overinvolved with their use, it may be possible to resolve the issue if the parents become involved as helping people.

The goal of crisis intervention is to offer help to the person in crisis so that the psychological equilibrium can be restored. The clinician tries to utilize all possible social network people who are important to the individual. The intervention should be as brief as possible and should focus on the immediate problem the person is facing. Some interventions may consist of one or two sessions. As soon as other significant (to the individual) people can be brought into the situation and these ties cemented, the crisis intervenor may assume a less active role and soon leave the situation.

Intervention models

1. Problem-solving partnership. Barrell discusses the problem-solving partnership model as one kind of intervention technique.[12] This approach emphasizes the following: (1) active involvement and participation by the intervenor and client in crisis therapy; (2) focusing and authenticating the crisis; (3) assessment; (4) generating an intervention plan; (5) implementation; (6) anticipatory planning, summary, and evaluation.

2. Crisis counseling. This model of crisis intervention may be contrasted to the traditional psychotherapy model. Crisis counseling is issue oriented; behavior difficulties of the past are not explored and are actively discouraged in the interview. In the initial interview, material is obtained relevant to the crisis and the events leading to it. The assessment issues are explored. The interview is directive and structured. The crisis is subsequently defined in the client's terms, and the degree of disruption to lifestyle is evaluated with the client. The goal of counseling is agreed to by the client and clinician. The plan for intervention is made and may continue with office visits or other techniques.[13]

3. Telephone counseling. The telephone, used as a crisis technique, is gaining acceptance as an intervention model. Suicide crisis centers have relied on the telephone to help talk people out of suicide. Alcoholics Anonymous uses the telephone to provide its members access to another human being in hopes of averting a drinking episode. The telephone is also widely used in pediatrics. The parent can call and talk with the pediatrician or pediatric nurse practitioner about a problem with the child. Health care centers use the telephone routinely to do follow-up on patients.

The telephone is especially useful in crisis work for several reasons. First, it provides relatively quick access to the person one wishes to contact. Second, the person in crisis does not have to seek out help, make the appointment to see the crisis worker, and travel to an office at her own time and expense — all when she is in a crisis state and is having difficulty making any decisions. Instead, the crisis worker initiates the intervention, seeks out the client, and offers the service. Third, the client has considerable power in the situation and can say if she wishes to talk or not. Fourth, the client is able to resume a pre-crisis life-style as quickly as possible. She does not have to disrupt her life further by adding office visits. Telephone counseling also reinforces the view that the person is considered "normal" instead of "sick"

---

[12]Barrell, "Crisis Intervention."
[13]Burgess and Holmstrom, *Rape.*

and in need of therapy. The client does not have to assume the sick role that therapy and the label of patient connote to many people. Fifth, it is cost effective. It uses fewer resources—time, energy, and money—than do many other intervention methods.

The nurse uses telephone counseling to assess the progress of the client. The nurse especially notes the symptom picture over time, that is, both physical and emotional symptoms and any other area of disruption to the person's life-style. The nurse can identify the crisis and counseling request and then respond to the request appropriately (see Chapter 22).

4. Home counseling. Home visits are an additional method of crisis intervention and can be used when telephone counseling does not suffice. Other reasons for using home counseling are to reach a client who does not have a telephone, to reach a client who is uncomfortable with the telephone and office visit, especially a child or family in crisis; to introduce oneself face-to-face as a member of a crisis intervention team; to obtain additional information by direct observation; and to facilitate group discussion within a family or social network. Visual observation may be the key factor as contrasted with telephone counseling or even office visit if an assessment of the social network is important.

Case illustration

A 28-year-old mother of three children called the crisis unit of a community mental health center. In a very distressed tone of voice she stated that her 5-year-old son had a "bad temper" and she could not control him. She described wanting to "hit and beat him" but was feeling guilty about having such feelings and needed help.

She related that one week previous her son was playing with a neighbor boy and wanted a toy the child had. He pushed the child who subsequently fell and hit his head. The boy's mother was very upset and told the client that she should discipline her son more and that there was "something wrong with him to do such a thing."

The nurse at the crisis unit listened to the client and concluded that the mother was in a situational crisis involving disciplining her 5-year-old son. Her normal coping skills were not available and she felt she would "lose control and beat the child." The nurse asked if she might make a home visit to talk further about the situation and also to see the child and together they could talk about the problem.

The nurse was unaware of the precipitating events and did not know the mother well enough to be able to identify her usual coping skills. However, the mother expressed her concern of losing control in the situation. The nurse made a visit to the home the next day and the following data were obtained:

The mother was verbal and easily discussed her feelings of frustration in dealing with her children all day long. Once during the conversation the 5-year-old son and 4-year-old sister started fighting over who was going to sit in the chair closest to the mother. The nurse observed the mother's becoming more tense, evidenced by her chain smoking and talking faster and louder. Her attempts to set verbal limits on the children were abortive. The nurse intervened and asked the son to sit on the couch with her. This action prompted some dialogue with the child. The sister quietly sat in the chair. After a few moments the children decided to go outside to play.

The dialogue continued with the mother's saying that she was upset over her fear she would lose control and beat her children. The nurse pursued this association, and the mother soon revealed that as a child she had witnessed her father murder her mother by physical assault. The mother was fearful that she was like her father and she sees herself in her son.

The nurse commented on this information by saying, "You are indeed concerned about your angry feelings and are fearful of them. It might be helpful to see how you can deal with these feelings when you are upset with your children so that you are not afraid of them."

This line of discussion led to talking about setting limits on the children's behavior, and the example of the fighting over the chair was used. The nurse helped the mother to see that talking about the fighting was an alternative to fighting. Other basic principles of setting limits on the children's behavior were discussed, such as how to intervene verbally as well as physically. Physical contact, such as holding one of the children to interrupt a fight was also discussed as a limit-setting action.

The nurse and mother agreed on the crisis issue: setting limits on the children's behavior. The stressor was the incident the week previous when the neighbor boy's mother suggested that something might be wrong with her son. The remark stirred up old conflicting feelings about how anger and aggressive feelings are handled within the family. Talking about this as the stressful event decreased the mother's anxiety and helped her to see that her son was not her father and that she also was not her father. The nurse said that she could help the mother with the techniques of parenting—that she realized that certain phases were more stressful than others. The nurse identified this as a crisis situation, but she also acknowledged that the incident involving her father and mother was an unresolved issue and that the mother might think of getting some help to talk that out sometime. The mother agreed but said she was more concerned with her day-to-day dealings with her children. The nurse suggested to the patient that she join a mother's group being run by the visiting nurse association in which issues of parenting were being discussed. The mother agreed to this and said that she wanted to get out and talk with other women. The social aspects of this treatment method were most necessary because the mother felt isolated within the confines of her home.

A 6-month follow-up of the crisis situation indicated that the mother was faithfully attending the mothers' group which helped her feelings of isolation. Her fears of losing control with her children had been faced and she was moving on to discuss other issues within the group.

5. Hospitalization. A crisis situation may be of such dimensions that hospitalization is necessary in order to provide additional support to the person. However, it is very important to evaluate how the impact of hospitalization (which is an external crisis) interacts with the existing developmental crisis. For example, hospitalization for an emotional disturbance during the first months following childbirth may trigger additional crisis reaction. Hospitalization usually separates the mother from her child and disrupts the task performance of mothering. One suggestion for intervention for this problem is joint admission of mother and child. As Grunebaum and colleagues emphasize:

> Joint admission was designed to resolve this conflict (of separation). Bringing the child into the hospital at some point during the mother's stay makes it possible for the mother to have the protection and support which the hospital provides while she resumes the maternal care which is so important to her child and to herself. In addition, the mother and her therapist are able to utilize in treatment important observations of her feelings and actions which would be unavailable if the baby were not in the hospital. If this aspect of the mother's treatment is neglected, when she returns home and resumes her maternal responsibilities, she must face, often without help, intense feelings of rage, guilt, jealousy, and ambivalence which may be overpowering.[14]

Evaluation

The best method of evaluating the effectiveness of crisis intervention is to match the verbal and behavioral response of the client in terms of the stated objective or goal. In the above example, the mother felt that she had returned to her pre-crisis state. Her behavior was consistent with her self-respect. She had not lost control of her anger. Instead, she was able to set realistic verbal and physical limits on all her children.

If the intervention is successful, the client is back to a precrisis life style. The client reviews her pre-crisis life-style, identifies the disruption caused by the crisis, and evaluates her current life-style. This should match the client and clinician's satisfaction.

Stalls in the intervention

Following are some stalls in the process of crisis work that clinicians should consider.

Direct interviewing skills   One may note an impending stall when the interview results in irrelevant monologues and when the reason why the client is seeking help seems vague. If the clinician does not pick this up, the clinician will present disorganized, unrelated information in which the crucial facts and details are missing.

The stall is corrected by asking the client questions that relate to his current situation. The crisis event rarely dates back more than several weeks, unless it is an unresolved crisis issue. Beginning crisis workers should receive careful supervision so that the supervisor may hear all cases and pick up stall situations. If the supervision is done in a group, each person

---

[14]Grunebaum, et al., *Mentally Ill Mothers*.

may learn from other cases presented. This increases one's experience in crisis work.[15]

Role anxiety   The beginner in any new work experiences a certain degree of anxiety. Wallace and Morley describe new role anxiety as being related to the issue of responsibility and accountability in which the pressure of assuming one's own case load is felt. Crisis work means that the crisis worker assumes responsibility, accountability, and authority. In crisis work, the clinician opens the case, does the crisis intervention and therapy, and terminates the case.

An impending stall occurs when the nurse wishes that the client were seeing a senior member of the staff or a member of another discipline instead of her. This stall potential subsides as soon as the nurse becomes comfortable and experienced in crisis work and can see the therapeutic value of helping people in distress.

Dependency issue   An essential principle of crisis work is the strengthening of the client's coping skills. The crisis worker is especially careful not to make the client dependent upon her. A potential stall should be considered when the client makes frequent telephone calls to the nurse, or vice versa, and when the client is not progressing to a pre-crisis life-style within a 4–6 week period.

Client's expression of feeling   Crisis situations are wrought with feeling. The clinician's role is to allow expression of feelings appropriate to the crisis. Sometimes these feelings are uncomfortable to hear and listen to. For example, in the previous example the nurse needed to listen to the mother talk about very intense, angry feelings, feelings that could have produced violent behavior. A stall situation would have resulted if the nurse had cut off the client's expression of feelings that needed to be discussed. Sometimes a client spontaneously and actively expresses feelings. The clinician must allow crying, screaming, and all forms of negative expression of feelings when it is in the best interests of the client.

SUMMARY   This chapter discussed the research and clinical development in the field of crisis theory. A typology of crises included developmental crises, which are the internal tasks that must be mastered as one progresses through the life-cycle, and external crises, which are situational events that may be anticipated, unanticipated, or victim experiences in origin. Assessment, intervention, and evaluation of crises and the stall factors in the process completed the chapter.

---

[15]Mary A. Wallace and Wilbur E. Morley, "Teaching Crisis Intervention," *American Journal of Nursing,* **70,** No. 7 (1970), 1485–87.

REFERENCES AND SUGGESTED READINGS

Aguilera, Donna C., Janice M. Messick, and Marlene S. Farrell (1974). *Crisis Intervention: Theory and Methodology*, 2nd ed. St. Louis: The C.V. Mosby Co.

Hall, Joanne E., and Barbara R. Weaver (1974). *Nursing of Families in Crisis*. Philadelphia: J. B. Lippincott Company.

Hitchcock, Janice Marland (1973). "Crisis Intervention: The Pebble in the Pool," *American Journal of Nursing*, **73**, No. 8, 1388–90.

Kuenzi, Sandra Hicks, and Mary V. Fenton (1975). "Crisis Intervention in Acute Care Areas," *American Journal of Nursing*, **75**, No. 5, 830–34.

Oberst, Marilyn T. (1973). "The Crisis-Prone Staff Nurse," *American Journal of Nursing*, **73**, No. 11, 1917–21.

Piero, Phyllis (1974). "Black-White Crisis," *American Journal of Nursing*, **74**, No. 2, 280–81.

Resnik, Harvey L. P., and Harvey L. Ruben (1975). *Emergency Psychiatric Care: The Management of Mental Health Crises*. Bowie, Md.: Charles Press Publishers, Inc.

Salerno, Elizabeth Meehan (1973). "A Family in Crisis," *American Journal of Nursing*, **73**, No. 8, 1388–90.

Wallace, Mary A., and Wilbur E. Morley (1970). "Teaching Crisis Intervention," *American Journal of Nursing*, **70**, No. 7, 1484–87.

UNRESOLVED GRIEF

24

lthough a variety of situations can lead to an emotional crisis, we believe that one particular situation—the process of grief—assumes unusual importance in clinical nursing. The process of grieving (mourning) is the reaction to loss that everyone must deal with during the course of one's lifetime. Those who manage the grief process successfully following a severe loss are able to resume their lives and may even gain in strength. Those who fail to grieve properly may suffer an impairment of function and possible psychiatric illness. In order to understand unresolved or pathological grief and its impact on people in the community, it is important to describe the process of normal grief.

THE PROCESS OF NORMAL GRIEF

Grief is a psychological process following a loss which allows one to cope in a gradual manner with an overwhelming loss so that the loss can be accepted as a reality. If the full impact of the loss were suddenly experienced, the person might be psychologically overwhelmed. In grief the existence of the one who is lost is prolonged so that the person gradually may come to terms with what has happened.

The initial reactions to learning of the loss are shock and disbelief. "It just could not have happened. I don't believe it." The denial of the event is illustrated by the bereaved's expectation that the lost person will appear or that he heard the voice of the dead person in the next room.

The bereaved experiences painful feelings of sadness and emptiness when he recalls the lost person. The psychological discomfort is often accompanied by waves of weeping, experiencing a feeling of tightness in the throat, or a choking accompanied by a shortness of breath and sighing. These waves or pangs of grief occur less frequently as time goes on, but they may be readily reawakened when memories of the lost person are recalled.

The bereaved is preoccupied with the image of the deceased and he reviews and relives many of the memories about the lost person as if to put the memories and the dead person to rest once and for all.

In the early phases of grief the bereaved often feels guilty. "Maybe there was something I could or should have done." There may be guilt for being the survivor, for not doing enough, or for never making peace with the dead.

The bereaved tends to be irritable and angry. Sometimes the anger is directed toward the dead person for not remaining alive, for leaving work unfinished, and for causing all the grief.

In normal grief the bereaved eventually frees himself from certain ties to the deceased by acknowledging and bearing the pain of the loss, by experiencing the feeling of sadness, and by recalling memories involving the deceased. When these tasks are handled successfully, the acute phase of normal grief lasts from 2 weeks to 2 months. Signs and symptoms of grief, however, may last for as long as 1 year. Establishing new relationships and interests, the ability to function as before the loss, and renewed capacity for pleasure are signs of the resolution of the grief.

Parkes, in his excellent book on bereavement, summarizes major aspects of grieving according to the following seven features:

1. A process of realization, i.e., the way in which the bereaved person moves from denial or avoidance of recognition of the loss toward acceptance.
2. An alarm reaction—anxiety, restlessness, and the physiological accompaniments of fear.
3. An urge to search for and to find the lost person in some form.
4. Anger and guilt, including outbursts directed against those who press the bereaved person toward premature acceptance of his loss.
5. Feelings of internal loss of self or mutilation.
6. Internalization phenomena—the adoption of traits, mannerisms, or symptoms of the lost person, with or without a sense of his presence within the self.
7. Pathological variants of grief, i.e., the reaction may be excessive and prolonged or inhibited and inclined to emerge in distorted form.[1]

GRIEF AS A SOCIAL PROCESS

Grief is a social process because it can best be handled when it is shared and assisted by others. Few people seem to be able to grieve entirely alone.

Various cultures and religions recognize grief as a social process and provide religious and social rules of conduct that assist the bereaved. These rules state who shall be with the bereaved before the burial, who shall say what during the burial, and the duration and kind of social interaction after the burial. The rules of conduct further describe on what anniversaries or religious holidays the bereaved will again meet with others to remember his loss.

For example, in Orthodox Judaism, after the initial period of grief, families go to the temple twice a day for 11 months to pray. Then 4 times a year they attend memorial services.

In the Irish culture the wake before to the funeral is a time for sharing

---

[1]Colin Murray Parkes, *Bereavement: Studies of Grief in Adult Life* (New York: International Universities Press, Inc., 1972).

grief through viewing the body, lamenting, and paying tribute through eulogies.

It becomes even more evident that grief is a social process when we view the rapid changes developing in contemporary society that are making it even more difficult for people to grieve.

1. As a result of technology, we are a mobile people without roots. Thirty percent of our population moves each year. Consequently, people who suffer a loss are likely to be far from the relatives and old friends who would be in the best position to help with the process of grieving. We have observed that people who are isolated from friends and relatives will seek out professionals (nurses, family physicians, psychiatrists) for assistance with their normal grief.

2. The "religious" rules of conduct traditionally in use when handling the process of grief are losing their importance because of the diminishing impact of religion in our culture. This is unfortunate since (religion aside) these rules comprise a wealth of psychological wisdom that our society can ill afford to lose.

3. The process of grief may also be obstructed because of hospitalization and medical technology. With people dying in hospital rooms and intensive care units instead of in the home, family are excluded or frightened away so that the process of dying is made into something unnatural and unreal. This inevitably hinders the normal grief process.

4. The growth of cities and the scarcity of space have resulted in overcrowded cemeteries that are of necessity difficult to reach and unappealing to visit. Some cemeteries have even been moved to make room for highways. In vanishing rural America the cemetery often occupies a scenic hill where children and adults may easily visit. Under these conditions, death is more likely to be seen as a natural part of the life cycle.

5. Because of the increased liberality of the abortion laws, with a total increase in abortions, there is an increased need to grieve. For many women the abortion represents a loss that must be dealt with psychologically. If the demand for abortions leads to impersonal procedures that ignore psychological needs, we may see pathological reactions arising from the failure to grieve.

Society will continue to change at an ever increasing rate and change will lead to psycho–social problems. Society may find new solutions to the problems created by change, but until it does, there will be psychological "casualties." We believe that the normal grieving process is one of the casualties of change. By understanding the social and psychological process of grief, one can have an important impact on large numbers of patients.

The ultimate impact on a bereaved person must also be viewed in social terms. For many, there is a deprivation of status, role, income, companionship, or sexual activity that may be irreplaceable. A 65-year-old childless widow talked of how she missed the pleasure of the nightly sexual intercourse that she had had with her husband for the entire 40 years of their marriage. She knew that despite her "successful grieving" it was highly unlikely that she would ever recapture this pleasure.

Many widows and widowers lack the ability to replace for themselves that which has been deprived. At the same time, they are discriminated against by society from achieving for themselves what they need and want. Parkes refers to the *stigma* or change in attitude toward the woman who becomes a widow that leads to her social isolation.

The ubiquitous nature of grief and the frequency of unresolved grief

THE IMPORTANCE OF GRIEF IN CLINICAL PRACTICE

Virtually everyone must deal with grief some time in his or her lifetime. These grief reactions may follow the death of grandparents, parents, siblings, children, friends, national leaders, or celebrities. Some people also appear to experience the process of grief following situations in which a person has not died. These include knowledge of one's own impending death, abortions, separations, divorce, aging in loved ones, loss of children's dependence, alteration of body image (through aging, surgery, wearing dental braces or glasses, growing bald, losing teeth), leaving a familiar neighborhood, giving up a life's dream, "giving up" neurotic behavior, even finishing a good book.

Most people are able to experience the grief process normally. There is no information on the percentage of people who experience pathological grief. From a clinical perspective, however, it has been our experience that in 10% to 15% of patients who request out-patient treatment, pathological grief plays a central role in their psychopathology.

The failure to grieve may lead to psychopathology

The most common reaction to unresolved grief is a mild, chronic depression. In most instances this reaction is hardly noticeable. The patient may withdraw from friends, stop going to church, feel guilty in various situations, and suffer various aches and pains. More severe reactions to failure to grieve include severe depressions, schizophrenic reactions, psychosomatic disorders, or acting out behavior. Under the stress of unresolved grief, the patient will regress according to his vulnerability.

WHY PEOPLE FAIL TO GRIEVE

We find it useful for the purpose of therapy to classify the causes of failure to grieve (or pathological grief) into social and psychological factors.

Social factors

Social negation of a loss

Pathological grief may result from situations in which the loss is not socially defined as a loss. This may occur following an abortion. The expectation is either that the person will keep the event a secret or that the woman should be grateful that the procedure is completed. The situation may be further complicated by the anger directed toward the woman for being "careless" and for inconveniencing others. Similar dynamics occur when a woman gives up an infant for adoption. With both adoption and abortions, there is grief work to be done, but social support necessary for the process is often inadequate.

Because of the number of patients who present for help following an abortion or giving up a child, we routinely inquire about these possibilities in all women of child-bearing age. The diagnosis is more certain when the presentation for help occurs, as it often does, on the anniversary of the loss.

A socially unspeakable loss
Pathological grief may result when the loss is so "unspeakable" that members of the social system of the bereaved cannot be of any help. As an example, a 24-year-old, bright, attractive young woman was found dead from an overdose of morphine. There was no prior history of drug abuse. It was never determined if the death resulted from foul play, accident, or suicide. Because of the uncertainty, no one would ask the bereaved mother the usual questions that facilitate the grieving process, for example, when did it happen? where did it happen? how did it happen? The mother failed to grieve and made a suicide attempt a month after the funeral in an attempt to "join my daughter." Following the suicide attempt, the patient was referred to a psychiatrist with whom the loss could be discussed. The patient was able to grieve successfully in 10 weekly visits.

Geographic distance from social support
Unresolved grief may occur if the person is away from his social supports at the time of mourning. In one situation, a mother decided not to tell her 20-year-old daughter of the father's death until college examinations were completed. By the time the daughter returned home, the family had completed their grieving. They were perplexed over the daughter's tears and provided little in the way of support for her grief. She sought psychiatric help the following year.

Sometimes, the bereaved is socially isolated from his family because of geographic distance or psychological alienation. Some people have neither family nor close friends. They hopefully seek help from clinics or mental health personnel.

Assuming the social role of the "strong one"
Some people are designated to be the "strong ones" by those around them. In family situations they are expected to make the arrangements for the funeral and be supportive to everyone else. Needless to say, these people miss the opportunity to deal with their own grief.

The "strong one" impasse also occurs outside the family setting. For example, an operating room nurse was seen crying by her physician and nurse colleagues. They insisted that she go to the psychiatric clinic for "therapy" even though they knew her best friend had been killed in an auto accident just two days before. Her social support system believed that operating room nurses—like Marines—are not supposed to cry.

Uncertainty over the loss
When the loss is uncertain, for example, a husband who is missing in action, both the wife and the social support system are unable to deal with the possible loss.

Psychological factors

Ambivalence toward the lost person
Unresolved grief may occur when the person has profoundly ambivalent feelings — intense love and intense hate — toward the dead person. The person is frightened to grieve for fear of discovering the intensely negative and unacceptable feelings. Obsessional people who have strict and rigid super-ego structures are likely to suffer from these psychological dilemmas.

Overcathexis of the lost person
A person may be so dependent on or place such a high value on the dead person that he will not grieve in order to avoid the reality of the loss. One patient said, "Mother was half of my ego. I would not be complete without her. She cannot be dead."

Overwhelmed by multiple loss
Some people who experience multiple losses, such as the death of an entire family, have difficulty grieving on two counts. First, the loss is too over-whelming to contemplate. Second, the family who supports the grief is no longer available. One patient experienced a multiple loss as a result of five miscarriages due to a uterine defect. In therapy, the patient grieved the loss of each fetus one at a time. The patient had a name and a set of hopes and dreams for each fetus.

The need to be strong and in control
Some people do not permit themselves to grieve for fear of losing control or appearing weak to themselves and to others. One patient said that if she began to cry, she feared that the tears would never stop.

Reawakening an old loss
Some people are reluctant to grieve because the current loss reawakens a more painful loss that has not yet been dealt with. The death of a distant aunt, for instance, may reawaken the death of a mother many years ago.

THE DIAGNOSIS OF UNRESOLVED GRIEF
The diagnosis of unresolved grief may be inferred from the following histori-cal data and interview observations:

1. If a patient fails to grieve following the death of a loved one, the diagnosis of unresolved grief should be considered. The patient may not have cried, may have absented himself from the funeral, and may have put thoughts of the deceased out of his mind.
2. Unresolved grief should be considered when the patient becomes symp-tomatic on the anniversary of a loss, when the symptoms recur the same time each year, or when symptoms occur during the holidays (especially Thanksgiving and Christmas).
3. Unresolved grief should be considered when the patient avoids visiting the grave and refuses to participate in religious memorial services of loved ones when these practices are a part of the patient's culture.
4. Unresolved grief should be considered when the patient develops a chronicity of normal grief symptoms, especially persistent guilt and lowered self-esteem.
5. Unresolved grief should be considered when the patient continues to search for the lost person after a prolonged period of time. Some patients

426

make the search while they are in fugue states. Others may wander from town to town and/or act as if they are expecting the dead one to return. They may even consider suicide to effect a reunion.

6. Unresolved grief should be considered when a relatively minor event triggers symptoms of grief. This event is psychodynamically connected to the original loss.

7. Unresolved grief should be considered whenever a patient is unable to discuss the deceased with relative equanimity. When the voice cracks and quivers and the eyes become moist, unresolved grief is likely.

8. Unresolved grief should be considered when an interview is characterized by themes of loss.

9. Unresolved grief should be considered when the patient experiences bodily symptoms similar to those of the dead person after the normal period of grief.

10. Unresolved grief should be considered when the patient's relationships with friends and relatives shifts for the worse following the death. This may represent a displacement of feelings from the dead person. For example, one patient, angry at a stillbirth "that almost killed me," found it difficult to love the next infant until the grief was resolved.

THE TREATMENT OF UNRESOLVED GRIEF

In order for a delayed or incomplete grief reaction to be successfully dealt with, the person has to experience the feelings and thoughts that were initially avoided. He is likely to cry, to have detailed recollections of the dead person, to dream more actively of the dead person, to reminisce. This process is often completed in 6 to 10 weeks. With a successful outcome, we have seen patients no longer have bodily aches that plagued them from the time of the loss. They experience positive and warm feelings toward the deceased, remembering them not as they were during their dying days and in the coffin but as they were in happier times. They experience a "sweet sadness" over the deceased, not a bitterness. One patient described feeling, after completing the delayed grief, that the axe was now out of her heart. There is sometimes a feeling that time had resumed after "standing still" ever since the loss occurred. Two patients treated commented that the New Year's Eve after the regrief work was very special. "I said goodbye 1974 and goodbye 1964 (the year of the loss)." After successful regrief work, people feel increased self-esteem, less guilt, and may resume church affiliation, if that was their pattern prior to the loss. They begin to visit the cemetery. Relationships that had been compromised because of a displacement of feelings from the dead person are changed in a healthier direction. One patient who failed to grieve a miscarriage of an 8-month female fetus had extraordinary difficulty relating to her next born daughter. After successfully dealing with the grief, the patient commented on how appealing and responsive her daughter had become.

How can one assist with the regrief process? Who can provide this assistance?

For the large numbers of people who fail to grieve because of the absence of an available and supportive social matrix, help can be easily provided. The therapeutic person needs only to gently encourage the patient to discuss the loss and then to bear with the bereaved during the grief process. He or she will be carefully but subtly scrutinized by the grieving person to see whether or not there is strength, respect, and kindness. It may be helpful to educate and reassure the person as to what is expected, what is all right. We reassure the bereaved, if necessary, that they will not cry forever, permanently lose control, or go crazy if they grieve. We have never seen these untoward consequences. To the contrary, these things may occur where there is a failure to grieve. If the person laments that the past is the past and should remain buried, we reply that the past is very much in the present because it has not really been buried. Grieving is necessary in order to put the past in its proper perspective.

For those people who experience considerable difficulty in grieving, especially those for whom there are psychological causes for failure to grieve, more active measures may be necessary. Special therapeutic skills may be necessary here. The clinician may help the bereaved reconstruct memories in order to elicit the feelings. "What did she look like?" "What happened the last time you talked with her?" "Where were you standing when you visited the hospital?" "Who else was in the room?"

When failure to grieve results from strongly ambivalent feelings toward the deceased, it is useful and necessary for the person to express the negative feelings. This must be done, however, not by confrontation but by a gentle and supportive approach. For instance, the bereaved may be reassured by the clinician of the strength of the positive feelings that he knows exist. Only then may the patient be willing to verbalize the negative feelings. Sometimes it is easier to assist the bereaved to discuss "disappointments with" rather than "anger toward" the dead person. In discussing negative feelings, it is often easier for the bereaved to use words such as "irritation," "annoyance," or "aggravation" rather than "anger."

With multiple losses, the bereaved will need to deal with them one at a time.

When there is an overcathexis toward the dead person, a firm therapeutic relationship may have to be established before the bereaved dares "give up" the dead person.

The overall response to regrief work is difficult to predict. We have seen no one get worse. We have seen most people improve to varying degrees. In the most dramatic cases we have seen people improve to their level of functioning before the death occurred, even if the event occurred 25 years before. In other situations, improvement is limited by pathological personalities which are not clearly apparent until the grief work is done.

In general, helping a person with regrief work can be a most gratifying experience for a helping person.

Subjective reactions

Several conditions may develop that would *interfere* with the nurse's ability to deal adequately with the patient's grief. These are:

1. If the nurse has not successfully grieved her own losses, listening to the patient's grief may reawaken and revive the nurse's pains.
2. When the deceased resembles one of the nurse's loved ones in age, sex, or other conditions, the nurse may be too pained in contemplating and fearing a similiar disaster to support the patient's grief.

Case illustration

Pam, a 21-year-old student, was presented at a psychiatric community clinic following referral from the Student Health Service. As she talked during the interview, she would periodically dig her fingernails into her palms and she acknowledged having cut her arm on several occasions.

Pam talked of having had feelings of "falling apart" and of not being able to control herself but that she currently felt more in control of her behavior. She felt that her difficulties were caused by her being away from home for the first time. However, she would become upset when she went home because "mother is so sad and father so old."

Pam almost immediately began talking about her sister's death six years previously. She did this with a great deal of intense emotion, explaining that it was very difficult for her to talk about it because they had been very close, with sister being a "mother" to her.

Historically, mother did not notice Pam's childhood problems, but her sister did and tried to help her. Pam views herself as having been a tomboy (because father had wanted a boy and Pam had tried to please him), fat, very self-conscious, shy, and ugly because of a severe acne problem. The sister began helping Pam by getting her to lose weight and was about to take her to a dermatologist when she was murdered.

The nurse asked Pam to describe the events relevant to the murder. The sister went to work as usual the morning after a holiday. The employer called the home around 10 A.M. to find out where she was. The family became concerned and called the police who felt it was not that serious a concern for alarm at 11 A.M. but stated they would begin a search. The father went to retrace the daughter's usual path to work. The father found his daughter strangled with her stocking in an isolated field that was part of a shortcut she often took to go to work.

Pam wept at this point and said that the feelings she had were of hatred and these feelings were difficult for her to think about as they upset her so much. The resentful feelings she had were toward the police department who wouldn't respond quickly to go to look for her sister and then when the father did find the body, they sent their rookies to "mess up the clues so that the murderer was never found."

The hatred feelings were also for the townspeople who made the family feel like "freaks" and forced them to withdraw, as a family, into their house "like strange animals in a cage." The family did receive a lot of crank calls and weird letters at the time and people continually talked about the incident in the town.

Pam saw this as the reason for her subsequent withdrawal from social contacts (she had one girlfriend) and for not dating in high school. Pam could recall feeling "numb" at the funeral and remembered looking at people to see their reaction. She then recalled her grandfather's funeral when she was seven when she did the same thing and they had to take her out of the church. She did not cry at the time of her sister's death but about two years later when a person whom she liked very much died, she cried with great feeling, realizing then that she was also weeping for her sister.

After the sister's death, Pam slept in her sister's bed (Pam's had been the lower part of a trundle bed) and she wore her sister's clothes. Her sister had been two years older than Pam.

Pam frequently had nightmares about a man coming in the window with a knife to stab her and had to receive medication from a local physician before these stopped. These nightmares developed into a fear that she has continued to have where she would not allow anyone to walk behind her. (She would not even allow her boyfriend to walk behind her.) She had been to her sister's grave only twice in the six-year period.

Case analysis of unresolved grief

One can readily make the diagnosis that the patient is suffering from unresolved grief for two reasons:

1. The patient is unable to discuss with equanimity a death that occurred six years previously. With a supportive listener, she immediately began to discuss the death with intense emotion.
2. There was a history of failure to grieve at the time of the death.

As to the reasons for her inability to grieve, the patient suggests that it was because they had been very close, with the sister being a "mother" to her. This closeness is further illustrated by the patient sleeping in the sister's bed and wearing her clothes. In addition, the patient has nightmares that she too is being murdered. It becomes clear that the failure to grieve is related to some quality regarding the relationship between the patient and her sister. The data suggest two hypotheses, First, although the patient verbalizes positive feelings toward the sister, she must have harbored many negative feelings toward someone who got from mother what the patient could not get. In effect, besides loving the sister, the patient hated her. The death consequently evoked too much guilt to let the patient grieve. Digging her fingernails into her palms and cutting her arm on several occasions is a means of relieving guilt. As an alternative hypothesis, it may be postulated that the patient was so attached to the sister, as the only one who cared, that to grieve would be to acknowledge that the sister really died. By not grieving, the sister is somehow still alive.

Whichever hypothesis is correct, the nurse must provide a supportive relationship which will allow the patient to mourn her sister. In the process, the nurse will discover and help the patient realize and understand the nature of the relationship to the sister that made the grief process so difficult.

SUMMARY Unresolved grief is an important clinical condition that nurses will assess and diagnose in their work within a community mental health setting. This chapter reviewed the normal grief process, why people fail to grieve, how one can make the diagnosis of unresolved grief, and the nursing management of unresolved grief.

REFERENCES AND SUGGESTED READINGS

Burnside, Irene M. (1969). "Grief Work in the Aged Patient," *Nursing Forum*, **8,** No. 4, 416–27.

Gerber, Irwin (1969). "Bereavement and the Acceptance of Professional Services," *Community Mental Health Journal*, **5,** No. 6, 487–95.

Hagen, Joan M. (1974). "Infant Death: Nursing Interaction and Intervention with Grieving Families," *Nursing Forum*, **13,** No. 4, 371–85.

Herman, Sonya J. (1974). "Divorce: A Grief Process," *Perspectives in Psychiatric Care*, **12,** No. 4, 108–112.

Jackson, Pat Ludder (1974). "Chronic Grief," *American Journal of Nursing*, **74,** No. 7, 1288–91.

Lindemann, Erick (1944). "Symptomatology and Management of Acute Grief." *American Journal of Psychiatry*, **101,** No. 1, 141–48.

Miles, Helen S., and Dorothea R. Hays (1975). "Widowhood," *American Journal of Nursing*, **75,** No. 2, 280–82.

Parkes, Colin Murray (1972). *Bereavement: Studies of Grief in Adult Life*. New York: International Universities Press, Inc.

431

THE ELDERLY
IN THE COMMUNITY

25

A statistical profile of the over 20 million Americans — 10% of the population — over 65 years of age showed an aggregation of poverty, sickness, loneliness, and powerlessness. Claire Townsend contributes the following observation in the Ralph Nader Study Group Report publication.

> The conventional injustices of the land bear down heavily on the elderly. Consumer fraud, inflation, fixed pensions and social security benefits, street crime, absence of mass transit, spiraling rents and housing costs, swelling medical and drug bills, and the virtual end of the extended family unit have a severe discriminatory impact on old people. But most gnawing and omnipresent is the psychological devastation heaped on the old by a society that lets them know in many ways, small and large, that they are no longer filled with life's potential and warmth — in short, that they are considered a drag.[1]

Dr. Howard P. Rome further describes this behavioral response generated by sociopolitical attitudes as *gerontophobia*.[2] He says that there is a truly morbid fear of aging and its ultimate consequences that prompts the shunning of the elderly.

MENTAL HEALTH OF THE ELDERLY We are at a point in time where the concepts of mental health, mental illness, and normality are still very vague. There are no clear-cut definitions. What is becoming clear is that mental health is influenced by age, sex, and ethnicity. People with various class and cultural backgrounds characteristically view health and mental health behavior differently. There are no norms established for what is considered useful or helpful mental attitudes and behavior for people at any life stage.

[1]Claire Townsend, *Old Age: The Last Segregation,* Ralph Nader's Study Group Reports (New York: Bantam Books, Inc., published jointly with Grossman Publishers, 1971), p. 29.
[2]Howard P. Rome, "Introductory Remarks," *Psychiatric Annals,* **2,** No. 10 (1972), 7.

Concept of leisure

One concept that plays a significant part in the mental health of the older person is that of leisure. Various definitions of the concept have been given. They range from classifying leisure as the absence of work to classifying leisure in more positive terms as including activity not related to obligations of family, work, or society and that the person selects at will for either diversion or relaxation and includes the free exercise of creative capacity.[3]

Doctors Charles Gaitz and Chad Gordon have proposed the following definition of leisure: "Leisure activity is a personal activity in which expressive meanings have primacy over instrumental meanings."[4] They also provide an ordering of objectives of leisure as the continuum of expressive involvement intensity. Their study of leisure activities, value preference, social attitudes, and various aspects of mental health was conducted on 1441 adults between the ages of 20 and 94 in Houston, Texas, in 1970.[5] Seventeen specific leisure activities were categorized as follows:

1. RELAXATION. Solitude, being alone, doing nothing, daydreaming.

2. DIVERSION. Spectator sports, watching sports live or on television, entertaining at home or going to a friend's home, reading, cultural consumption such as listening to music or looking at paintings, going to the movies, television viewing.

3. DEVELOPMENT. Organizations such as belonging to a social club or organization, travel for pleasure, not business.

4. CREATIVITY. Cultural production such as singing, painting, drawing, discussion groups, home activities such as sewing, mending, decorating, working in the yard, and cooking for family or friends.

5. SENSUAL TRANSCENDENCE. Participation in sports or exercise, hunting or target practice with guns, outdoor activities such as going to the country or beach for camping, dancing, and drinking.[6]

Age and participation in leisure activity

Four patterns of relationship of age and leisure activities were observed in the analysis of the participants in the study.[7]

1. There was a decline in frequency in seven activities with increasing age. These activities were dancing and drinking, outdoor activities, attending movies, traveling, reading, participating in sports or physical exercise and, for men, using guns for hunting.

2. Four of the leisure activities maintained a stable position across all age levels. These activities were entertaining friends, television viewing, cultural consumption, and cultural production.

3. Four of the activities show a pattern of high participation frequency until a

[3]Joffre Dumazedier, *Toward a Society of Leisure* (New York: The Free Press, 1967).

[4]Charles M. Gaitz and Chad Gordon, "Leisure and Mental Health Late in the Life Cycle," *Psychiatric Annals*, **2**, No. 11, 43.

[5]Ibid., p. 51.

[6]Ibid., p. 54.

[7]Ibid., 55–56.

peak near the middle of the life cycle and then a decrease in participation in the older age groups. Clubs and organization activities peaked at 40–54, home interests peaked early in maturity and again after retirement, discussion of issues was high at 55–64 for women and at 20–29 and 40–54 for men (double peak periods for men), and watching spectator sports peaked at 30–39 for both sexes.

4. Two activities showed an increasing participation in older ages — that is, solitude and for men only, cooking.

The significance of studies such as this one has to do with levels of health care and the role of the nurse in prevention of mental health problems in the elderly. Careful assessment should be done periodically with people starting at the middle years of life or earlier in order to identify leisure activities currently engaged in and those of potential interest.

Concept of retirement

A second important concept in the mental health of the older person is retirement. Various definitions are suggested for the concept of retirement. Dr. Dana Farnsworth has proposed the following definition: the organization of one's life with the goal of having as large a proportion of pleasant and rewarding experiences as physical, intellectual, and economic conditions permit.[8]

Retirement is not always planned. For some, it may be abrupt and seemingly arbitrary, and the person may feel victimized by the process. In the service of a person's mental health, this situation should be avoided. Therefore, it is suggested that people always keep in mind the possibilities of job disruption prior to their voluntary retirement as well as plans for the retirement period.

ALTERNATIVES IN RETIREMENT

Maintaining One's Life-style	Changing One's Life-style
Stay in familiar environment: strengthen family ties	Move to new environment: develop new associates
Stay in same line of work: supplement income	Change to new job or interest: explore new interests or hobbies; volunteer work
Providing for health care: familiar resources	Find new health resources: private care; clinic care
Kind of leisure activities: existing within the community	Adapt to new leisure activities: select new locale for new activities

Although there are many variables involved in making decisions about where to live during retirement, some attention must be paid to the health of the individual and to his economic independence. These two variables are major influences on the person's life-style.

[8]Dana L. Farnsworth, "Preparing for Retirement," *Psychiatric Annals,* **2,** No. 11 (1972), 16.

Stall factors in retirement

Disruption of any pattern of behavior has the potential to create a crisis. Such is the situation with retirement. The sudden or abrupt change from a work pattern to a nonwork pattern presents special dilemmas and issues for the individual. Confronting an entirely new routine, being forced to find new ways to meet basic needs, and developing a new circle of associates may precipitate a stall.

Suggestions to correct the stall are:

1. Planning or preparing for retirement by developing a wide range of interests early in life or certainly by the middle years. Such interests may be specific to one's life work or may be unrelated to employment or career.
2. Developing an attitude of readiness for change and welcoming it. Such an attitude needs to be developed over time and not at age 65.
3. Expanding friendships so that those lost through moving or death are balanced by new associates.
4. Maintaining contact with younger people as a means of passing along values and standards from one generation to another.
5. Learning how to use privacy and enjoy privacy as a way to reflect on the meaning of life.
6. Engaging in group discussions which specifically deal with the issue of leisure and retirement. Discussion groups may provide valuable insights for living in this period of the life cycle, and they may provide support through group membership for the emotional aspects of retirement.
7. Maintaining a sense of humor. This will provide an antidote to feelings of loneliness and suspiciousness.
8. Consistency in diet and exercise is a guiding principle for the retired person. Maintaining a homeostatic state is a major contributor to health maintenance.
9. Maintaining one's integrity. Much of the style of the person that has developed during one's early years carries with him in later years. Integrity may or may not have been a guiding personality trait; however, it is this characteristic that is a focus in the later years. Erik Erikson has defined this quality as follows:

Integrity is the acceptance of one's one and only life cycle as something that had to be, and that, by necessity, permitted of no substitutions . . . . is a comradeship with the ordering ways of distant times and different pursuits . . . Although aware of the relativity of all the various life-styles which have given meaning to human striving, the possessor of integrity is ready to defend the dignity of his own life-style against all physical and economic threats. For he knows that an individual life is the accidental coincidence of but one life cycle with but one segment of history; and that for him all human integrity stands or falls with the one style of integrity of which he partakes.[9]

Case illustration

The following case illustrates one couple and their attitudes toward retirement and health.

[9]Erik H. Erikson, *Childhood and Society,* 2nd ed. (New York: W. W. Norton, 1963), p. 268.

Arthur Mills and his wife differ in their attitudes toward retirement and health. Although retired for 8 years, Mr. Mills is not yet reconciled to retirement. Mrs. Mills, however, accepts retirement enthusiastically; she likes to refer to her husband and herself as a "retired couple" and is eager that both of them enjoy the privileges of retirement to the extent that their resources permit.

Mr. Mills is determined, even though he has ailments, to keep away from doctors. Mrs. Mills is resolved, even though she feels well, to seek medical attention.

Mr. Mills is 73, 2 years younger than his wife. They were originally from Canada, where their children were born and where the couple lived until they were in their 40s. Then they came to Boston 30 years ago, not planning to stay long, but they have lived here since. They have 9 children, 48 grandchildren, 12 great-grandchildren, and numerous siblings, cousins, nephews, and nieces.

Mrs. Mills is a Baptist and has been actively religious most of her life. Mr. Mills professes no religious affiliation. They rent a five-room apartment in a three-story tenement. With them lives a daughter, aged 32, and her three children. The daughter moved in with her parents several years ago after her husband left her.

The Millses own a car, radio, television, and stereo set. Household furnishings are old and worn but adequate. Although reticent about discussing their sources of income, they apparently get along comfortably. They own small properties in Canada which provide a little financial security and a great deal of emotional security. The daughter receives money from aid-to-dependent children.

A shipwright and carpenter most of his life, Mr. Mills retired 8 years ago from work at a shipyard. Although other older men interviewed differ in their ways of accepting retirement, the point is that they accept it at some level. Mr. Mills does not. He seems to regard retirement as an unpleasant interruption in his pattern of living instead of an irreversible alteration. He sees himself as a shipwright who is not working, not as a retired shipwright.

He does occasional odd jobs in carpentry for local householders and businessmen, and he busies himself in repairs in his own dwelling. However, he considers these things as not really constituting a man's work; for him, they are "just jigging around, just choring around a little." *Real* work for him consists of hiring out as a full-time worker for an industrial employer; it consists, in short, of his old job at the shipyard.

He has a driving need to keep busy. However, because of his way of defining work, odd jobs often succeed in frustrating instead of satisfying him. For instance, a householder asks Mr. Mills to repair a stairway. Mr. Mills is agreeable, provided that he be paid an hourly or weekly wage and that he be responsible for only two operations — (1) specifying the needed materials and (2) doing the actual work. Typically, however, the householder prefers that Mr. Mills also purchase the required materials and that payment be arranged by *contract* for the entire job. In a word, while Mr. Mills insists on defining his role as strictly that of skilled wage worker, the householder usually wants to deal with him as a contractor. Unable to accommodate to the "business" operations inherent in the contractor role, Mr. Mills turns down more proffered odd jobs than he accepts.

The Millses have married children in Canada and in the midwest and farwest of the United States. Mrs. Mills would like her husband and herself to devote more than half the year to visiting their children, most of whom are willing and able to underwrite the couple's travel expenses. Mr. Mills gave in and accompanied his wife on an air trip to California during the winter. He is now adamantly opposed to taking "vacation trips" in any season except the summer. He does not want to accept "charity" from his children; moreover, taking a long trip in any but the appropriate season for vacations would imply his tacit surrender to the status of "retired."

Mr. Mills believes that one should see a doctor only when one is sick. The question is, when is one sick? Mr. Mills has arthritis, which increasingly hampers his movements. Mrs. Mills has cataracts in both eyes, and her vision is progressively deteriorating. Both spouses, nevertheless, and Mr. Mills in particular, regard themselves as essentially healthy people, getting along in years but "better than average" for their age.

For Mr. Mills, health is dependent on work, and work is the hub about which life revolves. In other words, by working one stays healthy. Health, in turn, consists of the ability to work, eat, and sleep; ill-health is a breakdown in any of the three, particularly in the ability to work. Although arthritis handicaps his movements, he forcefully rejects the idea of seeking medical care; to do so would necessitate restructuring his concept of himself as a person normally able to work, eat, and sleep.

Mrs. Mills, however, says that although she feels remarkably well, she is determined to see a doctor about her cataracts. She has long put off "having something done" about them and is now resolved as a matter of virtue to have them removed. Over the years, she apparently learned to live amicably with her cataracts and seems not to regard them as a physical impairment. She now feels that they are a *moral* impairment. It is her duty as a good Christian, she says, to stop pampering herself and to submit the cataracts to surgery.

Mrs. Mills' dynamic issue is to be cared about and her main source of ego supplies are (1) interpersonal relationships within her ramified kinship circle and in the community and (2) church and religion. Mr. Mills' dynamic issue is to be successful, and his primary emotional investment is in *work* and how to define his role as a nonworker in a world of work.

Four of the Mills' offspring live in the Boston area, and Mrs. Mills in continually engaged in visiting or being visited by them. Each summer she and her husband take an auto trip to Canada. Significantly, Mrs. Mills likes the trip because of the kinfolk she will see. Mr. Mills, however, looks forward to such things as working out the mileage, stops, and schedules of the trip; at the same time he wonders what he will *do* after they have been in Canada a few days.

Even after 30 years in the same community, the Millses are unsure whether they are country folk who live in the city or city folk who originated in the country. Both regard the city as essentially an "immoral and wicked place," but react differently to this belief. Mrs. Mills deals with her immediate neighbors as though they were residents of a small village. She promotes much visiting back and forth and, in general, interacts at a high rate with the neighbors. In a sense, she has carved out for herself a small island of neighborliness apart from the wicked city.

For Mr. Mills, the community is a place where everyone wants something without working for it, where parents congregate in bars and children roam the streets. He makes no distinction between immediate neighbors and others — "they" are all city dwellers and equally bad.

This case may be discussed in various ways, for example, in terms of patterns of adjustment, health needs, and the problems this family faces as it progresses through the later stage of the life cycle.

MENTAL HEALTH CARE OF THE ELDERLY

Health care of the elderly in the United States receives low priority in national interests and even lower priority in the provisions for mental health care. Insurance coverage is necessary for prevention and for treatment of psychiatric concerns. Professionals are working with Medicare and Medicaid to insure adequate coverage for emotional illness.

Institutional response

There are many problems in delivering services to the elderly that may be classified as patterns of avoidance. Institutions establish criteria for admission, and they use these criteria to avoid dealing with a specific group of people. Many people are denied admission to state mental hospitals because they are diagnosed as having a social problem instead of a psychiatric condition. The family may say that they cannot manage the elderly person at home. The hospital, however, says that the symptoms are not of a psychiatric nature. In other situations, older people who are still confused or wandering in their behavior are sent home from general hospitals diagnosed as senile and not "ill." These are elderly people who have behavior problems resulting from the aging process. Such people may be suffering from reversible brain conditions caused by malnutrition, anemia, congestive heart failure, iatrogenic complications of tranquilizers, and infections. By failing to have such conditions properly diagnosed and a plan of care started, acute brain syndromes may become fixed and chronic in nature. Our society has not dealt with this developmental crisis situation as to where they may go, and who should care for them.

Reports indicate that people with other serious emergencies are also denied care. These people become increasingly depressed, preoccupied, and angry; they slowly take their own lives over time by refusing to eat, take medicines, or see physicians and nurses. No one is really interested in them and they are not regarded as dangerous to themselves. They refuse help and therefore are not considered eligible for legal commitment. In high-crime areas, the incidence of victimization of the older person is seen through robberies, beatings, and other criminal acts. The elderly do not report these crimes because they feel powerless and they fear reprisal. However, there is growing evidence that the nursing profession is identifying this as a crisis area so that nursing intervention may be utilized.

Transferring the mental hospital patient

A trend in community health has been to transfer long-term hospitalized patients out into the community in an attempt to equalize society's commitment to the care of its citizens. These patients have been transferred to halfway houses, nursing homes, and foster care homes where there is a paid authority person who watches over the groups of patients.

Many pitfalls involved in transferring patients have been identified. Critics of this trend state that the movement has often been precipitous, indiscriminate, and wholesale.[10] Critics do not deny the importance of alternatives to long-term hospital care, but they favor out-patient treatment, home care programs, and small-scale socio–medical residences for the older patient.[11] They argue that older patients are excluded from the mainstream of health care, research, and training and that patients receive inadequate evaluation and preparation for transfer.

Social policy issues

There have been many criticisms of the use of federal and state funding for the care of the elderly. Monies have been allocated for psychiatric–social care of the long-term and elderly patient. Critics of legislation point out that the federal money allocated has not resulted in high quality programs of health standards.[12]

Another public policy issue involves the question of who may receive payment for treating the elderly. Studies show that private psychiatrists see a very small group of the population and that this group is generally young, intelligent, and successful. Health insurance has historically granted rights only to the physician to receive payment; it has withheld funds from other health professionals who work with the elderly, specifically nurses. Psychiatric nursing groups in various states are proposing legislation for third-party payment for reimbursement of psychiatric-community mental health nursing services. Such legislation would permit psychiatric nurses to be more involved with the care of the elderly.

The concept of the right to treatment implies that the purpose of hospitalization, and specifically involuntary hospitalization, must be for treatment and not for custodial care or punishment. Judge David L. Bazelon stated, "The need for an individualized treatment plan cannot be overemphasized. Without such a plan there can be no evidence that the hospital has singled out the patient for treatment as an individual with his own unique problems.[13]

COMMUNITY MENTAL HEALTH AND THE ELDERLY The combination of increasing costs for health care and consumer demands for quality health care is having two important consequences. First, medical services are increasingly regarded as a right rather than a privilege. Second, there is a growing awareness that the delivery of health services is a system

[10]Robert N. Butlar, "Mental Health Care in Old Age: Conflicts in Public Policy," *Psychiatric Annals,* **2,** No. 10 (1972), 33.

[11]Ibid., p. 37.

[12]Ibid., p. 40.

[13]Ibid., p. 44.

rather than a component problem. Patients, nurses, physicians, social workers, psychologists, health counselors, nutritionists, and other members of the health team must be viewed as interacting components of a health system instead of as independent entities serving to fragment patient care.

People are recognizing the need to plan in a system context to ensure that proposed social legislation will lead to desired goals. New ways of managing health systems are being implemented in order to assure access of quality care for the elderly and a moderation of the inflationary spiral in medical care costs, at least partly by encouraging the use of varying levels of care appropriate to the health problem.

Health education

The elderly are encouraged to obtain the kinds of early diagnostic health services that will enhance the quality of life and reduce dependence on crisis health care which is often more stressful and costly. Prevention, through education of the individual and society at large, and governmental support and concern were expectations of the 1971 White House Conference on Aging. It was hoped that this conference would provide a major breakthrough in the field of aging.

One issue that was explored focused on the right to good health and the right to receive efficient methods of health services as an underlying principle of the Conference's "Declaration of Aging Rights."[14] Health education was identified as an effective tool for helping people meet their needs and improve the quality of their lives. Goerke and Stebbins[15] define health education as "that function of health and allied services which seeks to bring about change in health related behavior." All individual behavior is considered to be health related with some forms being health directed. Although many factors motivate behavior, to some, concern for health appears to be of relatively minor importance.

According to Goerke, health education "is a form of planned intervention attempting to influence largely unplanned, natural processes in such a way as to bring about an improved health status."[16] Dolfman refers to health as a family of concepts which in operational contexts may be equated with the concepts of function, stress, and adaptation.[17] To elaborate, this encompassing health concept enables the individual to function in his environment and make progress toward achieving goals and objectives; it eliminates stress laden forces which may be harmful to the person; it improves an individual's ability to adapt, to cope, and to interact; and it concentrates his attention on acceptable or normal limits.

[14]Thomas Hickey and Claire T. Davies, "The White House Conference on Aging: An Exercise in Policy Formation," *Aging and Human Development,* Vol. 3, 1972.

[15]Lenor S. Goerke and Ernest L. Stebbins, *Mustard's Introduction to Public Health* (New York: Macmillan Co., 1968), p. 44.

[16]Ibid., p. 412.

[17]Michael L. Dolfman, "Health Planning—A Method for Generating Program Objectives," *American Journal of Public Health,* March, 1973, pp. 238–39.

Communication of health knowledge is not sufficiently motivational to bring about change in health related behavior. In order for the needs of the elderly to be more effectively responded to, an analysis of their way of life, of their emotions and aspirations, of their beliefs, of their levels of education, and of their perception of their own personal and group needs should be evaluated.

Studies strongly urge that health professionals engage in human dialogue so that they will be able to take into account the activities, thoughts, and feelings of senior citizens and so that they will be able to seek out reliable and valid information. This will help to reduce the sociocultural distance between the health professional and the community being served.

Assessment

In working with all three levels of health care (health maintenance, health restoration, and health reorganization), one must be familiar with community resources available to the elderly, review problem areas specific to aging, understand the interpersonal relationship issues with the elderly, be aware of their spiritual needs, dietary considerations and susceptibility to particular illnesses, and know the resources for medical help and the issues of housing, economics, and transportation for the elderly.

Essential attributes of the clinician are being a good listener and sensitive observer. These skills are conducive to data gathering and promote optimal clinician–citizen contact. Several interviews might be needed to ensure a frank discussion of health concerns. The elderly person may not be able to clearly distinguish between symptoms of illness and symptoms that they attribute to the aging process; thus, the clinician should see the person periodically in order to clarify certain points.

The interview process with the elderly person has special considerations inherent in it, specifically the assessment of the hearing capacity, the visual capacity, and the comprehension capacity of the person.

Hearing capacity Hearing and seeing are very real concerns of the elderly; therefore, when interviewing them, the interviewer must physically be within an easy hearing distance. Face-to-face contact is essential; the person must be able to see the lips of the interviewer. Also, the elderly person may say that one ear is better for hearing, and he may prefer to sit in a certain position. The best rule of thumb is to ask if the person can hear you talking to him.

Visual capacity The vision of the elderly is an equal concern for the interviewer, and the clinician should be aware of the two most common eye conditions of the elderly, cataracts and glaucoma. If the person has either of those two conditions, the interviewer may have to sit closer to the person in order to be seen.

Comprehension capacity The aging process often slows down the ability of the person to receive information and promptly interpret it in order to be able to answer a question. The interviewer must adjust the technique of asking questions in order to compensate for this capacity in the interviewee. Techniques which facilitate and increase the comprehension capacity of the interviewee include rewording long sentences into shorter ones so that the person may understand more clearly. Speaking slowly will increase comprehension. Too many questions may confuse the elderly person. It is also essential to clarify the purpose of the interview so that the person will not become alarmed by the questions being asked.

Stall factors   Signs of an impending stall in the interview are diminished attention span, physical tiring which may be due to a physical illness or medication, shutting the eyes during the interview, watching a television program during the interview, turning the head away from the interviewer, and fidgeting with items or clothing. When the interviewer sees these signs, he should terminate the interview; if the questions have not been sufficiently answered, the interviewer should try to arrange another interview.

Assessment and case formulation

The following interview guide was devised to assess the health of the elderly person.[18] It may be used in total or in part when talking with any older person about his health.

Assessment guide

Identifying data   Name, address, age, sex, place of birth, marital status, education, occupation.

Health data   How would you describe your health: good, fair, poor?

What does being healthy mean to you?

In general, how would you describe your health in comparison with most people your age: better, the same, poorer?

Do you have any of the following? If so, is it handicapping?

Diabetes	Hypertension
Arthritis	Cardiovascular difficulty
Emphysema	Circulatory difficulty
Asthma	Parkinsonism
Chronic bronchitis	Gastrointestinal difficulty

What have you been told about your health condition?

How do you feel about your physical condition?

Do you have a family physician? Last visit? Frequency of visits? Does he make home visits in emergencies?

Are you on any medications? If yes, what kind and how often do you take them?

Do you have any difficulty hearing? (Observe)

[18]Cecile Therese Couture, "Health Needs of the Aging," unpublished paper, July, 1974.

Do you have a seeing problem? Last eye checkup?

Do you go to a dentist? Last visit? Do you have dentures?

Do you see a podiatrist? Any foot difficulties, such as painful corns, bunions, callouses?

How do you take care of your medical expenses? Do you receive any medical or financial assistance?

Have you been tested for diabetes? Have you had a pap smear?

Activities at home: mobility

Do you have pain or stiffness in your joints?

Do you have difficulty walking? Climbing stairs?

Have you fallen in the past year?

Are you physically active each day? Are you more active than necessary?

How do you arrange for housecleaning?

Do you have a breathing problem?

What is your sleeping pattern?

Eating

Can you shop for groceries without physical difficulty?

Can you prepare your own meals? With whom do you eat?

Are you on a special diet suggested by a physician?

Is your appetite good?

Do you have any problems with elimination?

Do you have some of the following foods every day?

> meat or fish; eggs or cheese
> bread, rice, potato, cereal, or macaroni
> milk or dairy products
> fresh or canned fruit
> green and yellow vegetables

Can you manage eating utensils?

What is your present weight? Is this your normal or usual weight?

Outside activities

Do you know your neighbors well enough to socialize with them?

Where do your close friends live?

Are there members of your family with whom you keep in close contact?

Do you belong to or participate in any church or club activities?

What do you do in your leisure time? What are your hobbies?

Do you ever feel lonely? How do you handle the feeling?

Do you feel that transportation in this area is adequate for you?

Are you familiar with any of the community services available in your community? Do you use any of these resources?

Economics

What is your major source of income?

Do you have an additional source of income?

Is your income adequate per month?

Attitudes and
opinions

What do you like most about your life now?

What troubles you most about your life now?

What recent changes have taken place in your life?

How do you feel about your personal contacts with your family and friends?

In what way do you think your present life could be improved?

How do the next 5 years look to you?

Case illustration

The following case illustrates how two interviews provide data for formulation of a health plan:

Mr. Philip Dean is 73 years old and is a widower. He retired from his job 10 years ago, shortly before his wife died. His address for the past 5 years has been a rooming house in which he lives alone in a shabby second-story room. Informed years ago by a physician that he has low blood pressure, he admits also to suffering from rheumatism in neck and shoulder, increasing short-windedness, and impaired hearing and vision. He is without teeth. On income provided by Old Age Assistance and occasional aid from his married sons, he subsists in chronic poverty. Although two married sons live in the area, he sees them only at irregular intervals; his youngest son, unmarried, has been out of touch with him for years.

It would hardly be surprising if, for Mr. Dean, old age were a lonely existence and empty of meaning. In point of fact, however, it is not. In a universe centering around his rooming house, his days are full of things to do and people to see. He is a busy man. He is "too busy" to visit his sons for more than a few days at a time; he was "too busy" to talk with the nurse for more than two interviews; and, though admitting that a thorough physical examination would be a good thing, insists that he has been "too busy" during the past several years to have it done.

Mr. Dean is Irish, Catholic, and a life-long resident of the community in which he now lives. One of four children, he left school in the sixth grade to go to work after his father died. In 1926, at the age of 30, he married a neighborhood girl. Three sons, of whom the first two were twins, were born to the couple in the next 4 years. Before and after marriage, he worked at a variety of semi-skilled jobs, completing his work career with 20 years of employment in a pharmaceutical firm. He is a semi-skilled handyman, competent in a variety of trades but a skilled specialist in none.

When his wife suffered a heart attack in 1956, Mr. Dean gave up his job to stay home and care for her. Retirement was apparently not a severely traumatic experience for him. Although he found himself at loose ends for a few weeks, he soon became absorbed in looking after his wife's sickbed needs and in doing miscellaneous carpentry, plumbing, and painting repairs in the apartment. His wife died several months after falling ill, and Mr. Dean moved out of the seven-room apartment in which he had spent most of his married life.

During the next few years, at their urging, he lived in succession with each of his married sons. He still finds it painful to discuss the latter experience: "I nearly went crazy. You're always in the way of the daughter-in-law. Even if you go to your room and sit there, you go crazy; you're still in the way. They say if you live with your own daughter, it's different—she's on your side. But a daughter-in-law, she's not on your side. How can she be? Your're just an old man, and no matter what you do, you're in the way." Mr. Dean was intensely aware that no matter what he did, his sheer presence created multiple strains in the families of his daughter-in-laws. In addition, living with his sons triggered feelings of social uselessness.

Over the objection of his sons, both of whom live in the suburbs, the father moved back to the city. He obtained a room in his present rooming house where he has now lived for 5 years. During that time he succeeded in making a comfortable adjustment to the rooming house's patterns of activity, human interactions and facilities.

On a typical day he wakes at 5 A.M. and boils water for tea on his electric plate. Outside his door he finds a copy of the previous evening's newspaper left for him by a roomer who has read it the evening before. With his tea, Mr. Dean reads the newspaper and smokes his first cigarette. He then tidies the room and listens to the radio news. Out of consideration for adjoining roomers who work, Mr. Dean waits until they have gone before visiting the common bathroom to wash and shave.

During the day he performs a number of voluntary chores about the house. He empties trash baskets, cleans up yard litter, and occasionally mows a small grassy area. He sometimes does light plumbing or carpentry repairs. In the winter he clears snow from the house steps. He looks after the house in the absence of the proprietress and her husband. In the late afternoon, when roomers return from work, he looks forward to gossiping with them about sports, politics, or rooming house affairs. With paint purchased by his son, Mr. Dean is in the process of repainting some of his room furniture and is planning to paint the room itself.

He has numerous acquaintances in the neighborhood; during the warm weather months he spends hours in "passing the time of day" with them. Most of his relationships are superficial, in that none of them involve a heavy emotional investment on his or the other's part.

His evening meal is his main one. Occasionally, he eats at a nearby cafeteria, where he maintains first-name relationships with most patrons and a joking relationship with the counter man. On his last visit, the counter man told him, "You know, Phil, you'd be a good looking fellow if you had teeth."

Usually, however, he prepares his evening meal in his room. Although his electric plate is an inexpensive single-unit type, he has learned to use it with remarkable efficiency. On the evening prior to the interview, Mr. Dean prepared a meal consisting of two lamb chops, mashed potatoes, string beans, spinach, a slice of bread, tapioca pudding, and two cups of tea. Preparation time for the meal, a somewhat more substantial one than he ordinarily eats, was one hour.

He lacks teeth. Years ago he had them extracted, expecting to return one day to the dentist to be fitted with new dentures. Somehow, the day never came. At present, he is satisfied with his hardened gums and accommodates to their limitations by avoiding difficult foods.

Unlike some elderly people, Mr. Dean has no difficulty in referring to himself as "old." Indeed, because he is "old," he regards his ailments neither as preventable not curable but as part of the normal insults of aging.

Formulation of a health plan

A major concern of the elderly is their fear of having a "spell of illness." Interviews with the elderly have revealed that they are concerned about not being able to find a physician in times of need, and they are especially aware of the decrease in home visits that physicians make. As a result, often the person must go to the hospital emergency room where there may be long tedious hours of waiting. The elderly have many concerns about acute medical illnesses, for example, the high cost of hospital services, the fear and apprehension associated with being taken to the hospital by ambulance, and the additional financial implications for residents who wish to be taken to hospitals outside the ambulance zone.

Careful consideration should be given to the pitfalls in this procedure in the event that the person is not sufficiently ill to warrant hospital admission. Often the individual must return weary, weak, ailing, confused, and alone to an empty apartment without assistance or follow-up care. For many, this is a traumatic experience. Also, the elderly who live alone fear being locked up in their apartments at night "in case something might happen," but they do not dare leave their doors unlatched because "you never know who might come in."

Further complaints of the elderly are that they are forced to wait one, two, or even three months for an appointment only to receive a superficial examination, a new drug prescription (without evaluation of the medication now being taken by the patient), and little psychological support. Such remarks as "What do you expect at 72?" "Go home and stop worrying," "I can't perform miracles," or "That's just old age" have turned off the aged and have led to serious, irreversible physical and psycho–social problems stemming from neglect to report legitimate symptoms of ill health for fear of appearing ridiculous.

It is acknowledged that there is a shortage of physicians, but Finch and Egeberg[19] point out that this shortage is made even worse because of the increasing number of physicians who are not actually engaged in patient care. Not only are physicians scarce, but many will not accept Medicare or Medicaid patients. And, again, the medical services that are actually performed may come too late if the client has waited too long.

Nursing is becoming more involved in the care of the elderly precisely for this reason. Research into nursing interventions are going on in the attempt to define ways to better deliver health services. Nurse–practitioners are setting up screening clinics in life center homes where the elderly live in

[19]Robert Finch and Robert Egeberg, "Report to the President," *U.S. News and World Report,* July 21, 1969.

units. Nurses are able to diagnose and treat minor conditions and screen for those conditions that require medical attention.

Intervention

Since families are becoming less capable of meeting the demands of this community concern, it then becomes a concern for the care givers in the community. Thus, community mental health centers and community health centers have felt an increasing need to explore their resources in an attempt to deal with this issue.

In the area of primary prevention, community resources are establishing drop-in centers for the elderly, Golden Age clubs, and other similar groups in order to meet the social needs of the elderly. The groups participate in other community projects and make significant contributions to society. For example, the elderly in some communities become foster grandparents to children in mental retardation institutions or in orphanages.

Secondary prevention involves direct services to the elderly. An important intervention is based on the concept of time. In the aging process many physical, emotional, and social abilities decline. Taking this into account, one learns to pace therapeutic activities in order to spend more time with the geriatric patient. For example, providing adequate lighting helps the older person compensate for decreased visual acuity; speaking slowly and clearly gives the older person more time to process the communication and to respond; allowing enough time for teaching the patient health care habits or how to use equipment to complete the activities of daily living, such as eating, dressing, and moving from activity to activity, are essential.[20]

During an acute health situation that requires hospitalization, nurses must diagnose the common behavior problems of the elderly that are not related to their illness. Nurses who work with elderly patients need to differentiate between the behavior of a patient with a senile psychosis (see Chapter 18) and a patient along the behavioral continuum who is forgetful or momentarily mistakes the nurse for someone else. This latter behavior is due to the aging process of the brain which makes recall of current information much more difficult than recall of the past. The nurse intervenes by reorienting the patient to the hospital environment. Dealing with this behavior in a calm and human manner is reassuring to the patient who is easily frightened and upset in finding himself in an unfamiliar setting.

The tertiary level of nursing intervention involves the health reorganization process. For this intervention, the elderly person may be in an extended care facility or in the home environment.

The visiting nurse or community mental health nurse is often the liaison agent between an acute care facility and an extended care facility. The nurse must be involved in the patient's care from the moment he is admitted to the

---

[20] Virginia Stone, "Giving the Older Person Time," *American Journal of Nursing,* **69,** No. 10 (1969), 2124–27.

hospital so that she may learn the level of functioning that the patient may be able to reach after he has been treated for the acute phase of the illness. The nurse then usually works with family members in order to understand their perception of the problem and their requests in the health reorganization process.

If the family cannot adequately handle the relative after the acute phase of treatment (health restoration), community services should be considered. The nurse would work as the liaison between the hospital and the community services in order to maintain continuity of patient care. Following the after-care phase, the family may then be able to care for the patient, and, of course, the nurse or health worker would be involved in this period.

Health leadership

To produce changes in working with the elderly, mental health professionals must assume a leadership role in defining the resources for the aged in the community. Colleague and collaborative relationships with other health professionals must be fostered. Health education at the individual and small group level, program evaluation, planning and implementation, assisting at interdisciplinary conferences, participation and application of research findings, and participation in the cooperative effort are strategies to help initiate change. The nurse often plays the critical role in bringing about change by presenting issues and by representing organizational support. Actively working with community groups on their feelings and attitudes toward the elderly and confronting the community with the issue of gerontophobia are first steps. If people are able to express their fears and confront the issue, they may be freer to support services and programs that bring the elderly into the mainstream of community life.

Drop-in clinics in housing units are an excellent resource for the elderly. The basic goal of the drop-in clinic is to maximize client health. Outreach through personal interview or telephone interview provided by a 24-hour telephone service makes social contact possible and dispels feelings of isolation and loneliness experienced by the elderly, especially in the evening and morning hours. A drug and treatment monitoring service, follow-up on doctor or clinic appointments, planned transportation, accurate referral information and follow-up, and the availability of the nurse-physician team in case of unforeseen illness (not serious enough for hospitalization but necessitating nursing care) would be beneficial and would appreciable reduce the cost of health maintenance.

Evaluation

Evaluation of the effectiveness of a community program is very important. Indicators of success are the acceptance and active support given by the community to programs for the elderly. Narrowing the gap between gerontophobia and the actual facts of aging will greatly relieve people's misapprehensions. Harry Hepner put the issue well when he said,

The majority of older people are not "problems," do not die in institutions, do not depend upon the state. Indeed, according to the 1970 census, 88 percent of those 65 years and older reside in the community. The majority of the older generation are constructive, active, thinking human beings who have much of value to teach us—they are a real source of ideas about life . . . .[21]

A successful community program for the elderly would be one that truly provides meaning to the individual in terms of optimal physical and mental health and the maintenance of the independence of the person according to his requests and needs.

SUMMARY Geriatrics presents a growing problem because of the new social forces. People are living longer, technology is providing a faster pace of living, and the evolving structure of the nuclear family relegates the grandparents and relatives to insignificant positions. These three factors increase feelings of alienation, loneliness, and isolation in the elderly citizen of the community. The elderly often feel that they are powerless and at the mercy of outside forces which control their personal and social rewards. They are estranged from the activities of society.

These problems result from the many dilemmas which the elderly must face: (1) As the pace of life in our society increases, the elderly are experiencing a slowing down. (2) At a time when the elderly need more involvement, the family structure has changed. The honored role once held by the aged has been radically changed to a superfluous role which makes many families wonder, "What shall we do with him now?" (3) Technology increases the span of life but the quality of life is ignored.

REFERENCES AND SUGGESTED READINGS

Burnside, Irene M. (1969). "Touching is Talking," *American Journal of Nursing,* **73,** No. 12, 2060–62.

Calnan, Mary F., and Jane B. Hanron (1970). "Young Nurse—Elderly Patient." *Nursing Outlook,* **18,** No. 12, 44–46.

Clark, Margaret, and Barbara G. Anderson (1967). *Culture and Aging.* Springfield, Ill.: Charles C. Thomas.

Gunter, Laurie M. (1969). "A New Look at the Older Patient in the Community Through the Eyes of Nursing Students," *Nursing Forum,* **8,** No. 1, 50–63.

Levine, Rhoda (1969). "Disengagement in the Elderly—Its Causes and Effects," *Nursing Outlook,* **17,** No. 10, 28–30.

Scott, M. Louise (1973). "To Learn to Work with the Elderly," *American Journal of Nursing,* **73,** No. 4, 662–64.

[21]Harry W. Hepner, *Retirement: A Time to Live Anew* (New York: McGraw-Hill, 1969).

ALCOHOLISM AS A COMMUNITY PROBLEM

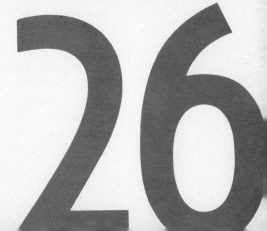

26

John A. Renner, Jr.

When an individual's behavior is viewed as deviating from socially designed patterns, it becomes a community concern as well as a concern for the individual and his family. Alcoholism is such a problem. Its treatment also requires a community centered approach.

ALCOHOL ABUSE

Case Illustration: "Do you think I am an alcoholic?"

Bill, a 23-year-old high school graduate, worked for a construction company after high school and did not like his work. He enlisted in the service and was sent to Vietnam. He was shot during a company assignment of night patrol and sustained a leg injury that resulted in his right leg's being two inches shorter than his left. Poor body alignment and back pain resulted in shortening the left leg 1 inch. Bill is currently in a surgical unit of a Veterans' Administration hospital for correction of the leg variations.

While he has been in the hospital, Bill has been frequently known to drink until he blacks out. Notations on his chart state that he is an alcoholic. Bill asks the nurses, "Do you think I am an alcoholic?"

This case illustration points up how many variables (age, circumstances, war, injury, hospitalization) influence one's behavior. This young man defended against his psychological and physical pain through action behavior (drinking). The question he raises (and the medical chart states) is his diagnosis of alcoholism. To discuss the question, the medical, psychological, social, and behavioral factors need to be more fully understood by both patient and nurse.

THE ALCOHOL PROBLEM

To view alcohol abuse in a social context defines it as more than an addiction, a toxic state, a disease, a bad habit, a criminal or spiritual offense. The problem is a social one since it concerns the person's family, the physician, the nurse, health team, the anthropologist, sociologist, legislator, jurist, crim-

John A. Renner, Jr., M.D., is Director of the Alcohol Clinic and Drug Treatment Program at Massachusetts General Hospital. He is an Instructor in Psychiatry at Harvard Medical School.

452

inologist, penologist, lawyer, welfare worker, and economist. Drinking behavior has broad social implications and always affects the person's social life in some way. The relationship between drinking behavior and the social context of drinking customs is best understood by considering the nature of alcohol, its action in the human body, its impact on human behavior, and its historical patterns.

The nature of alcohol

An intoxicating beverage has been defined as one that may produce a state of abnormal behavior and a blood alcohol concentration of 0.15% or more. Levels above 0.2% correspond to moderate-to-severe intoxication and blood levels of 0.5% may be fatal. A concentration of 0.15% blood alcohol is established as a legal test for inebriation in many states and countries.

Action in the human body

Alcohol is mostly absorbed from the small intestine and distributed into all tissues. From 2% to 10% of the alcohol is excreted through lungs, kidneys, and the skin. The rest, depending on the amount of intake, is broken down largely in the liver. Alcohol can enter the brain, which can oxidize and degrade it, but there are insufficient data on these central biochemical changes. Alcohol is a central nervous system depressant with possibly slight excitatory effects on respiratory centers. The stimulating qualities are felt to be the result of release of inhibition. In larger doses, alcohol is a severe depressant of respiratory centers.

Physical symptoms during early intoxication are vascular dilation of the skin with a flushed and sweaty face, increased pulse, and deepened and accelerated respiration. Gastric secretion is increased. In ordinary drunkenness the excitation phase is often followed by somnolence and sleep. Simple intoxication does not last longer than 12 hours, and then a hangover may develop. With increasing intoxication, cerebellar ataxia with unsteadiness of gait and dysarthria appear.

Impact of alcohol on human behavior

The outstanding behavioral effect of alcohol is a decrease in inhibition, or what is called the release effect of alcohol. This effect leads to the transient feeling of well-being and increases the likelihood that the individual will fulfill some of his inhibited and conflicted needs. The individual variance in effects is caused by the differences in physiology, in basic personality patterns, and in current situations.

Suspicion and fear may be relaxed, love shown more openly, and dependence expressed more freely. The sedating function of alcohol also varies. Some people become drowsy; others become stimulated. Alcohol adversely influences psychomotor performance and decreases reaction time. The decrease in motor skills, reaction time, and judgment, as well as an overestimation of one's abilities, are responsible for many traffic accidents caused by intoxicated drivers.

Historical perspectives

The attitudes and practices of drinking behavior in America reflect many customs brought here from different countries and are influenced by many cultural orientations.

The English colonists who settled in America considered the use of alcohol important to their religious, medical, and dietary needs, but religion directed against excessive use of alcohol. Alcohol quickly became a marketable item and a prominent component of the colonial economy.

The continued immigration of unattached males whose drinking was unrelated to family or religious sanctions soon began to make its impact. This factor, coupled with the Revolutionary War, led to a change in drinking customs. The consumption of alcohol increased markedly, the communities began to have less structure, and the family structure was changed when men went to war. This change continued following the war.

Social concern regarding alcohol became apparent in the form of the temperance movements in the latter half of the eighteenth century. By the end of the eighteenth century the temperance movement had enough support to influence the first congress, which, in turn, imposed prohibitive tariffs on the import of distilled spirits.

The temperance movement remained relatively consistent and had strong support from religious organizations, national and federal legislature, farmers, businessmen, schools, and some hotels that would not offer spirits for sale. The goal of the movement focused on the major problems inherent in alcohol as they were defined by the society.

By the middle of the nineteenth century changes of goals occurred in the temperance movement. The emphasis shifted from excessive drinking to moderation to abstinence. Temperance philosophy also shifted from the moral persuasion to proposals for legal enforcement of total abstinence.

When women were admitted to membership, the leadership quietly shifted from professionals and businessmen to women. This change soon identified the movement with programs for women's rights, especially suffrage and higher education. With the addition of these emotional and controversial issues, the movement tended to lose sight of total community or society goals.

Legislative support of the prohibition of manufacture, distribution, and sale of alcoholic beverages came in the 1850s when one-third of the states enforced the law; in the 1880s eight more states enforced the law; and in 1919 twenty-five states participated in the Prohibition Amendment, which was not repealed until 1933.

The impact of the temperance movement and its goal of total abstinence still have influence in some states, as shown by the age limit for legal drinking. Its impact is also seen in treatment goals that often are aimed at total abstinence.

Neglect of the alcoholic

Social attitudes toward drunkenness help to explain in part why the health care system has tended to neglect services for the alcoholic. There are between 6 and 9 million alcoholics in the United States, and another 30 million relatives and friends are adversely affected by their disease. Alcoholism is the third ranking public health problem in America, and it costs this country $20 to $25 billion in medical expenses, lost wages, and reduced productivity;[1] yet most health insurance policies exclude coverage for alcoholism and less than $218 million of the federal health care budget is directed toward alcoholism. To make the situation worse, the rapid increase in drinking among young Americans suggests an even greater need for alcoholism services in the future.

Unfortunately, many health care programs have avoided any commitment to the alcoholic. Despite a statement by the American Psychiatric Association in 1955 that alcoholism is a "disease," some professionals retain the prejudicial view that this is a moral weakness and attempt to deny any responsibility for such dubious "patients." Others avoid responsibility by claiming that the alcoholic is untreatable. Nonetheless, large numbers of individuals seek help for alcohol related problems at hospitals and community mental health centers. In some areas, as many as 40% of new males admitted to mental hospitals have been diagnosed as alcoholics. The situation at Boston State Hospital in 1967 was not atypical. A survey done at that time showed that 28.8% of all males on first admission were diagnosed as alcoholic, and a total of 48.7% were probably alcoholics; yet in a 2500-bed hospital, there were no beds set aside for specialized alcoholism treatment.[2] It is no accident that many psychiatric facilities have failed in their treatment of these patients. Aside from the failure to deliver primary alcoholism services, the diagnosis itself is often missed. This is a particularly serious issue; failure to adequately diagnose a patient's alcoholism may lead to the failure of other treatment plans, since adequate treatment for other major medical and psychiatric illnesses may be impossible unless a related drinking problem is also under control.

Despite the large number of potential patients, this is one area in which effective treatment is not impossible, even in an era of dwindling funds, particularly if nurses and other mental health professionals make use of existing paraprofessionals and community resources. The lack of an adequate treatment system for alcoholism is a real tragedy since the potential for rehabilitation for most alcoholics is good. They can benefit greatly from treatment in already existing programs (Alcoholics Anonymous, alcohol clinics, and outpatient psychiatry clinics) if appropriate mechanisms for case finding and referral can be developed and if existing agencies can be encouraged to make their services available to alcoholics. Nurses can play a particularly important role in early case finding and referral. Since the majority of alcoholics

[1] "Teen Age Drinking Rising Sharply," *American Medical News,* July 22, 1974, p.1.
[2] W. F. McCourt, A. F. Williams, and L. Schneider, "Incidence of Alcoholism in a State Mental Hospital Population," *Quarterly Journal of Studies on Alcoholism,* **32,** No. 4 (1971), 1085–88.

are employed and already have health insurance, a self-supporting care system can be developed once the limitations on insurance coverage are eliminated. Given the major role of Alcoholics Anonymous and its relative lack of cost, the possibility for developing a truly effective system for caring for most alcoholics is not unrealistic.

THE TREATMENT NEEDS OF THE ALCOHOLIC

The primary focus in this discussion will be on the 95% of American alcoholics who do *not* reside on skid row. In approaching the treatment needs of the alcoholic, it is important to recognize that you are dealing with a chronic condition whose treatment requires a wide variety of medical, psychiatric, social, and paraprofessional services. Effective treatment requires a *system* that links these various services. There are five primary areas of need: (1) crisis intervention and emergency medical care; (2) detoxification; (3) medical or psychiatric in-patient care; (4) halfway houses; (5) aftercare. In most communities, this is a fragmented system involving general hospitals, private physicians, community mental health centers, Alcoholics Anonymous, detoxification facilities, halfway houses, alcohol clinics, and social welfare agencies. The patient may enter the system at any point, depending on the stage of his illness; yet, he is rarely referred to other appropriate elements of the system. Patients seen in hospital emergency rooms for lacerations may not be referred for detoxification; Alcoholics Anonymous may not be mentioned to a patient being treated for cirrhosis on a medical ward; a depressed alcoholic seen at a detoxification facility may not be sent for out-patient psychiatric treatment. Because of the diversity of the patients' medical, psychiatric, and social needs, it is clearly impossible for any one agency to provide all of the needed services. In addition, the proven effectiveness of Alcoholics Anonymous makes it inappropriate for health care agencies to see themselves as the *primary* resource for the long-term treatment of most alcoholics.

In putting together a program for the alcoholic, it is important to recognize that traditional mental health approaches have rarely been successful with this population. An innovative program is necessary and the nurse may find that her most useful role lies in referral and the coordination of services rather than in the direct delivery of care. For the majority of alcoholics, the services provided within the formal mental health system may play a secondary role to rehabilitation services provided by Alcoholics Anonymous and other community agencies. In fact, the long-term burden for the successful management of these patients may indeed fall on agencies presently outside the traditional health care system. However, the nurse will still have to care for those alcoholics who do require specialized medical and mental health treatment.

In relation to traditional mental health services, the treatment of the alcoholic is also unique, since the role of the paraprofessional is clearly established and represents an obvious challenge to the more traditional professional treatment modalities. The nurse must learn to work with paraprofessional agencies if coordinated treatment programs are to be established. Alcoholics frequently seek help initially for medical or psychiatric problems; this may be the patient's only point of entry into the care-giving system. If appropriate linkages to paraprofessional aftercare facilities do not exist, opportunities for successful intervention are often lost. The nurse can play an effective role by facilitating referrals between intake points (general hospital wards, emergency wards, psychiatric crisis centers, alcohol detoxification centers) and long-term treatment facilities (Alcoholics Anonymous, out-patient clinics, halfway houses).

Detoxification

In most hospitals the medical ward or the psychiatric ward will be used for the detoxification of alcoholic patients. Some communities have also established free-standing detoxification facilities. Regardless of where detoxification is carried out, it must be recognized that this is not a "treatment" for alcoholism, it is only the first step in treatment. All patients must be referred either to Alcoholics Anonymous or to other aftercare programs.

Out-patient psychiatric services

Treatment for alcoholics is available in either psychiatrically oriented alcohol clinics or in general psychiatric clinics. These programs seem to be a better alternative for individuals who are uncomfortable with the A. A. approach. This is often the case with both lower-class and upper-class patients.[3] Many people who perceive their problems as having psychological determinants will specifically request psychotherapy. In addition, individuals in the early stages of alcoholism may find this a more acceptable alternative than the requirement that they identify themselves as "alcoholics" and join A. A. This is especially true of patients who wish to reestablish a pattern of social drinking. Individuals with schizophrenia, depressions, or other psychiatric conditions requiring drug therapy can only be successfully managed within the context of a psychiatric clinic whether or not they also participate in A. A.

In many cases, evaluation will show that the patient's drinking is secondary to an obvious problem with the spouse or a problem involving other family members. Couples therapy or family therapy is clearly indicated in these cases. This situation can be best handled by an out-patient psychiatric clinic, although the alcoholic may also be referred to A. A. as an adjunct to other therapy.

Disulfiram (Antabuse ®) is also used in the treatment of alcoholics. Disulfiram inhibits the enzyme acetaldehyde dehydrogenase and causes elevated blood levels of acetaldehyde when alcohol is consumed. This precipitates an extremely unpleasant reaction marked by nausea, vomiting, sweat-

[3]"Patient Differences Should Influence Choice of Therapy, Researchers Say," *Alcohol and Health Notes,* April 1974, p. 2.

ing, flushing, and a sensation of warmth on the upper part of the body.[4] Many individuals find that fear of this reaction helps them avoid drinking; in fact, a severe reaction can produce hypotension, shock, and death. Disulfiram works best within the context of a supportive home situation where a relative can oversee the daily consumption of the drug and as part of an organized treatment relationship with a concerned therapist who will see the patient on a regular basis. It is of no use when prescribed in a setting in which the therapist does not follow the patient closely or when the patient has low motivation.

Industrial alcoholism programs

Some of the most effective approaches to alcoholism have been programs developed by companies to treat their employees. The loss of employee time because of excessive drinking has been a chronic problem to employers. Federal legislation has taken an active role in this area by establishing a federal civilian employee alcoholism program.[5] Alcoholism is defined as an illness and thereby can be treated from the medical standpoint. Nurses will assume a key role in this kind of program.

When Congress set up programs for the alcoholic, it emphasized that the following policies be implemented:

1. Alcoholism is defined as an illness in which the employee's job performance is impaired as a direct consequence of the abuse of alcohol.
2. An employee having an illness or other problem related to the use of alcohol will recieve the same careful consideration and assistance that the company extended to employees having any other illness.
3. The employing agency is not concerned with an employee's use of alcohol except as it may affect his job performance or the efficiency of the service.
4. No employee will have his job security jeopardized by his request for counseling or referral assistance under the program.
5. Medical records of employees with drinking problems will be preserved in the same degree of confidence as all other medical records.
6. Sick leave will be granted for treatment or rehabilitation on the same basis that it is granted for other illness.
7. Employees who suspect that they may have an alcoholism problem are encouraged to seek counseling and information on a confidential basis from the individuals who are designated to provide such service.

Alcoholics Anonymous

Because A. A. is the prime resource for the rehabilitation of most alcoholics, all nurses should understand how it works. A. A. is a group process, and individuals are comfortable within it only if they can identify with other

[4]E. Jacobsen, and D. Martensen-Larsen, "Treatment of Alcoholism with Tetra-ethylthiuram Disulfide," *Journal of the American Medical Association,* **139,** No. 4 (1974), 918–922.
[5]"Public Law 91-616 and the Civil Service Commission," *American Journal of Nursing News Report,* **71,** No. 11 (1971), 2088.

members.[6] Officially, A. A. is uncomfortable about labeling individual groups as having any particular social or economic orientation and will insist that the common identity of being an alcoholic is all that is necessary for an individual to fit into any A. A. group. However, discussions with many people who have never been able to adjust to A. A. suggest that for some people these other elements of group identity are extremely important.

Ideally, a person should be referred to an A. A. group that is compatible with his race, social class, and employment background. In every large city there are many A. A. groups and usually a central office that will help with referrals. A. A. is the original self-help program, in which sober alcoholics, by their support and example, help the active drinker achieve sobriety. Emphasis is placed on remaining sober "one day at a time," and the alcoholic is required to acknowledge his disease and his inability to control it. Total abstinence is felt to be the only acceptable goal; this requirement is an issue that many would-be social drinkers use to justify their refusal to participate in A. A. The program consists of frequent group meetings in which members describe how alcohol affected them and how they learned to control their illness. Strong support is given to members who are still struggling to achieve sobriety. A. A. is basically a middle-class organization with a strong religious/philosophic orientation. It has not always been a successful treatment modality for lower-working class individuals, and it is not acceptable to some members of the upper middle class and upper class. As with all long-term treatment plans, it is vitally important that contact with A. A. be made prior to the patient's discharge from any in-patient setting. Ideally, patients should be visited by a member of A. A. while still hospitalized.

In addition to their program for the alcoholic, A. A. has two affiliated organizations that can be extremely helpful in managing a problem drinker. *Alanon* is a group support program for the spouses or important other people involved with the alcoholic. *Alateen* provides similar services for the children of the alcoholic. Both groups are very supportive to family members and are helpful in relieving the guilt these people often feel about their relatives' drinking problem. Helpful guidance is given on how to respond to an active drinker in ways that will encourage rather than subvert sobriety. This program is extremely effective in many situations; the nurse can refer relatives to these groups even if the alcoholic patient refuses to go to A. A. or to get other help.

Halfway houses

Halfway houses are a vital element in the rehabilitation of the severe alcoholic. When individuals no longer have any stable social situations, jobs, or homes, it is impossible to reestablish them in society without a 2- to 4-month

---

[6]M. A. Maxwell, "Alcoholics Anonymous: An Interpretation in Society" in *Culture and Drinking Patterns,* D. J. Pittman and C. R. Snyder, eds. (New York: John Wiley & Sons, Inc., 1962).

stay in a halfway house. Most halfway houses are strongly oriented to A. A. which provides out-patient support after they leave the halfway house. For individuals who cannot accept the A. A. approach, a halfway house should be located that does not insist on participation in A. A.

Evaluation and referral of the alcoholic

The nurse is often in a position to detect the early signs of alcoholism in her patients. These signs may include recurrent gastritis, blackout spells, early morning drinking, drunk driving arrests, episodes of violence, family quarrels, or poor job performance due to excessive drinking. Because of the wide variety of treatment approaches available, it is extremely important that nurses know how to evaluate alcoholics and how to determine which patients can best be treated at psychiatric clinics or general hospitals and which should be referred to A. A. or other facilities.

The diagnosis of alcoholism is often missed because the patient does not label the problem when seeking help and does not fit the stereotype of the skid row alcoholic. Since less than 5% of the alcoholic population are derelicts, nurses may miss the majority of individuals with alcohol related problems unless they recognize that *anyone* may have serious alcohol related problems. Extensive research over the last 30 years has failed to identify a specific personality type or psychiatric diagnosis that is unique to the alcoholic.[7] Each patient is an individual with his or her own special needs and must be evaluated on that basis. There are few common denominators, except for a history of inadequate care if they have been previously labeled as alcoholic. It is important that this situation change and that the identification of an alcohol problem lead not to discrimination and exclusion from care, but to the delivery of appropriate rehabilitative services.

Evaluation of the alcoholic clearly demonstrates the usefulness of the four conceptual models of psychiatric care (see Chapter 3): the medical, psychological, behavioral, and social. These models permit us to appreciate the broad manifestations of alcoholism. This is far from an academic exercise, since successful treatment is dependent on the recognition that the patient may have problems in many areas and that a coordinated and broad based treatment program dealing with all of these areas is necessary in order to achieve successful results.

The *medical* aspects of the patient's disease are usually fairly obvious. Does the alcoholic metabolize alcohol in an abnormal manner? Is detoxification the patient's immediate need? What other health problems may occur secondary to alcoholism and has adequate treatment been instituted? Alcoholics may also suffer from a variety of other psychiatric conditions, such as schizophrenia or manic–depressive disease; effective management of the alcoholism may require the psychopharmacologic treatment of other under-

[7]J. F. Oxford, "Personality Factors in Alcoholism: A Psychological Approach," *Update*, (June, 1972), 1371–78.

lying conditions. In addition, Disulfiram (Antabuse ®) may be an appropriate medical tool in the treatment of some alcoholics.

From the perspective of the *psychologic* model, several questions are appropriate. What psychodynamic issues have initiated the patient's drinking behavior and have permitted this behavior to continue over a period of time? How will these psychodynamic issues affect the patient's participation in treatment and does a treatment program need to be developed to compensate for the patient's particular psychological make-up? Finally, what are the immediate psychological precipitants that have led to the patient's request for treatment?

When viewed from the *behavioral* perspective, alcoholism presents a unique issue. Drinking is clearly a learned behavior that has strong reinforcing qualities because of alcohol's ability, at least initially, to relieve anxiety and to alleviate depression. This raises the question of whether total abstinence is necessary for effective rehabilitation. Is it possible to help the patient develop new coping devices and more appropriate behavior when he continues to drink and receive reinforcement from that behavior? Often, successful treatment is dependent on our ability to supply adequate alternative sources of gratification so that the patient can give up his or her dependence on alcohol.

In defining the *social* aspects of the patient's problem, it is important to recognize that serious functional impairment is often associated with alcoholism. It is rare for a patient to have a significant drinking problem that has not had an adverse effect on his family or his job. These situations need to be fully evaluated; treatment often requires specific services for the family or spouse as well as adequate educational and vocational rehabilitation services for the patient. Abstinence may require a complete change in the patient's social activities.

Successful treatment requires a coordinated and comprehensive plan that is based on all four conceptual models. The nurse must also go beyond the patient's stated request for help. Patients may ask for assistance with only the most obvious medical problem, such as detoxification. Often, they are too depressed or discouraged to articulate their other less obvious needs. It is incumbent upon the nurse to explore these issues in detail with the patient.

Treatment, however, must start by meeting the patient's primary request whenever possible. Successful results depend on a program that can begin at a point that is acceptable to the patient. Nurses must be careful not to drive a patient away from treatment by pressing for complete abstinence at a time when the patient is unable to accept this as an appropriate goal. As long as the patient acknowledges that he or she has a problem and expresses a wish to deal with it in a meaningful fashion, then the nurse should attempt to satisfy his request. Ultimately, a more comprehensive treatment plan can be negotiated with the patient, but often this will occur at a later stage when the patient is more willing to accept the major commitment to therapy and rehabilitation that is required. Failure in treatment may occur whenever treatment plans have ignored any major patient need.

Once an alcoholism problem has been identified, the nurse will find that special techniques are needed to manage the patient in either a medical or a psychiatric setting. The first goal must be to help the patient acknowledge that he has an alcohol problem. Dealing directly with the issue shows that the nurse is not afraid to hear what he has to say.

If the nurse is hesitant about directly discussing the issue because of her own previous experiences and feelings about alcoholics, she should autodiagnose her feelings first.

As the nurse discusses the issue with the patient, he may deny the problem, make excuses, become angry, feel remorseful, be dishonest, or make promises never to drink again. These are all ways of defending himself against his feelings and behavior of drinking.

If the patient is able to respond to the question of why he drinks, the nurse may find that his answers are not at all difficult to understand. The patient may say drinking relieves tension, helps him to be sociable, combats boredom, helps him unwind, makes him feel good, drowns his sorrows, and makes him feel free. His reason for drinking is no different from the reason why any person drinks.

The difficult question that the nurse may wish answered is, "Why do you drink in view of the fact that it is ruining your life in a physical, emotional, social, economic, and personal way?" This is the issue that needs exploration if the patient is to gain any understanding of his behavior and of his present style of life.

Nurses can stall the interview with the alcoholic in several ways. Sometimes nurses apologize for having to ask the questions, sometimes they become involved in a moral discussion of man's right to drink, or sometimes they merely advise. Such advice as "You probably are drinking too much" or "You should just drink on weekends with your friends" is what he hears from friends and relatives. The nurse is offering no new alternatives to the drinking problem.

The scare approach ("You'll get an enlarged liver") will often lead to a stall situation. The patient may well react by telling the nurse that his grandfather lived to age 96 drinking a quart of liquor a day.

The way to correct the stall situation is to use the therapeutic tasks of setting a goal such as talking about how the alcohol has created difficulties to him personally and to his family. How he perceives this situation and how he intends to deal with this issue will determine the nurse's intervention. Encouraging dialogue, listening carefully, and helping him to bear the painful feelings that he must express are essential tasks for the nurse.

The attitude and personality of the nurse are most important. Authoritarian, pessimistic, cynical, and moralistic attitudes will not be helpful to the patient. The attitudes of compassion, understanding, nonjudgmental feelings, and acceptance will be helpful. An affirmative therapeutic relationship with the nurse is the most positive motivation for the patient to change his behavior pattern.

After the patient has come to accept his problem and the need for treatment, the nurse may assist in referral to A. A. or other appropriate treatment agencies.

In some situations, it may be possible for the nurse to continue working with the patient on a regular basis. If she becomes the patient's primary therapist, the following issues must be considered.

Therapeutic optimism

As in any other form of treatment, successful alcoholism therapy is dependent on the nurse's attitude toward the patient. One of the major ingredients of success in A. A. is their willingness to accept the active alcoholic and the high degree of therapeutic optimism conveyed by A. A. members. Acceptance and optimism are necessary for successful treatment because the patient usually begins at a point where he or she feels hopeless and perceives himself or herself in a very negative fashion. Strong support is needed from the nurse if the alcoholic is to continue in treatment.

Appropriate treatment goals

Because of their failure to develop appropriate treatment goals, many nurses become easily frustrated while working with the alcoholic, and thus they subvert what might otherwise be a successful treatment approach. Nurses may become demoralized because of recidivism and an allegedly high failure rate. This often produces hostility that is inappropriately directed toward the patient. If nurses can appreciate that they are dealing with a chronic relapsing illness and can learn to expect a prolonged treatment course that is sometimes interrupted by recurrences of drinking and if they can see control of the illness as a reasonable goal rather than total cure, then they are better able to sustain an optimistic attitude toward the patient and can avoid this stall. Thus, for each patient, appropriate and attainable goals must be developed. Evidence of improvement in relation to these goals is usually adequate to sustain the nurse, particularly if she is able to give up fantasies about a "cure" dependent on permanent abstinence. Other problems that present major stalls are the depression and demoralization that can affect anyone working with difficult chronic patients. While working with such patients, it is important that the staff support each other during periods of frustration and therapeutic difficulty.

Although there is evidence to suggest that some alcoholics can return to a pattern of social drinking, it is difficult to identify these patients at the start of therapy, and nurses are advised to recommend abstinence for all alcoholics.[8] Nonetheless, patients who wish to return to a social drinking pattern should not be rejected from therapy.

[8]E. X. Freed, "Abstinence for Alcoholics Reconsidered," *The Journal of Alcoholism,* **8,** No. 3 (1973), 106–110.

Nurses must also be willing to accept a patient back in treatment at whatever time the patient presents himself. Whenever a patient returns to therapy after a relapse, the therapist is in a good position to negotiate a more realistic and often more demanding therapeutic contract. It is important that the nurse be sympathetic and understanding of the patient's difficulty, but she must persist in pointing out the problems, regardless of the patient's efforts to deny them. A therapist can avoid arguments about whether or not the patient is an alcoholic without denying that he has problems with alcohol. Many serious alcoholics will accept this as the initial step to treatment, whereas they will avoid treatment altogether if it is demanded that they begin by accepting the diagnosis of alcoholism. At this stage, however, many individuals resist accepting the label of "alcoholic" and any insistence on their accepting the diagnosis might needlessly keep them out of treatment.

Dependency issues

Many traditionally trained therapists have great concerns about the alcoholics' dependency and their demands for extra attention from a therapist or an agency. Successful therapists as well as A. A. have learned that excessive dependency is the norm in the early stages of recovery and that it can be tolerated without any detrimental effects to the patient. Constructive responses to the patient's dependency needs may in fact be necessary in order to successfully engage the patient in treatment. Thus, the nurse must be willing to respond with extra attention when necessary and to reach out to the patient in times of need. One of the major reasons for the effectiveness of A. A. is their availability on a 24-hour basis and their realistic knowledge that patients with serious problems such as alcoholism cannot confine their therapeutic needs to a 9:00 to 5:00 schedule. The appropriate key to managing dependency is not to reject the patient's needs during the early stages of treatment, but to assist the patient in such a way that he is gradually able to become more independent and can eventually come to terms with his dependency needs.[9]

Dealing with intoxicated or violent patients

The intoxicated patient presents a special problem. These patients may be separated into two categories. If an individual presents himself in a crisis situation requiring immediate care such as detoxification or treatment for a suicide attempt or a psychotic episode, he obviously should be treated regardless of his intoxicated condition.

If, however, an individual being followed for long-term psychotherapy or supportive counseling appears intoxicated at the time of a regularly scheduled meeting, it is probably best that the session be canceled unless there are extenuating circumstances. The patient should be told to call back

[9]S. S. Jordy, "Dependency Problems in Alcoholism Treatment," *Connecticut Review on Alcoholism*, **23**, No. 1 (1971), 1–2.

within 24 hours to schedule another appointment and that he will be seen again when he is sober. The patient should be helped to understand that it is difficult to do productive work on his problems when he is intoxicated. Experienced therapists have learned that individuals rarely remember discussions that occurred while they were intoxicated. Such discussion may provide some interesting material for the therapist, but it is rarely of any benefit to the patient. It may also be counterproductive because it may reinforce the patient's drinking; the patient may learn that appearing intoxicated is a way of gaining extra attention.

Other patients who may present problems are those who become violent when intoxicated. Such individuals must be handled through firm limit setting. Nurses must be discreet in dealing with the hostile, provocative patient and must be in touch with their own hostile feelings and be able to manage such patients without losing control themselves. In dealing with these patients, it is important to be supportive and to avoid any hostile or provocative action toward them. Potentially violent patients are best seen in larger rooms where they do not feel closed in and where it is possible for them to leave without feeling that they are being trapped by the nurse. It is equally important that the nurse have easy egress from the room should the patient become violent. In such situations, some male patients may be dealing with unconscious homosexual fears. For that reason, a nonthreatening nurse may be more effective in dealing with the patient than a group of threatening security men or male staff persons. If it does become necessary to subdue a violent patient, it is important that three or four staff members be assembled and that steps be taken immediately to control the patient in order to protect him, staff members, and other patients. Appropriate techniques are available that provide little risk to the staff and little danger of injury to the patient.

Work with community agencies

Despite the secondary role that the traditional health care system may play in the long-term treatment of many alcoholics, nurses can serve this patient population in a major way through their work with other community agencies. In the community situation, the technique of crisis intervention is especially effective in dealing with the acute phase the alcoholism. The nurse can be instrumental in trying to gather all available resources for help for the patient. Family and friends, as well as organizations and community resources, can all assist in trying to aid the patient to rechannel his energies. Detoxification facilities, A. A., and A. A. oriented halfway houses can provide extremely effective care. It is important that professionals acknowledge this and recognize their obligation to support the development and growth of such indigenous self-support systems. Paraprofessionally run programs are usually pleased to have professional back-up for consultation and treatment of their clients. Nurses can help to establish appropriate linkages so that referrals can be made easily from the paraprofessional organizations to the community mental health center or to community hospitals. If paraprofessionals and indigenous self-support systems like A. A. are dealt with in a patronizing manner, this will guarantee hostility and further separate the elements of a potentially effective treatment network. In light of the professional community's neglect of the alcoholic, acknowledged hostility for such patients, and relatively poor success rates in the past, there is little reason to justify a patronizing attitude toward the obviously successful program of A. A. Acknowledgement of our past neglect of these patients will do much to reopen the channels of communication with such paraprofessional groups.

In order to reach the public, the nurse may organize primary prevention programs in the schools and in the community. Educational methods regarding the nature and use of alcohol have in the past tended to emphasize the evils of its use rather than to promote more responsibility for drinking behavior on the part of those who drink. Educational programs should be geared toward encouraging responsible drinking behavior as well as toward facilitating understanding and acceptance from those who abstain. The focus of such programs should be on attitudes regarding drinking, one's responsibility for his or her behavior, and teaching appropriate skills for making decisions.

Alcoholics with special problems

An ongoing difficulty in the management of many alcoholics is the problem of polydrug abuse. Particularly with younger patients, the custom of mixing alcohol with barbiturates, other sedatives, and marijuana is becoming widespread. Current patterns in adolescent drinking suggest that in the future alcoholism as an isolated entity may disappear and be replaced by polydrug abuse. It is important for nurses to recognize that all alcoholics have a high potential for the abuse of other sedative drugs, especially sleeping tablets and minor tranquilizers. While medications such as Chlordiazepoxide and Diazepam have an appropriate role in alcohol detoxification, they are inappropriate for long-term management of such patients. One rarely does an alcoholic a service by detoxifying him and then introducing him to a minor tranquilizer that can become his new drug of abuse. For patients with severe anxiety, low doses of major tranquilizers, such as Trifluoperazine and Thioridazine, offer effective control of symptoms and have minimal abuse potential. Antidepressants or combined antidepressants and antianxiety agents such as Doxepin HCl also may be useful for alcoholics and may be more appropriate than sedatives or minor tranquilizers. Whenever possible, an alcoholic should be handled without medication; all drugs should be withdrawn as soon as the individual can function without them. Whenever medications are prescribed, they should be given in relatively small quantities with nonrefillable prescriptions. If an individual does require medication, it is important that he or she be seen on a weekly or biweekly basis for adequate medical management.

Skid Row alcoholics

While comprising less than 5% of all alcoholics, skid row alcoholics are highly visible and have very specialized needs. They are rarely able to make effective use of A. A. or psychotherapy, but they do require shelter, food, and medical care.

In dealing with the chronic alcoholic, nurses must recognize that some individuals will not respond to treatment and that domiciliary or shelter-type facilities are needed. If alcoholism is indeed a disease, then these individuals are incurables who deserve as humane and decent a standard of care as any other patient. Facilities are needed which provide adequate shelter and meals without requiring abstinence and which have a high degree of tolerance for the life-style of the derelict. Although some chronic alcoholics may be salvaged as a result of their care at such a facility, this may be the permanent alternative care system for most of these unfortunates.

Adolescent problem drinkers

Finally, a word about the growing number of young people who are showing signs of early problem drinking. A study released in 1974 by the National Institute on Alcohol Abuse and Alcoholism placed 36% of high school seniors in this group. These statistics are probably low since they do not include high school dropouts who are likely to have an even higher incidence of alcohol abuse.[10] These findings can be contrasted with a national survey done in 1964 and 1965 which classified 24% to 26% of the population over the age of 21 as heavy drinkers.[11]

We are now seeing youngsters below the ages of 20 who are presenting with full-blown d.t.'s and other symptoms of alcoholism, the result of 6 to 8 years of chronic drinking. Special techniques are needed to deal with these individuals. Some A. A. groups for young people are now available, and they should be referred to such groups. They may also be treated effectively in some drug treatment programs if the programs are designed to work with younger people, have more flexible treatment techniques, and have eliminated the more paramilitary aspects of some of the earlier heroin oriented programs. An important role for the community nurse is to educate teachers and other individuals working with youth to identify adolescents with alcohol related problems and to guide them into treatment as early as possible. It can be predicted that alcoholism will develop at an earlier age in this population and that they will present an even broader range of psychiatric, social, and economic difficulties than our current population because the developmental tasks of adolescence have been interrupted at an earlier age.

[10]Jordy, "Teen-Age Drinking Rising Sharply," *American Medical News,* July 22, 1974, p. 1–2.
[11]D. Cahalan, I. H. Cisin, and H. M. Crossley, *American Drinking Practices* (New Brunswick, N.J.: Publications Division, Rutgers Center of Alcohol Studies, 1969).

SUMMARY Social problems pertain to human relationships and to the value contexts in which these relationships exist. They are defined as problems when they deviate from the socially accepted or morally designed pattern of the society. A major community problem discussed in this chapter was alcoholism.

REFERENCES AND SUGGESTED READINGS

Estes, Nada J. (1974). "Counseling the Wife of an Alcoholic," *American Journal of Nursing,* **74,** No. 7, 1251–55.

Ferneau, Ernest W., Jr. (1967). "What Student Nurses Think about Alcoholic Patients and Alcoholism," *Nursing Outlook,* **15,** No. 10, 40–41.

Gelperin, Abraham, and Eve Arlin Gelperin (1970). "The Inebriate in The Emergency Room," *American Journal of Nursing,* **70,** No. 7, 1494–97.

Gillespie, Cecilia (1969). "Nurses Help Combat Alcoholism," *American Journal of Nursing,* **69,** No. 9, 1938–41.

Greenberg, Leon (1959). "Alcohol in the Body" in *Drinking and Intoxication,* ed., R. G. McCarthy. New York: Free Press of Glencoe, Inc.

Kimmel, Mary E. (1971). "Antabuse in a Clinic Program," *American Journal of Nursing,* **71,** No. 6, 1173–75.

Lucia, Salvatore P. (1963). *Alcohol and Civilization.* New York: McGraw-Hill Book Company.

Mueller, John F. (1974). "Treatment for the Alcoholic: Cursing or Nursing," *American Journal of Nursing,* **74,** No. 2, 245–47.

Pittman, David J., and Charles R. Snyder (1962). *Society, Culture and Drinking Patterns.* New York: John Wiley & Sons, Inc.

TREATING THE DRUG ABUSER

27

John A. Renner, Jr.

T reatment models for drug abuse problems have been difficult to establish. One method that is now being used is the self-help program. The encounter group techniques used in self-help programs have also been adapted for use in more traditional psychiatric programs.

Case Illustration: "I'm a Heroin Addict"

Marc, age 23, graduated from high school with academic honors and received a football scholarship to a well-known university. He enlisted in the military, served in Vietnam, and is now a hardcore addict. Before this current hospital admission for treatment, his habit cost him $100 per day for which it was necessary for him to push narcotics to maintain his habit. This is not his first attempt to kick the habit, but only one of several.

For the past 8 weeks, he has been in a detoxification program and has not had medication of any kind. Sleep is short, averaging 2–3 hours per night.

Marc participates in individual therapy with his "shrink" twice weekly and in a group with other addicts (veterans) led by a nurse and an ex-addict. The group meets daily for 2 hours. Marc is very supportive of other members in the group and appears to be one of the strong members of the group. Marc is free to leave the program at any time, but he realizes that if he leaves, he will go back on heroin because the streets are full of junkies and addicts whom he knows well and who know him.

In this case example, the problem of the hardcore addict is obvious, that of not being able to be free of the addicting habit. Marc is actively trying various treatment models in order to "kick" his habit. Time will tell how successful these treatment models are for him.

HISTORICAL PERSPECTIVES China was the first major nation to experience problems of opium abuse. Despite the futile attempts of the emperors of China to enforce restrictions, there was a significant struggle (the Opium War, 1840–1842) between the Chinese and British in which the British defeated the Chinese army. By a

John A. Renner, Jr., M.D., is Director of the Alcohol Clinic and Drug Treatment Program at Massachusetts General Hospital. He is an Instructor in Psychiatry at Harvard Medical School.

treaty involving $6 million, the British established themselves in the British Crown Colony and the great Far East port of Hong Kong. Opium importation doubled and then tripled until 1911 when the British and Chinese governments agreed to restrict trade from India and to discourage the cultivation of the opium poppy in China.

In America it was not until the isolation of morphine that addiction became an identified problem. The social influence that magnified the addiction problem was war. The uncontrolled use of opium and morphine in military medicine led to the problem that became known as the "soldiers' disease." The American Civil War (1861–1865), the Prussian–Austrian War (1866), and the Franco–Prussian War (1870–1871) all had this problem of addiction among its men.

In 1874 little attention was paid to a chemical modification of morphine (called heroin) that was being developed in England. When it was discovered that heroin was ten times more potent than morphine, interest in and addiction to this new chemical substance increased.

During the nineteenth century, drug addiction in the United States was treated strictly as a medical problem. In the first decades of the twentieth century, control methods shifted to law enforcement approaches and addiction was seen as a crime rather than a disease. Under the Harrison Narcotic Act of 1914, drug maintenance clinics were closed and most medical personnel abandoned any efforts to treat addicts. In 1930 the Federal Bureau of Narcotics was established. In 1948 the newly created United Nations adopted a Narcotic Protocol and placed the authority for control with the World Health Organization. Since World War II the emphasis has again shifted to the medical treatment of the addict. Contemporary American society is highly drug oriented, and there has been a steady increase in the number of drug abusers. During the 1970s heroin abuse changed from a raging epidemic into a slowly increasing pandemic which may again become a serious problem. There is a core of heroin abusers in most major cities, and the potential for increased abuse exists, depending on supply and demand factors and economic conditions.

The major shift in patterns of drug abuse over the last 10 years has been the increased abuse of all drugs, including alcohol and marijuana. There currently seems to be a trend away from heroin and back toward alcohol abuse, but now in combination with barbiturates and other sedative–hypnotic drugs. A recent study on a university psychiatric in-patient unit revealed that 34% of the patients, regardless of diagnosis, were using nonprescribed psychoactive medications.[1] Because sedatives and hypnotics are less expensive and can be more easily obtained through legitimate medical channels, they have not been associated with crime and therefore with the hysteria that has been connected with heroin abuse.

There is now less of a tendency for the individual drug abuser to stay with a given drug and more of a tendency to use combinations of drugs. It is

[1]Thomas J. Crowley, David Cheslak, Stephen Dilts, and Robert Hart, "Drug and Alcohol Abuse among Psychiatric Admissions," *Archives of General Psychiatry,* **30**, No. 1 (1974), 13.

unclear whether the abuse of hallucinogens such as LSD has really leveled off or whether the users of these drugs have become more sophisticated and are less likely to be seen in psychiatric or medical settings because of "bad trips" or other adverse reactions. The other major change in patterns of drug abuse is a steady downward drift in the age when individuals first experiment with drugs. Because of this, there is at least the possibility that the next generation of serious drug abusers will manifest even greater psychological difficulties than those of the present, because of the earlier age at which they became seriously involved in drugs and the concomitant "dropping out" of society before they have accomplished many of the developmental tasks of adolescence. It is certainly clear that heavy drug abuse is incompatible with the maintenance of a normal life-style. While the debate about the relative safety of marijuana remains unresolved, millions of Americans have experimented with this drug and are now using it on a regular basis. For a small percentage of this group, chronic marijuana use will be associated with an amotivational syndrome. It is unclear whether individuals demonstrating this kind of behavior will continue to use marijuana or will drift back to alcohol or to other drugs of abuse.

Drug dependence

ASSESSMENT FACTORS The official diagnostic term *drug dependence* avoids the confusion associated with the precise meanings of *addiction* and *habituation*. The term implies habitual use or clear evidence that the patient has an emotional need for the drug.

Addiction is defined as a state of chronic or recurrent intoxication from the use of a drug characterized by:

1. *Psychological Dependence.* This implies emotional dependence, desire, or compulsion to continue taking the drug.
2. *Tolerance.* The doses required to obtain the desired effect gradually increase, and there is a definite tendency on the part of the addict to increase the amount that he takes.
3. *Physical Dependence.* This is manifested by the appearance of withdrawal symptoms (abstinence syndrome) when the drug is not taken.

All of the above factors are necessary for true addiction. However, the term *addiction* is loosely used and may be applied to situations in which only psychological dependence is present. Some confusion in terminology results from the fact that narcotics legislation covers some drugs that are not addicting and does not include others that are.

The problem of drug dependence may come up unexpectedly in the course of medical management of other conditions, for example, accidents, hepatitis, malnutrition, venereal disease, pneumonia, tuberculosis, skin infections, and pregnancy.

It is difficult for anyone to give up pleasure. The essence of addiction lies in the irresistible and insatiable need for gratification in a person with low tolerance of pain, frustration, tension, and anxiety. There is also an added difficulty: Addicts seek not only pleasure through the drug process but also the security, attention, and authoritative structure entailed in the punishment process.

Evaluation of the drug user

The first step in the evaluation of a patient and his drug problem is to try to establish a trusting relationship. Even when dealing with a medical emergency, remember that drug abusers may be fearful of contact with the police and may be reluctant to give the correct facts. Patients need to be told that what they tell you will be held in confidence and that their request for treatment will not lead to criminal action. Addicts have come to expect rejection and hostility from "straights"; initially, they may be very defensive and will need to be reassured of your genuine desire to help.

Assessing the need for medical treatment

Before looking more closely at the drug abuser, it will be helpful to briefly go through the major categories of drugs with an emphasis on those situations requiring immediate medical attention. Patients should be questioned carefully regarding their drug use, but it is important to remember that more accurate information may be obtained by interviewing their parents or friends or by physical examination and blood and urine toxicology.

The following questions should be asked of all drug abusers:

1. What drug or drugs are being used?
2. For each drug, note:
   a. the quantity used on a daily basis
   b. the frequency of such use
   c. how long such drugs have been used
3. Is alcohol used in combination with other sedative–hypnotic drugs?

It is sometimes necessary to check the belongings of comatose patients for evidence in order to identify the drugs they have ingested. Adequate evaluation of the kind of drugs used is vital to the development of an appropriate treatment plan.

Sedative–
Hypnotics
This is a large group of drugs including alcohol, barbiturates, and barbiturate-like drugs such as Meprobamate and Glutethimide. Minor tranquilizers, such as Chlordiazepoxide and Diazepam, and sedatives, such as Flurazepam, are in this group. All of these drugs have a potential for physical and psychological dependence and will produce tolerance leading to increasing dosage. Acute withdrawal will produce seizures. Overdoses can cause coma and death. Overdoses and acute withdrawal from these drugs are medical emergencies and require hospitalization. It is sometimes difficult to assess

whether an abuser of these drugs is physically dependent, especially since users have a tendency to *underestimate* the amount of sedative–hypnotics they are taking. As a general rule, it takes 800 mg or more a day of Seco-barbital for more than 5 weeks to produce physiologic addiction. Equivalent doses of the other drugs in this group are listed in the table on page 476.

Marijuana Marijuana is also classified as a sedative–hypnotic; it can produce moderate psychological dependence, but it has a low abuse potential since it produces neither tolerance nor physical dependence. The psychic effects depend on the quantity consumed, which in turn is dependent on the substance used, strength of the preparation, and route of consumption. The most common effect is a "dreamy" state usually characterized by euphoria, hilarity, and an intense, excited inner feeling of well-being. Thought is rapid, voluble, and at times disjointed. This leads to impairment of memory and judgment. Thoughts may take on new or special meanings. Mood and behavior vary according to the environmental stimuli. In other words, if the user is alone, he may become drowsy or moody, but if he is in the company of others, he may become restless, gregarious, and garrulous. Perception of space and time seems distorted and extendable. Higher doses cause a subjective experience of lowered sensory threshold, hallucinations, and delusions. Panic reactions sometimes occur in the naive user, but these are rare and usually can be alleviated by reassurance that the effects are drug related and will soon end.

Narcotics The narcotic group includes opium, heroin, morphine, meperidine (Demerol®), codeine, methadone, and a variety of other synthetic compounds. With the exception of codeine, all of these drugs are highly addictive and rapidly produce tolerance, physical dependence, and psychological dependence. As a general rule, an individual can become addicted to narcotics in less than a week if they are used on a daily basis and in regularly increasing dosages. However, because of inadequate information on the quality of the drugs being used or the pattern of drug use, addiction to narcotics can never be fully documented unless withdrawal signs are observed or the individual is challenged with a narcotic antagonist. In the mild abstinence syndrome, symptoms resemble a common cold or an allergic reaction with sore throat, rhinorrhea, lacrimation, sweating, and slightly elevated temperature. In the more severe cases the patient appears ill. Dilated pupils with a decrease in reactivity to light, gooseflesh, muscular twitches and muscle and joint pain, insomnia, increased blood pressure, and marked restlessness are symptoms in the very severe cases. These symptoms start 4–48 hours after the last drug is taken. Heroin and methadone overdoses are life-threatening emergencies and require immediate medical care. Withdrawal states, while quite uncomfortable, are not dangerous. Methadone detoxification is the preferred method of handling withdrawal from narcotics, but some patients prefer to do it without medication ("cold turkey"). For most narcotic addicts, the major issue is not only detoxification but also whether they should be placed on methadone maintenance or should enter a drug-free residential self-help program.

Central nervous system stimulants

These include drugs of low abuse potential, such as caffeine and nicotine, and the more dangerous cocaine and amphetamines. Some authorities question whether amphetamines are truly addictive; however, they clearly produce tolerance and psychological dependence. Amphetamines have effects similar to those of ephedrine: constriction of peripheral blood vessels, stimulation of heart and increased blood pressure, relaxation of bronchial and intestinal muscles, and a decrease in appetite. Trade names for stimulants are Benzedrine, Dexedrine, Desoxyn, Methedrine, Preludin. These drugs are used as mood elevators in depression and as an appetite depressant in obesity cases. The drug also combats drowsiness and simple fatigue. The drug dependence is high. It is usually taken orally, but it may be taken intravenously.

Psychologic dependence may develop even on therapeutic doses, probably because the patient needs to maintain the feeling of well-being after the medical regime is completed. With continued doses, tolerance develops and daily doses may be raised to several hundred times the therapeutic level. As tolerance develops, the lassitude and depression between doses increase. The sense of well-being is increasingly blurred by apprehension, and an increasing emotional lability characterized by hostile impulsiveness develops. The physical signs are increased pulse and blood pressure, fine tremors of the extremities, headache, anorexia, nausea, and dilated pupils with decreased reactivity to light.

Methampheta-mine

Methamphetamine ("speed") is frequently used intravenously, and chronic use can be very destructive both physically and psychologically. Chronic amphetamine use or acute overdoses can produce a toxic paranoid psychosis that requires hospitalization. Less intense paranoid reactions can be managed on an out-patient basis. Withdrawal from amphetamines usually causes depression and somnolence but rarely represents any physical threat to the individual or requires any specific chemical treatment. Nonetheless, such individuals may become suicidal and may require psychiatric hospitalization.

Cocaine

Cocaine is used medically as a topical anaesthetic. It is usually sniffed as a powder or used intravenously. More rarely it is chewed. If taken in sufficient quantity, it induces euphoric excitement and hallucinatory experiences.

The drug is rarely taken alone; almost all cocaine addicts also take opiates. A combination of heroin and cocaine is called a *speedball*. Cocaine causes a strong psychologic dependence, but physical dependence and withdrawal phenomenon have not yet been demonstrated. Tolerance does not develop, presumably because the drug is rapidly destroyed in the body. The

Hallucinogenic drugs

nursing care is to withdraw the drug abruptly because no abstinence symptoms occur and to provide a protective environment if delirium occurs.

The hallucinogenic drugs do not produce physical dependence, but they can produce psychological dependence and mild tolerance. This group includes LSD, mescaline, psilocybin, and tetrahydrocannabinol (THC), the most potent active ingredient in marijuana. THC is a very unstable compound and is never available on the street. If an individual claims to have used THC, he probably has been using LSD or anticholinergics such as atropine or scopolamine.

LSD is a synthetic derivative from the ergot fungus. Mescaline is an alkaloid contained in the buttons of certain cactuses found in Mexico. Psilocybin is isolated from the "sacred" mushroom found in Mexico. Cactus buttons and mushrooms have played significant roles in religious rites of some Indian groups in Mexico and the U.S.A. Morning glory seeds provide an active principle similar to LSD in chemical structure and effect.

The tolerance to LSD and psilocybin comes and goes rapidly and the tolerance to mescaline develops more slowly. The most characteristic effect of these drugs is the kaleidoscopic visual hallucination of vivid colors and forms. Auditory hallucinations are common. Tactile hallucinations occur less often. Illusions and distortions of perception and body image are common. Usually, the person is preoccupied with his own thoughts and perceptions. Mood may be ecstatic, but it may alternate with uncertain anxious and depressive feelings. Feelings of depersonalization and estrangement are common. Long-term periodic or chronic use may cause intellectual changes, such as looseness of associative processes, vagueness of formulations, and difficulty with coherent communication. The major problems with these drugs are acute panic reactions ("bad trips") and flashbacks, a transient reoccurrence of part of a prior psychedelic drug experience.

ADDICTIVE DOSES OF SEDATIVE–HYPNOTICS

Trade Name	Generic Name	Dependency-Producing Dose (Mg per Day)	Number of Days Necessary to Produce Dependence
Librium ®	Chlordiazepoxide	300–600	60–180
Valium ®	Diazepam	80–120	42
Noctec ®	Chloral hydrate	2000–3000	
Equanil ® Miltown ®	Meprobamate	1600–2400	
Doriden ®	Glutethimide	200–3000	
Seconal ®	Sodium secobarbital	800–2200	35–37
Nembutal ®	Sodium pentobarbital	800–2200	35–37
Sopor ® Quaalude ®	Methaqualone	2100–3000	21–28[a]

[a] "Methaqualone: Dangerous New Drug Fad Sweeping West?" *Connection*, **1**, No. 1 (1972), 1–5.
Adapted from G. R. Gay, D. E. Smith, D. R. Wesson, and C. W. Sheppard, "A New Method of Outpatient Treatment of Barbiturate Withdrawal," *Journal of Psychedelic Drugs*, **3**, No. 2 (1971), 81.

Evaluation of the patient's rehabilitation needs

After assessing the pattern of drug abuse and the need for immediate medical treatment, the next requirement is a thorough evaluation of the patient. With whom are you dealing? Avoid the stereotype of the hardcore street "junkie." This individual may be easily recognized as a drug abuser, but he may represent only a small proportion of the drug abusing population. Remember that many barbiturate addicts are suburban housewives, and amphetamine abusers can be college students or truck drivers. Is the patient an experimenter who has gotten into trouble because of a single adverse reaction to a drug used on a casual and naive basis, or is this an individual who has been using drugs regularly but has not become addicted? Are you dealing with a social user who uses marijuana or other sedative–hypnotics in a social setting on weekends with his or her peers? Many young people will be brought to treatment agencies because of parental concern about such behavior. They need to be carefully assessed to determine whether or not their drug use presents significant psychopathology. Most experimenters and casual social users do not require treatment and are rarely seen at treatment centers. However, there is a danger that they will go on to become drug dependent. Some counseling may be indicated to make them more aware of the risks (legal and otherwise) inherent in their drug use.

Rehabilitation of the serious drug abuser is a major problem and will tax the resources of anyone committed to working with this population. It is important to realize that such individuals often have multiple psychiatric problems. As with the alcoholic, there is little evidence to suggest that a specific personality type or psychiatric diagnosis is associated with addiction or serious drug abuse. Nonetheless, these individuals are usually depressed, impulsive people who, while often intelligent, have little ability to cope with the stresses of life and have found drugs to be an easy escape from their difficulties. In the real world of the drug addict, there is little distinction between the drug dealer and the addict. Do not be put off if the patient you are treating admits to dealing in drugs. In the value system of the streets, most addicts feel that it is less disreputable to deal in drugs than it is to steal, and this will often be their preferred way of supporting themselves and their habit. Few heroin addicts can support their habits for long without becoming involved in drug trafficking.

The notion of the non-using drug dealer is a fantasy supported by politicians seeking to gain support for repressive drug legislation. There are indeed a few non-using drug dealers at the very top of the distribution system. These dealers are the only ones who make any real profit out of the system; yet they are almost never affected by the law, and they certainly are unlikely to ever show up in the treatment system.

A complete evaluation of the drug abuser will be greatly aided by using the four conceptual models.[2] The most immediate problem is a *medical* assessment of the patient's condition, whether it be intoxication, overdose,

[2]See Chapter 3.

or withdrawal. Idiosyncratic reactions, such as "bad trips," acute anxiety reactions, or allergic phenomena, can occur in any individual, not necessarily an addict or a serious drug abuser. Using the medical model, there are two possible treatments for narcotic abuse: methadone maintenance and narcotic antagonists. There are no comparable medical treatments for barbiturate abuse.

In evaluating the patient from the perspective of the *behavioral* model, it is important to recognize the extraordinary reinforcing capacity of the opiates and amphetamines as pleasure-producing agents and as escapes from internal and external psychic stress. Some patients may make contact with medical or psychiatric facilities only when their drug supply has been exhausted. They may not be seeking rehabilitation, and they may be only looking for alternative sources of drugs to relieve their physical craving. Nonetheless, they present a challenging opportunity to the nurse who may be able to use this crisis to encourage them to get help for their problems.

In regard to the *psychological* model, it is clear that many individuals are driven to use drugs because of unconscious psychological conflicts. Addicts may request help for a drug problem without acknowledging their more basic need for psychological help While they may indeed be motivated to change and get help, they may find it much easier to present their problems in terms of adverse drug reactions rather than admit to their psychological inadequacies. Even when such individuals are not motivated to change, they may be genuinely desirous of a respite from their current existence, and thus present care-givers with an opportunity to work on their more basic problems.

Lastly, all addicts should be evaluated from the *social* perspective. They frequently seek help only when external pressures from family, job, or court force them to do so. These individuals may represent excellent candidates for successful treatment. Recent data suggest that such patients may do almost as well as individuals who enter clinics and community based programs on a purely voluntary basis.[3] For all patients, it is important to recognize why they have sought help at this particular point in time. This will provide effective clues for good nursing management. Since drug abuse tends to be a chronic problem, it is inadequate to suggest that they are simply there for help with drugs; something has changed in their life situation which has led them to seek help.

A successful treatment plan must take into account all of these various perspectives regarding the patient and the particular drugs being abused. If a patient is to be successfully engaged in treatment, his most pressing request must be responded to whenever this is possible and appropriate. The crisis which has forced such patients into treatment presents an excellent opportunity to effect long-term rehabilitation.

[3]William F. Wieland and Janet L. Novack, "A Comparison of Criminal Justice and Non-Criminal Justice Related Patients in a Methadone Treatment Program," *Proceedings: 5th National Conference on Methadone Treatment,* March 17–19, 1973, pp. 116–22; Louis Lieberman and Leon Brill, "Rational Authority," in *Major Modalities in the Treatment of Drug Abuse,* eds., L. Brill and L. Lieberman (New York: Behavioral Publications, 1972), p. 67.

After the immediate medical problems have been handled, where do you refer the drug abuser? Which agency or program is best for which patient? In terms of long-term rehabilitation, which patient needs in-patient psychiatric care, day care, self-help residential care, psychotherapy, or methadone maintenance? These issues can be best discussed in reference to the kind of drug abuse.

Drug experimenters

If no other serious psychological problems are present, experimenters do not need to be treated. However, they should be told about the possible medical and legal consequences of drug use. Parents may need reassurance that their child is not an addict and should be referred for counseling if they appear unable to cope realistically with the situation. Parental overreaction may inadvertently reinforce a child's drug use. With some adolescents, such drug use may reflect family oriented problems; they should then be referred for family therapy. Individuals who have come into conflict with the law because of experimentation with drugs frequently do well under supervision by the probation officer. If the nurse has any question about the "experimenters' " potential for more problems, they can be referred to a peer counseling center or a community outreach program. They should not be referred to a psychiatrist or to an addiction treatment program unless there is evidence of serious problems.

Social users

Social users of marijuana or individuals who occasionally combine alcohol with other sedative drugs in a social setting do not need to be referred for treatment. However, if these individuals show evidence of *any* significant psychological problem (other than their drug use), they have a potential for more serious drug abuse. They should be referred to an out-patient psychiatric clinic. If their psychological problems are not severe, they might also be referred for out-patient counseling or groups run by self-help programs. The nurse should be aware of the quality and appropriateness of such programs in her community.

Drug abusers and addicts

Most serious drug abusers require residential care and should be referred to a self-help program. These programs can be effective, regardless of the kind of drug being abused, and work equally well with voluntary and court referred clients. The best programs have flexible time limits, provide both encounter groups and individual counseling, and have eliminated the more paramilitary elements that were present in the original Synanon program. Look for programs that provide educational and vocational counseling to help their clients return to society. The staff should be a mix of ex-addicts and professionals, and there should be an active citizen board that supervises the program. The State Drug Abuse Authority can be helpful in identifying the best self-help program in your area.

Unfortunately, these programs cannot be recommended for individuals with poor ego boundaries. Drug abusers who are psychotic, manic–depressive, or have severe borderline character disorders cannot tolerate the stress of these programs. They will do better if managed by a community mental health center, either in in-patient or out-patient treatment. Methadone maintenance is a useful alternative for older opiate addicts with more serious character disorders. However, all addicts should first attempt a trial of treatment in a drug-free self-help program, even though this approach seems to work best with younger (under age 25) addicts or highly motivated older addicts. Narcotic antagonist programs are available in a few metropolitan communities, but they are primarily research programs and appear to be effective with a relatively small proportion of addicts. There are no comparable chemical treatments available for the abusers of barbiturates and other sedatives.

Establishing relations with new patients

Regardless of whether the patient is being dealt with on an in-patient ward or in a crisis intervention unit, the basic elements of managing the drug abuser during an acute crisis are the same. Such patients are frightened and need considerable support and reassurance. If such support is not made available, they will make excessive demands for drugs. Many addicts are frightened that they will get severely ill during detoxification; the nurse should give them specific reassurance that the staff understands their medical problems and is skilled in managing them. It is equally important that patients feel accepted and recognize that they are being treated with respect as people who require help, and not with the prejudice and hostility that they have come to expect from medical personnel. Most patients initially present a defensive, hostile veneer because of their expectations that their requests will be denied and that they will be dealt with in a prejudicial manner. Once they recognize that the staff is genuinely concerned about them, this hostility will disappear. Nonetheless, many of them present severe characterological problems and they may persist in "testing behavior," in which their provocative hostility is used to test the limits of the nurse's concern about them. The nurse must also be prepared to deal with the patient's denial of psychological problems. Such patients may present their needs as being strictly medical and deny the psychological factors underlying their addiction. The nurse must learn how to tactfully confront such patients with the seriousness of their problems and their need for long-term treatment.

Treating the "bad trip"

These are acute anxiety and panic reactions that occasionally occur among naive LSD users who have not been adequately prepared for the physical and psychological sensations associated with psychedelic drug use. Psychedelic drugs usually produce alterations in visual and other sensory perceptions. Ordinarily, the user is aware that these perceptions are drug induced. At some point during the "trip," however, the user may forget that the illusions are drug induced, or the individual may panic and become frightened that the illusions will last forever. Auditory hallucinations are rare and suggest an underlying psychotic process.

Patients on a "bad trip" should be placed in a quiet room, either with a trusted friend or with one staff person who can spend several hours to "talk them down." Techniques to be used include quiet reassurance that what they are experiencing is drug related and will shortly disappear and that they will not incur any permanent damage from the drug. Any distortions of physical or psychological reality that are verbalized must be countered with effective reality testing. The nurse must be careful not to upset or threaten the patient; anything she does will be altered because of his distorted perceptions. A hostile comment can easily set off an extreme panic reaction.

Medication should not be used unless the nurse is unable to calm the patient by talking him down. Chlordiazepoxide (25 mg) or Diazepam (10 mg) will calm most patients if needed. Phenothiazines (Chlorpramazine 50 mg orally) should be used only in severe cases in which the nurse can no longer communicate verbally with the patient.[4] This dose can be repeated hourly if necessary. Intramuscular medications should be avoided unless the patient's behavior is a threat to himself or to others.

Flashbacks

These are transient reoccurrences of part of a previous psychedelic drug experience. There are primarily three types. The most common is a reoccurrence of *visual distortions* and pseudo-hallucinations (intense colors, "trails," micropsia, seeing geometric forms in objects, etc.). Some individuals experience *emotional flashbacks* where they relive an intense emotional experience (panic, joy, loneliness, etc.) that had occurred during the original trip. Least common are *somatic flashbacks* consisting of feelings of pain or paresthesias. Flashbacks are more likely to occur after an initial "bad trip," especially if it was interrupted by a traumatic experience such as hospitalization rather than being treated by being "talked down."[5] Flashbacks may occur after one or any number of uses of psychedelics and have been reported occurring as long as eighteen months after the last drug use. In general, they are best treated by supportive counseling and, if necessary, Chlordiazepoxide or Diazepam (10 mg. t.i.d.), though these drugs should not be used unless absolutely necessary. Patients should be reminded that the continued use of psychedelics or other mind-altering drugs, including marijuana and alcohol, will cause a perpetuation of their flashback symptoms. If they wish the symptoms to disappear, it is absolutely mandatory that they stop all drug use. Symptoms may also occur at a time when patients are undergoing unusual stress or at the point of falling asleep. Anything that

---

[4]David E. Smith, "The Trip—There and Back," in *Major Modalities in the Treatment of Drug Abuse,* eds., L. Brill and L. Lieberman (New York: Behavioral Publications, 1972), p. 267.

[5]G. Schoener, "Flashbacks or Flashes," *STASH Capsules,* **5,** No. 4 (1973).

alters the usual state of ego control can cause such symptoms to develop. In general, reassurance and explanation of these phenomena will help most patients manage these experiences.

Amphetamine psychosis

Severe paranoid reactions can occur in amphetamine abusers either after prolonged use (in high or low doses) or after a single overdose. The violent and paranoid amphetamine abuser is the only drug user who is likely to be dangerous. It is best to approach the patient in as calm and as non-threatening a manner as possible, but talking him down is rarely successful. Temporary hospitalization and treatment with phenothiazines are necessary if the toxic psychosis persists. Symptoms will usually clear completely within 48 to 72 hours.[6]

Long-term treatment of the drug abuser

As with alcohol abuse, many individuals who become seriously involved with drugs may be most effectively treated by agencies outside of the usual mental health system. Nonetheless, there are many times when such individuals will come in contact with mental health agencies or may have particular problems that require specific medical or psychiatric management. When dealing with serious drug abusers or addicts, specialized techniques are necessary. The usual psychiatric approaches of hospitalization or out-patient psychotherapy are rarely of any use to this difficult patient population. Hospitalization may be needed at points of crisis, such as suicide attempts, and medical care may be needed as a result of overdoses or detoxification needs, but long-term rehabilitation can best be carried out by self-help programs.

Out-patient psychotherapy

Individual psychotherapy may be of some use to individuals who have *completed* a paraprofessional treatment program, and have had several months or a year of drug abstinence. These people may find that there are particular psychological issues that they can work on in psychotherapy that were not dealt with sufficiently in the encounter groups found in most drug rehabilitation programs. These individuals may well be appropriate patients for long-term out-patient psychotherapy.

Nonetheless, I would caution against placing addicts in individual psychotherapy until they have had a fairly lengthy period during which their drug use has been under good control. Unless the psychotherapist has had intensive experience dealing with drug abusers, it is unlikely that treatment of this nature will be successful.

Group therapy may also be useful for some addicts, but this can be more easily obtained through drug counseling programs. However, most

[6]Smith, *The Trip.*

addicts find it difficult to gain adequate control of their drug problem, and any therapy which involves only 1 or 2 hours per week is rarely adequate to meet their needs.

Day care

Day care may be a viable treatment modality for many addicts. This may be particularly helpful if they have other major psychiatric symptoms. If they are adolescents or individuals with characterological problems, they may find it extremely difficult to identify with the patients in the typical psychiatric day care facility, and thus they would not do well in such a program. Some community mental health centers have developed day care programs specifically for drug abusers. These would be appropriate for individuals who are unwilling to enter residential facilities.

Methadone maintenance

It must be remembered that methadone maintenance is useful only for heroin and opiate addicts and that it has no role in the treatment of barbiturate or polydrug abuse. Methadone maintenance treatment can be provided only under rigid federal guidelines; these limit the treatment to individuals over the age of 18, who have been addicted for more than 2 years and have a history of one failure in detoxification treatment. Many drug programs recommend that all addicts, regardless of their history, be encouraged to make a serious effort at residential, self-help treatment before they are placed on methadone maintenance. A day or two in a residential program or participation in a methadone detoxification program not followed by a realistic effort at rehabilitation should *not* be considered adequate justification to place an individual on maintenance.

There has been a major shift in thinking on the goals of methadone maintenance since it was first pioneered by Dole and Nyswander in 1964 at the Rockefeller Institute.[7] While this was initially perceived as a treatment that responded to permanent drug induced changes in the nervous system, many programs have now learned that methadone maintenance can be an effective tool leading to a drug-free state. After 6 to 18 months of methadone maintenance, some addicts who have achieved a satisfactory job and social adjustment can be slowly detoxified and have a good chance of remaining drug-free. Programs that do this effectively, however, must deliver high-quality rehabilitation services in addition to providing methadone. Methadone alone is rarely of any therapeutic value. An adequate methadone maintenance program should deal with a small number of patients and should have a high staff–patient ratio. It is important that supportive services, counseling, vocational, and educational rehabilitation services be pro-

[7]Vincent T. Dole and Marie Nyswander, "A Medical Treatment for Diacetylmorphine (Heroin) Addiction: A Clinical Trial with Methadone Hydrochloride," *Journal of the American Medical Association,* **193,** No. 646 (1965).

vided, and that a program be sought that encourages a "family" type atmosphere and whose philosophy is geared toward eventual detoxification.[8] The ideal program should have no more than 25 patients, although programs with fewer than 50 patients can be recommended. Unless there is a high staff–patient ratio, large programs are often ineffective and can be devices for social control rather than rehabilitation. Methadone maintenance treatment can be recommended for older addicts, for those who are less motivated and have failed in other treatments, as well as for those individuals with family responsibilities that prevent their participation in residential treatment programs.

Working with self-help drug programs

The role of the mental health professional in the long-term rehabilitation of most serious drug abusers is a secondary one, aside from methadone detoxification and maintenance programs. Out-patient psychiatric services are indicated only for individuals with relatively minor drug problems or for those with such serious psychopathology (major psychosis, manic-depressive disease, etc.) that they cannot be managed by most paraprofessional agencies. The most effective and the primary treatment for most addicts will be residential self-help programs. Medical professionals should therefore foster the development of such indigenous self-support care systems. Some nurses have worked as paid or volunteer staff for self-help programs. The nurse can also act as liaison between such paraprofessionally run programs and other agencies in the "straight community" which may find it extremely difficult to understand the role of these programs or their legitimate place in the treatment system. The self-help movement is very broad based and heterogeneous. If a nurse wants to establish good working relationships with these programs, it is important that these differences be recognized. Many self-help programs, particularly those engaged in outreach work, drop-in counseling, and crisis intervention, are typically staffed by young people with a middle-class background who are not ex-addicts. Some are college graduates and many have very idealistic social goals. Many of them have gone into this work because of their concern about society and their desire to change things. They may see their role in a broad, political context and may put a great deal of effort into political organizing as a tool for drug prevention. If a nurse is going to work well with these groups, it is important that she be sensitive to their concerns and recognize the broader social contexts in which they see treatment activities. Many of them are unduly sensitive about professionals as being representatives of "the establishment," and the nurse may initially have to work hard to establish her role not as an exploiter, but as someone who is concerned and has real services to offer to people in trouble. Working with groups that put emphasis on political activity is a new experience to many nurses, and it requires the careful thinking

[8] Frederick B. Glaser, Freda Adler, Arthur D. Moffett, and John C. Ball, "The Quality of Treatment for Drug Abuse," *American Journal of Psychiatry,* **131,** No. 5 (1974), 598–601.

through of the nurse's own philosophic position on the scope of her own activities in this area.

Ex-addict staff members of self-help residential programs frequently have a very different background. Most of them are more lower-middle class in background and have come up through treatment programs as clients. Nurses may be more comfortable with their orientation, which is usually directed to the rehabilitation of single individuals and has fewer political overtones. While their treatment techniques may be very different from those of traditional psychiatry, their emphasis on the individual and their relatively lesser degree of interest in social and political activities is an approach that is comfortable for most mental health professionals. They tend to be more rigid about the use of drugs, including alcohol and marijuana, than do other paraprofessionals who may be very liberal about some social drug use, although they eschew the use of opiates and barbiturates.

For one to survive many years on the street as a heroin addict, one is required to have a great deal of intelligence, cunning, and manipulative skills. If there is a hierarchy on the street, the heroin addict is clearly at the top. He or she has to be a successful crook, a successful drug dealer, and a shrewd judge of people to survive in this milieu. Individuals who have come this route and then have gone through successful treatment are frequently extremely bright and capable. Nurses will do themselves a disservice by not recognizing the caliber and competence of some of these ex-addicts. If treated with genuine respect, many ex-addicts and other paraprofessionals will be very willing to work comfortably with professionals.

SUMMARY   Much of the frustration in dealing with addicts is centered around the management of the chronic treatment failure. The natural history of addiction suggests that many individuals who have previously failed in treatment may suddenly respond to a new treatment opportunity or may spontaneously stop using drugs.[9] What combination of social, biological, and psychological factors contributes to this reversal of their previous history of failure is unknown. Nonetheless, the nurse must always maintain an optimistic attitude toward patients and recognize that many addicts will eventually mature out of their illness and that this present treatment encounter might be an opportunity for effective rehabilitation. The nurse also must be tolerant of the chronic nature of the disease and willing to start again with patients who have failed or previously dropped out of treatment. These failures must not be held against the patient, and they must not be used as excuses to prevent re-entry into programs. Staff morale and effectiveness can best be maintained if treatment goals for each individual patient are realistic. Goals must be developed in complete cooperation with the patient and, in many situations, must represent small progressive steps rather than demands for the

[9]George E. Vaillant, "Twelve-Year Follow-up of New York Narcotic Addicts," *New England Journal of Medicine,* **275,** No. 23 (1966), 1282.

achievement of major personality and social changes over short periods of time. In dealing with these patients, it is important that programs set consistent limits and that they respond immediately whenever there is any indication that the patient is having difficulty. Many addicts have a strong unconscious need to manufacture recurring failures in their lives. This is usually done by setting very unreasonable goals which they are guaranteed not to achieve, and thus they continue to support their depression, low self-esteem, and sense of failure.

Although drug abusers may be extremely difficult and frustrating, they present a real therapeutic challenge. The gratification of successful treatment of these patients is a major reward for individuals working in this field.

REFERENCES AND SUGGESTED READINGS

Caskey, Kathryn, Enid Blaylock, and Beryl Wanson (1970). "The School Nurse and Drug Abusers," *Nursing Outlook,* **18,** No. 12, 27–31.

B., Elaine, Clare M., June S., and Janet A. (1974). "Helping the Nurse Who Misuses Drugs," *American Journal of Nursing,* **74,** No. 9, 1665–71.

Fink, Max, Alfred M. Freedman, Arthur M. Zaks, and Richard B. Resnick (1971). "Narcotic Antagonists: Another Approach to Addiction Therapy," *American Journal of Nursing,* **71,** No. 7, 1359–63.

McDermott, Sister Raphael (1970). "Maintaining the Methadone Patient," *Nursing Outlook,* **18,** No. 12, 22–26.

Morgan, Arthur James and Judith Wilson Moreno (1973). "Attitudes toward Addiction," *American Journal of Nursing,* **73,** No. 3, 497–501.

Russaw, Ethel H. (1970). "Nursing in a Narcotic Detoxification Unit," *American Journal of Nursing,* **70,** No. 8, 1720–23.

Yolles, Stanley F. (1970). "The Drug Scene," *Nursing Outlook,* **18,** No. 7, 24–26.

PERSPECTIVES

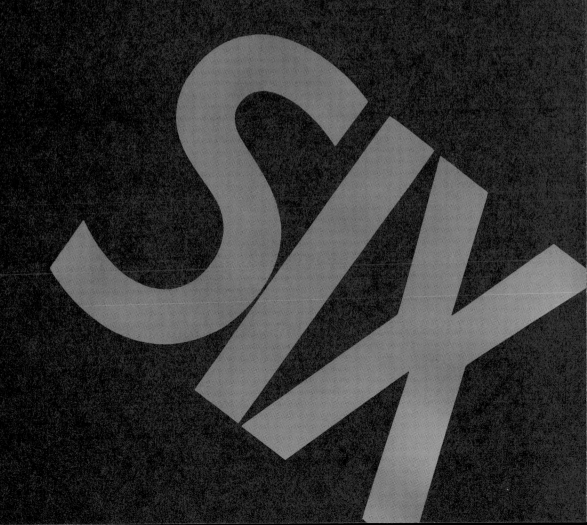

History and theory are two essential components of any systematic study of a discipline. The heritage and substantive content provide the foundation for the profession to proceed with its challenge and direction.

Psychiatric nursing not only has a theoretical basis but also has a historical evolution of practice. In the last chapter we will discuss the historical and theoretical perspectives of psychiatric nursing.

Chapter 28 Perspectives in Psychiatric-Mental Health Nursing

The mystical model of mental healing describes the historical thread from primitive times through the eighteenth century. The custodial model of care traces the thread through contemporary times. The evolution of psychiatric nursing includes the current role parameters of practice.

The basic theoretical foundation for this text is the humanistic theory of people. In conjunction with this, the contributions from the fields of psychoanalysis, social theory, medical theory, learning theory, the existential school of thought, and nursing are so identified.

Standards of Nursing Practice are included in the appropriate sections of the chapter.

PERSPECTIVES IN PSYCHIATRIC-MENTAL HEALTH NURSING

28

In order to provide a perspective for psychiatric nursing practice today, the historical evolution of mental healing should be considered. It is often surprising that what is considered contemporary frequently has its roots centuries back and that which was considered poor and antiquated practice then still exists today.

The practice of mental healing has been a chronic problem for society to face and a challenging one for nursing to confront. Attitudes held centuries ago still prevail in some communities.

One view for the value of the historical perspective may be seen in the following example:

> A psychiatric nurse–clinician was listening to several undergraduate nursing students discuss something new they wanted to try out in the clinical setting. The nurse said, "You ought to do some reading on it. Several years ago they tried to do that here."
>
> One of the students threw up her hands and said, "Why is it that someone has always done what we want to do?"

Although this example points up some of the frustrations in attempting to be creative in a clinical setting, it also implies that the historical aspects are important in moving ahead and trying out ideas. The past often determines the future of a project. Scientific knowledge is history and giants do stand on the shoulders of giants.

Psychiatric nursing will advance in proportion to the clinical research that it is able to conduct. Many productive clinical research projects are going on in nursing and there needs to be more support for them. As more nurses do research, they will increase their sensitivity to the problems inherent in the research process and, in turn, will be further developing the nursing body of knowledge.

Standard XIV specifically emphasizes the importance of research.[1]

[1]Congress for Nursing Practice, *Standards of Psychiatric-Mental Health Nursing* (Kansas City, Mo.: American Nurses' Association, 1973), p. 7.

STANDARD XIV

CONTRIBUTIONS TO NURSING AND THE MENTAL HEALTH FIELD ARE MADE THROUGH INNOVATIONS IN THEORY AND PRACTICE AND PARTICIPATION IN RESEARCH.

RATIONALE: Each professional has responsibility for the continuing development and refinement of knowledge in the mental health field through research and experimentation with new and creative approaches to practice.

Assessment Factors:
1. Studies are developed, implemented and evaluated.
2. Responsible standards of research are used in investigative endeavors.
3. Nursing practice is approached with an inquiring and open mind.
4. The pertinent and responsible research of others is supported.
5. Expert consultation and/or supervision is sought as required.
6. The ability to discriminate those findings which are pertinent to the advancement of nursing practice is demonstrated.
7. Innovations in theory, practice and research findings are made available through presentations and/or publications.

THE MYSTICAL MODEL OF MENTAL HEALING

The story of mental healing starts with the history of people. To early humans mental life was something either supernatural or something to be ignored.

The concept of mystical or supernatural causes accounting for the destiny of a person is not uncommon today. Many superstitions lend credence to this concept. "Whatever will be will be" or "that was meant to be" are examples of such beliefs when tragedy strikes.

The historical origins of this mystical model of viewing mental illness go back to ancient or even prehistoric times. Primitive man viewed disease as an evil spirit that took possession of the body as punishment for an offense against the spirit world. When man offended the demons of nature, he invited their revenge. This revenge might strike down an individual, his family, the village community, or an entire tribe. Therefore, the primitive art of mental healing was the art of driving hostile spirits away. The possibility of dying a natural death was unknown to primitive people. To them death was caused by the spirit world.

This view of illness was believed to be in effect around 2500 B.C. and was dominated by attitudes of fear and superstition. It became evident that mental patients were turned out into the hills. Skulls with trepa (drilled holes) were found far from the rest of the village. Restraints or actual physical rejection were the only care afforded these unhappy victims.

Undoubtedly, the primitive world had its share of psychiatric problems. Epileptics, the eccentric individual, or the psychotic often were the witch doctors of the village. They were able to capitalize on the weakness or power, as it were, of their minds. The supernatural cause of illness was a major influence during this period.

From the fifteenth to the seventeenth century the mentally ill were legally prosecuted and burned as witches, for they were thought to be the agents of evil spirits. Since these people were supposedly endangering the community, they had to be put to death.

Physical rejection of the mentally ill was seen not only in ancient times but also in the early days of the colonies, but, fortunately, some of these communities did nothing as drastic as executing anyone who was mentally ill. When community resources were unavailable, mental illness was the responsibility of the immediate family. In this situation some of the handicapped and mentally ill were often turned out to wander as vagrants and others were imprisoned in their rooms. In the days when communities were being settled, social values were placed on work productivity. Care could not be spared for nonproductive members of the society, and no provisions were made for those who could not meet work requirements. Mental illness was not viewed as having a cause or needing treatment. If the person improved or was able to work, he was allowed back into the family. The attitude during colonial times was punitive and the care was often sadistic.

An example of the mystical model of mental healing in current medical practice is the use of placebo medicine. The prestige of the professional stance can be quite useful at times. The patient is given sugar and water as a method of medication treatment. In effect, a "jelly bean" has helped the patient, although in most cases the patient is not usually aware of such placebo medicine. He is helped by his "belief" in the professionals caring for him. The attitudes of the physicians and nurses toward the medicine and power they hold over the patient have an effect on the recovery.

The description of magical cures, generally called "miracles," frequently are reported in the newspapers. Everyone has read of cases in which people have survived fatal diseases or have recovered from serious illnesses without any aid or benefit from medical treatment. When people are faced with serious illness, they usually hope for an unexplained or supernatural model of care.

The concept of magic strategy is prevalent among children. When young children fall down, they generally hurt their pride more than they hurt themselves. If they have Bandaids applied to their minor scrapes and bruises, tears and complaints will mysteriously disappear. The children think that magic has taken away their hurts.

This kind of thinking may carry over into adulthood. When a physical symptom occurs, many people will employ the magical idea that the symptom will disappear. They quite vehemently deny the existence of the symptom. Or when serious illness or tragedy occurs, people automatically ask themselves, "Why me?" or "What did I do to deserve this?" These archaic beliefs seem to be indestructible.

The historical origins and treatment models of custodial care, the second evolutionary model of care, can be traced back to Greek and Roman times. The enlightened attitudes of humane treatment and concern were obvious. The care included sedation with opiates, music therapy, good physical hygiene, and humane management of the patient's daily activities. This concept, however, was abandoned when the Roman Empire deteriorated and the supernatural concept again existed until the eighteenth century.

In the nineteenth century the mentally ill were collected together and someone was paid to watch over them. This model developed out of necessity because families could not bear the full responsibility of guarding or tending to the mentally ill person. Thus developed the model of custodial care, supported financially by private and community efforts. Mental difficulties at this time were considered irreversible and, therefore, protecting society from these deranged individuals took precedence over treatment models.

The institutions operated on the concept of detention rather than treatment. State hospitals rapidly became too large and overcrowded. These institutions were, and still are, the only source of psychiatric help for many citizens. The social–psychiatric problems inherent in this system and the organization of patient care are the concerns of mental health specialists today. Patient care services have developed markedly in many state hospitals, but severe problems still remain.

The mental hospital assumed this custodial role early in American psychiatric history. This goal was to keep the patient safe, to guard him, and to manage him because he was incapable of managing his own life.

Mental hospitals at this time functioned in an autocratic way, rendering patients helpless by their treatment. The patient was seen as defective, incompetent, and potentially dangerous. His rights were denied him and he was considered an incapable citizen in our society. The patient was forced into an institutional mode of behavior. Families were not allowed to take an active role in the treatment process and, in many instances, were even discouraged from visiting. The stigma of being a mental patient was communicated to the patient. There was a continual increase in social isolation and an increasing pattern of conformity to the needs of the institution.

The institution did provide "custodial care." Shelter, rest, and food were provided for the patient. Under the existing conditions, however, this was not the most effective treatment. Losing more and more of his options, interacting mainly with other psychotic patients, and dealing with a non-trained and frequently punitive staff, the mental patient became more institutionalized, more chronic, and less able to return to his family and community.

Where these conditions still exist, the possibility of change must be raised by the community. The attitudes and social consciousness of people are what make the difference in care models. Until a community feels concern and responsibility for the mental illness of its people, change cannot occur.

THE EVOLUTION OF PSYCHIATRIC NURSING

It is difficult to document exactly when the caring of the mentally ill by nurses actually began because the history we have available is incomplete. However, it is known that the mentally ill were treated very kindly by members of religious orders during the Middle Ages. The first attempt to provide special training for this kind of work was made in 1645 by Madame Le Gras at the Petite Maison in France. Students were recruited by the Order of St. Vincent de Paul. William Pinel organized the "Filles de Services" for convalescent and recovered patients, but after a few decades of trial in France, Holland, and other European countries this system gradually failed.

The first psychiatric training school in the United States began in 1882 at the McLean Hospital in Belmont, Massachusetts, by Edward Cowles, the medical director. The value of this school was so quickly appreciated that within 10 years there were 19 American institutions providing psychiatric training programs.

Certificates were given to the students at McLean upon completion of the course and in 1886 the hospital took another step forward by making an affiliation with the Massachusetts General Hospital whereby credit for a full nursing course was given upon completion of the senior year at the hospital. In England a similar program was in effect and a certificate was given to these graduates from the Medico–Psychological Association.

Many difficulties were encountered in the development of psychiatric nursing in America. The greatest was that there seemed to be little demand for the so-called "asylum-trained" nurse. By 1916 half of the mental hospitals in the United States still had no school for their nurses. These hospitals employed attendants at very low wages and provided them with very poor living conditions. It is no wonder that nursing of the mentally ill was so slow starting and catching on.

In 1935 only half of the then existing diploma schools of nursing offered psychiatric nursing in their curriculum. Psychiatric nursing was not a requirement for state registration until 1952.

The initial inroads of psychiatric nursing were most dramatically made in the 1940s and 1950s. The pioneer nursing leaders at this time primarily worked with the long hospitalized psychotic patient. This was the patient population left untreated or even unattended in some institutions. These nurses provided human services for the mentally ill with minimal financial return. Wages were extremely low and many nurses with advanced academic education were glad to get room, board, and uniforms. But this is the heritage and the backbone of the kind of nurse who aided in mental healing in the first half of the twentieth century.

The major impetus in the field of psychiatric nursing resulted from a study by the National League for Nursing in 1950 which concluded that special training was required for psychiatric nursing. This report coincided with the renewed interest precipitated by World War II in psychiatric care. The National Mental Health Act of 1946 had had a dramatic effect on education for psychiatric disciplines and on the development of patient care. It also provided federal funds to improve, expand, and initiate training programs in the mental health professions.

In the last decade the role dimensions of the psychiatric nurse have greatly expanded. The psychiatric nurse's role currently encompasses a broad range of services. The nurse may assume the traditional role of working as a team member in a psychiatric hospital. Here the nurse manages the milieu and patient care over the 24 hours. The psychiatric nurse's leadership role function is emphasized in Standard XII as a significant trend.[2]

STANDARD XII

LEARNING EXPERIENCES ARE PROVIDED FOR OTHER NURSING CARE PERSONNEL THROUGH LEADERSHIP, SUPERVISION AND TEACHING.

RATIONALE: As leader of the nursing team, the nurse is responsible for the team's activities and must be able to teach, supervise and evaluate the performance of nursing care personnel. The focus in on the continuing development of each member of the team.

Assessment Factors:
1. Leadership roles and responsibilities are accepted.
2. Team members are encouraged to identify strengths and abilities. A climate is provided for the continuing self-development of each member.
3. A role model in giving and directing nursing care is provided for the team.
4. The supervisory role is used as a tool for improving nursing care.
5. The client's needs, as well as the abilities of each member of the nursing team, are evaluated and assignments are based on these evaluations.

The trend toward interdisciplinary collaboration and the role of the nurse in the community is spelled out in Standard XI.[3]

A very important trend in psychiatric nursing is that of independent practice. This concept was discussed earlier in relation to counseling patients. Concurrent with this trend is the work in progress on certification, which is the professional recognition of the nurse who is qualified to practice advanced psychiatric–mental health nursing.

The curriculum design in psychiatric nursing affords the nurse increasing opportunities in the delivery of psychiatric–mental health services. The

[2]Ibid., p. 2.
[3]Ibid., p. 6.

STANDARD XI

NURSING PARTICIPATES WITH OTHER MEMBERS OF THE COMMUNITY IN PLANNING AND IMPLEMENTING MENTAL HEALTH SERVICES THAT INCLUDE THE BROAD CONTINUUM OF PROMOTION OF MENTAL HEALTH, PREVENTION OF MENTAL ILLNESS, TREATMENT AND REHABILITATION.

RATIONALE: In our contemporary society, the high incidence of mental illness and mental retardation requires increased effort to devise more effective treatment and prevention programs. There is a need for nursing to participate in programs that strengthen existing health potential of all members of society. In this effort cooperation and intervention and continuity of care are essential in planning to meet the mental health needs of the community. The nurse uses organizational, advisory or consultative skills to facilitate the development and implementation of mental health services.

Assessment Factors:

1. Knowledge of community and group dynamics is used to understand the structure and function of the community system.
2. Current social issues that influence the nature of mental health problems in the community are recognized.
3. High risk population groups in the community are delineated and gaps in community services are identified.
4. Community members are encouraged to become active in assessing community mental health needs and planning programs to meet these needs.
5. The strength and capacities of individuals, families and the community are assessed in order to promote and increase the health potential of all.
6. Consultative skills are used to facilitate the development and implementation of mental health services.
7. The needs of the community are brought to the attention of appropriate individuals and groups, including legislative bodies and regional and state planning groups.
8. The mental health services of the agency are interpreted to others in the community. There is collaboration with the staff of other agencies to insure continuity of service for patients and families.
9. Community resources are used appropriately.
10. Nursing participates with other professional and nonprofessional members of the community in the planning, implementation and evaluation of mental health services.

nursing student is taught the fundamentals of the nurse–patient relationship in her basic nursing education. At the graduate level, intensive training in interviewing and the psychotherapeutic concepts and techniques are taught so that the nurse is prepared to do individual and group therapies. Skills in consultation, collaboration, and primary care practice are included. Doctoral nursing clinical programs continue to build on this foundation and enable the nurse–therapist to further expand the parameters of the role.

In acknowledgement of this trend in the profession, Standard XIII cites the need for the nurse to assume responsibility for continued education.[4]

STANDARD XIII

RESPONSIBILITY IS ASSUMED FOR CONTINUING EDUCATIONAL AND PROFESSIONAL DEVELOPMENT AND CONTRIBUTIONS ARE MADE TO THE PROFESSIONAL GROWTH OF OTHERS.

RATIONALE: The scientific, cultural and social changes characterizing our contemporary society require the nurse to be committed to the ongoing pursuit of knowledge which will enhance professional growth.

Assessment Factors:
1. There is evidence of study of one's nursing practice to increase both understanding and skill.
2. There is evidence of participation in in-service meetings and educational programs either as an attendee or as a teacher.
3. There is evidence of attendance at conventions, institutes, workshops, symposia and other professionally oriented meetings and/or other ways to increase formal education.
4. There is evidence of systematic efforts to increase understanding of psychodynamics, psychopathology and avenues of psychotherapeutic intervention.
5. There is evidence of cognizance of developments in relevant fields and utilization of this knowledge.
6. There is evidence of assisting others to identify areas of educational needs.
7. There is evidence of sharing appropriate clinical observations and interpretations with professionals and other groups.

THEORETICAL PERSPECTIVES We have attempted to describe throughout the book the ways in which effective nurses work with patients. We described how the theoretical approach varied according to the treatment setting, the patient's request, and other important variables. The future may provide one unified theory of human behavior that will satisfy everyone, but until such a theory is proposed we will have to take into account several theories as we view each patient.

This section will take an overview of the various theoretical frameworks that have been described in earlier chapters. In clinical practice, the problem is not deciding which approach is good and which is bad; the prob-

[4]Ibid., p. 7.

lem is deciding what combinations of theoretical approaches are best for a given patient in a particular clinical situation.

Humanistic framework

Much of our outlook in this book is the result of a general humanistic approach to humans: an approach that deems people worthy of such human considerations as respect, caring, understanding, patience, and concern. Different theoretical systems in psychiatry have translated these needs into technical terms, but we feel that it is essential to recognize that this humanistic theoretical perspective is broader than any particular theory.

Two basic assumptions of the humanistic approach are: (1) The potential helping quality of all people. It becomes important, therefore, to maximize those "helper" attitudes in the nurse by enabling her to find what is human within herself. (2) The worth of all those needing help. Unless one feels that all people are worthy of maximal therapeutic efforts, then all attempts, no matter how technically sophisticated, will fall short of the mark.

We have said that talking is a human characteristic. By encouraging meaningful dialogue through interviews that deal with matters of the heart rather than irrelevant intellectual issues, the nurse reaches the human goal. In effect, she talks person-to-person rather than person-to-thing.

Even when a person has not had the experience of talking sincerely about what really matters to him, the nurse tries to teach the patient that he can express his feelings. The goal is to let the patient know that his feelings and what he has to say are important.

Although we acknowledge that the humanistic approach is basic to our philosophy, we also realize that this approach by itself is not enough. We as professional helpers must have technical knowledge. For this reason, we shall now discuss the several different conceptual frameworks and schools of thought that have contributed to the nursing care of psychiatric patients.

Psychoanalytic school of thought

Psychoanalytic theory is an important conceptual framework used throughout the book. Much of psychoanalytic theory, it should be noted, has become a part of the everyday vocabulary of mental health workers and even lay people. The "Freudian slip," the unconscious, and defensive techniques such as projection, rationalization, and displacement are but a few examples.

Contributions from social theories

The major thread of Part Five, the Community, is based on the sociological concepts of the individual, society, and culture and their interrelationships.

The individual has a life cycle in which he develops a style of life through his socialization process and learning. He learns to behave in certain ascribed and achieved ways that may be integrated or in conflict and that may afford him a particular status in reference to others. He may, at any given time in his life, be healthy or ill, and he may face equilibrium or crisis. His concept of self is acquired through association and communication in intrapersonal and interpersonal situations. He may experience anxiety or loneliness, even alienation or happiness.

The individual lives within a society and culture that provide him with norms of behavior and group life. Within the society are groups, families, and communities, each with political, economic, and legal systems. Professions, ideologies, and institutions add to the social systems within which members of the socially stratified society function. Society too changes and with its changes often come social problems.

Society cannot exist without individuals; individuals cannot live apart from society. Both constantly interact with and influence each other. This must be considered as all of the above concepts become woven into the fabric of community mental health nursing.

Contributions from medical theories

Part of the nursing heritage is the medical approach which focuses on (1) careful observation of signs and symptoms which assist the physician in the diagnosis of diseases, (2) treatments by medical techniques such as the administration of drugs and electroconvulsive therapy, (3) the observation of side effects of any of the above treatments.

Contributions from learning theory

The format of this book has as its basic foundations the goals of education and learning theory described by Alfred North Whitehead, who said that education is learning the art of utilizing knowledge. His philosophy is built upon two forms of instruction: the teaching of content and the teaching of attitudes and modes of approaches. The teaching of content is often the less difficult of the tasks for it involves presenting subject matter (data and facts); the basic rules and principles of scientific methodology and techniques, the do's and don't's; and the opposing views and information with which to combat ignorance. The teaching of attitudes and modes of approaches, which is a harder task, is essential if there is to be a high-level of performance in the practice. Nursing requires both goals of teaching.

The principles of teaching people by presenting alternatives and helping them with their decision-making process will result in people's feeling responsible and involved in their own fate. This method is felt to be superior to the method of teaching by telling the individual only the negative aspects of the issue instead of both the affirmative and negative aspects of the issue in order for him to make the decision.

Another contribution from learning theory that we utilized is conceptualizing psychotherapy as a learning process. The nurse can reward those behaviors that are approved of by showing warmth, giving emotionally, and by a nod of the head. She reinforces positive behavior by giving an affirmative response to what the patients tell her.

Contributions from the existential school of thought

The search for meaning is a basic component of the existential framework. It is one of the important aspects of psychiatric nursing. Meaning in this particular sense denotes the connection of an unknown with the known. The behavioral symptoms (described in Part IV) that the patient presents, coupled with an understanding and a comprehension of the patient's problems, are what provide meaning in mental healing.

Much of the difficulty the person with an emotional disturbance experiences is his inability to communicate clearly his distress with another human being. This failure produces feelings of estrangement along with the feeling that he is not properly understood. The nurse's task becomes one of helping to bridge the gap between the symptoms the person describes and the meaning and understanding he is requesting.

The existential framework implies that the process of living is an art. It is the most important and at the same time the most difficult and complex art practiced by man. A person's choice is not necessarily between life and death, but rather an alternative between a meaningful or a nonrelevant life. As discussed in the chapters dealing with psychotherapeutic approaches, the nurse uses therapeutic skills to help the patient deal with alternatives to life's situations. If alternatives to an intolerable situation are not offered to a patient, particularly a suicidal patient, he may choose to die.

SUMMARY This chapter described the treatment models related to a historical evolutionary thread. The mystical model of mental healing traced primitive man's view of mental illness and healing and the custodial model traced its focus from Greek and Roman times to the nineteenth and twentieth century practice. The evolution of mental healing by nurses was traced from its first attempts in 1645 to the current psychiatric nurse's role. Perspectives were identified as stated by the Standards of Nursing Practice.

Theorectical perspectives of the text were identified. Overall philosophy is the humanistic approach to the patient. Nursing particularly lends itself to the humanistic dimension of caring because the nurse has traditionally cared for the patient on a 24-hour basis.

Many contributing theories, concepts, and schools of thought were presented in this chapter, such as the psychoanalytic, the social, the medical, the learning, and the existential. All of these contributions should be viewed in terms of how useful the concepts are in a particular setting.

One does not have to accept all the theories. It may be more useful to accept parts of them rather than the whole. The essential goal, however, is to give the patient the human care that he deserves in order to show him that human life really does matter—that his life really matters.

REFERENCES AND SUGGESTED READINGS

Briggs, Paulette Fitzgerald (1974). "Specializing in Psychiatry: Therapeutic or Custodial." *Nursing Outlook,* **22,** No. 10, 632–35.

Clemence, Sister Madeline (1966). "Existentialism: A Philosophy of Commitment," *American Journal of Nursing,* **66,** No. 3, 500–505.

Flynn, Beverly C. (1974). "The Effectiveness of Nurse Clinicians Service Delivery," *American Journal of Public Health,* **64,** No. 6, 604–11.

Fromm, Eric (1966). *The Art of Loving.* New York: Harper & Row, Publishers.

Georgopoulos, Basil, and Luther Christman (1970). "Clinical Nurse Specialist: A Role Model," *American Journal of Nursing,* **70,** No. 5, 1030–39.

Gordon, Marjorie (1969). "The Clinical Specialist as Change Agent," *Nursing Outlook,* **17,** No. 3, 37–39.

Jacox, Ada (1974). "Nursing Research and the Clinician," *Nursing Outlook,* **22,** No. 6, 382–85.

Jordon, Judith D., and Joseph C. Shipp (1971). "The Primary Health Care Professional was a Nurse," *American Journal of Nursing,* **71,** No. 5, 922–25.

Kalisch, Beatrice (1975). "Creative Nursing Research," *Nursing Outlook,* **23,** No. 5, 314–19.

May, Rollo, Ernest Angel, and Henri Ellenberger (1958). *Existence: A New Dimension in Psychiatry and Psychology.* New York: Basic Books, Inc.

McElroy, Evelyn, and Anita Narciso (1971). "Clinical Specialist in the Community Mental Health Program," *Journal of Psychiatric Nursing,* **9,** No. 1, 19–26.

Meldman, Monte, Bernard Newman, Donna Schaller, and Paul Peterson (1971). "Patient's Responses to Nurse Psychotherapists," *American Journal of Nursing* **71,** No. 6, 1150–51.

Mereness, Dorothy (1970). "Recent Trends in Expanding Roles of the Nurse," *Nursing Outlook,* **18,** No. 5, 30–33.

Rohde, Illdaura (1968). "The Nurse as Family Therapist," *Nursing Outlook,* **16,** No. 5, 49–52.

Stachyra, Marcia (1969). "Nurses, Psychotherapy and the Law," *Perspectives in Psychiatric Care,* **7,** No. 5, 200–13.

Whitehead, Alfred North (1963). *The Aims of Education (1929).* New York: The Macmillan Company.

GLOSSARY

Acting out: Expressing certain kinds of unconscious conflicts through behavior.

Addiction: Physical and/or psychological dependence on alcohol or drugs.

Adversary: Antagonist, opponent, enemy, foe.

Affect: The feeling tone specific to an idea or issue.

Affective psychosis: A psychotic reaction in which the predominant feature is a disturbance in emotional feeling tone, usually depression or elation.

Aggression: A feeling or action that may be self-assertive, forceful, or hostile.

Agitation: The psychomotor expression of uncomfortable feelings (pacing, picking at the skin, restless movement of the hands or legs).

Alienation: Belonging or pertaining to another.

Ambivalence: Simultaneous conflicting feelings or attitudes toward a person or object.

Amnesia: A dissociative experience in which the person's recollection is lost or split off from conscious recall. May be functional or organic.

Anaclitic: Characterized by dependence, a leaning on.

Anxiety: A state of uneasiness, apprehension, or tension caused by a non-specific danger or threat. There is the subjective sense of impending doom that is accompanied by autonomic symptoms of rapid pulse, increased respiration, and perspiration.

Apathy: A state of indifference.

Assault: A violent attack which may be physical or verbal.

Association: Connecting one thought or feeling with another.

Attitude: The position taken on an issue.

Autism: An absorption, in fantasy, to the complete exclusion of reality as in hallucinations and day dreaming.

Autoerotic: Sensual self-gratification as through thumbsucking, stroking, masturbation.

Behavior: The actions of an individual or persons.

Blocking: The sudden arrest in the train of a thought.

Blunting: A dullness of emotional response.

503

Castration: Literally, the loss or damage of the genital organs. Symbolically, a state of powerlessness or psychological impotence.

Cathexis: The emotional investment in a person, an object, or an idea.

Character: The personality traits or behavioral style of an individual.

Circumstantiality: The quality of being circumstantial; minuteness of detail.

Cognitive: The mental processes of thinking, memory, comprehension, and reasoning.

Community: A population within a geographic area engaging in social interaction and having common ties.

Complex: A group of associated ideas that have a strong emotional tone and generally are unconscious.

Compulsion: An act resulting from an uncontrollable impulse.

Concussion: A condition of impaired functioning of a body organ, especially the head, following a forceful blow.

Confabulation: The filling in of memory gaps with made-up stories. The patient believes the stories to be true.

Conflict: A clash largely determined by unconscious forces between two opposing emotional forces. Conflict is basic in psychic life and fundamental in the etiology of psychological disorders.

Confusion: A state of disordered orientation.

Congenital: Inherent at birth.

Consciousness: Being aware of one's environment and one's self.

Constitution: The psychological and physical endowment of an individual; his potential or physical inheritance from birth.

Consumer: One who utilizes services.

Conversion: An unconscious process by which an emotional conflict is expressed as a physical symptom. For example, the psychogenic paralysis of an arm prevents its use in an aggressive manner.

Coping: Problem-solving efforts in a stressful situation.

Counter-transference: The feelings and reactions of the therapist toward his patient that are derived from his early experiences.

Crime: Conduct that is in violation of the law.

Crisis: A crucial situation which, in turn, causes a disequilibrium to an individual's life-style.

Crisis intervention: Short-term treatment that attempts to assist the patient in the settlement of a crisis.

Culture: The social characteristics of a particular group of people, often more narrowly defined as the normative aspect of society, the prescriptions about what one should do and the proscriptions about what one should not do in a given society.

Customer: One who purchases some commodity or service.

Defense mechanisms: Processes by which the mind seeks relief from emotional conflict.

Deja vu: A feeling of familiarity with a place or situation that one has never actually been to or been in.

Delinquent child: A person under a specific age who has violated a law.

Delirium: A state of mental disturbance caused by organic conditions and characterized by disorientation, confusion, and often hallucinations.

Delirium tremens: Delirium induced by prolonged and excessive use of alcohol.

Delusion: A false, fixed belief that cannot be changed by logic.

Dementia: An irreversible deterioration of mental capacities.

Dementia praecox: An obsolete term for schizophrenia.

Denial: A defense mechanism by which the mind refuses to acknowledge a thought, feeling, wish, need, or reality factor.

Dependency needs: Essential needs for mothering, love, affection, shelter, protection, security, food, and warmth that begin at birth.

Depersonalization: The experiencing of feelings of unrealness about the self or the environment.

Depression: A psychiatric term to describe morbid sadness, dejection, or melancholy. It is distinguished from grief which is realistic and proportionate to what has been lost.

Deprivation, emotional: Lack of adequate human or environmental experience.

Deprivation, sensory: Lack of adequate perceptual stimuli such as may occur to a confined prisoner.

Descriptive psychiatry: A system of psychiatry based upon the study of observable phenomena; to be differentiated from dynamic psychiatry.

Deterioration: A progressive decline.

Diagnosis: A careful examination of evidence to determine an opinion as in the nature of a traumatic or diseased condition.

Discrimination: Unfavorable treatment of groups of people on arbitrary grounds.

Discrimination: To separate one person or group from another by the use of preferential characteristics.

Disfranchise: To deprive of a right, privilege, or power.

Disorientation: Loss of awareness of the position of self in terms of time, space, or other people.

Displacement: A defense mechanism whereby a feeling is transferred to a more acceptable substitute object.

Dissociation: A mental defense of separating one item from another item.

Dream: Mental activity during sleep that is dissociated from the self and consciousness of the waking state.

Drive: Motivation or basic urge in man; to be distinguished from the purely biological concept of drive.

Dynamic: Forceful and active.

Dynamic psychiatry: The study and interpretation of emotional processes and the changing factors in human behavior and its motivation.

Dynamics of behavior: The understanding and significance of a person's behavior.

Dysmnesia: An impairment in the ability to retain and recall information.

Eclectic: Selecting from various systems.

Ego: That part of the pscyhic structure that deals with reality.

Egocentric: Concern with self.

Ego ideal: That part of the psychic structure that represents the ideal aims and goals of the individual.

Electroconvulsive therapy: Electric treatments to produce a grand mal convulsion in an individual.

Electroencephalogram: A tracing by an electroencephalogram to record electrical discharges in the brain.

Emotion: A subjective feeling, such as fear, anger, joy, love, surprise, etc.

Empathy: The capacity for participating in or a vicarious experience of another's feelings, volitions, or ideas.

Empirical: Based upon experience or observation. Capable of being confirmed, verified or disproved by observation or experiment.

Encopresis: Fecal soiling.

Enterprise: An undertaking that involves activity, energy, and courage.

Enuresis: Incontinence of urine; bed-wetting.

Epilepsy: A neurological disorder of consciousness that is often accompanied by a convulsion.

Euphoria: An exaggerated sense of well-being.

Exhibitionism: (1) The act or practice or behaving so as to attract attention to oneself; (2) display of one's genital organs in public.

External crisis: A crisis event that is externally imposed (as contrasted with a developmental crisis).

Extroversion: Behavior, thoughts, and feelings that are directed outward from the self.

Fabrication: Made-up events to fill in gaps of memory.

Fantasy: A sequence of imagined events as in day dreaming.

Fainting: Temporary loss of consciousness.

Fear: An emotional response to perceived danger; to be distinguished from anxiety that does not necessarily identify the danger.

Feminist movement: A social movement organized on the behalf of women's rights.

Fixation: Psychoanalytic term to indicate an arrest at a particular stage of psychosexual development.

Flight of ideas: The rapid succession of ideas that are not necessarily related to each other.

Free association: A psychoanalytic technique whereby the patient must say whatever comes into his mind.

Fugue state: A dissociative state characterized by amnesia and actual physical flights from an intolerable situation.

Functional mental illness: Illness of an emotional origin in which organic change cannot be demonstrated.

General paresis: A psychosis caused by a chronic syphilitic infection in the central nervous system.

Gerontophobia: A morbid fear of aging.

Ghetto: A section of a city in which members of a social group are segregated.

Globus hystericus: A symptom in which there is a sensation of having a ball in the throat; an hysterical spasm of the esophagus.

Grandiose: A term referring to delusions or feelings of power, fame, splendor, magnificence.

Grief: A normal emotional response to recognized loss; self-limiting and gradually subsiding within a reasonable time.

Group dynamics: The study of the process of small groups.

Hallucination: An imaginary sense perception.

Heterosexual: Sexual attraction between members of the opposite sex.

Homosexual: Sexual attraction between members of the same sex.

Homosexual panic: Acute and severe feelings of anxiety based upon unconscious homosexual conflict.

Human: That which is characteristic of people.

Hyperactive: Increased behavior.

Hyperkinesis: Increased muscular movement.

Hypochondriasis: A strong and abnormal preoccupation with one's state of health.

Hypnosis: An induced dissociative state.

Hysteria: A neurotic behavior disorder that includes a wide variety of physical symptoms without organic changes and which uses the defense of conversion and dissociation.

Id: A psychoanalytic term to identify that part of the psychic structure that is unconscious, contains primitive drives, and operates on the pleasure principle.

Ideas of reference: The incorrect interpretation of incidents as having direct reference to the self.

Identification: An unconscious psychological mechanism whereby an individual endeavors to pattern himself after another person.

Illusion: The misinterpretation of an actual sensory experience.

Incorporation: A psychological mechanism whereby a person symbolically takes in a part of another person to be part of his self. For example, the infant fantasizes that mother's breast is part of him.

Indigenous worker: Liaison community person who facilitates health care.

Infertility: Inability to conceive a pregnancy after one year of sexual relations without contraception or the inability to carry a pregnancy to a live birth.

Insight: Self-understanding and a major goal of psychotherapy. This includes the individual's understanding of the nature, origin, and mechanisms of his thoughts, feelings, and behavior.

Instinct: Inborn drive.

Insulin shock: A somatic treatment in which a coma is induced by the injection of insulin in prescribed dosage.

Intellectualization: A defense mechanism that employs reasoning and logic to defend against uncomfortable feelings.

Intelligence: The power or act of understanding; the intellect or mind in operation.

Internal crisis: Developmental or maturational crisis situations.

Interview: To question or have a conversation with, especially in order to obtain information.

Intrapsychic: That which takes place within the mind.

Introjection: A mental mechanism in which one incorporates and accepts patterns, attitudes, and ideals of others.

Introversion: Preoccupation with one's self; the opposite of extroversion.

Involutional psychosis: A psychiatric disorder occurring during that period of life referred to as menopausal, climacteric, or involutional.

Issue: A matter on which there exists two or more points of view.

Juvenile delinquency: A legal classification of children's behavior that violates the law.

Kleptomania: Compulsive stealing.

Labile: Rapidly shifting emotions.

Latency period: A psychoanalytic term for the developmental phase between childhood and adolescence, usually ages 7 to 10.

Law: Rules of conduct formally recognized as binding by authority.

Lesbian: A female homosexual.

Liaison: Coordination of activities.

Libido: A psychoanalytic term meaning the vital force or psychic energy.

Litigation: A suit of law.

Malinger: A deliberate endeavor to use an illness to avoid an uncomfortable situation.

Manic-depressive psychosis: A major emotional illness characterized by severe mood swings alternating from depression to elation.

Megalomania: A psychiatric syndrome characterized by delusions of great self-importance, wealth, or power.

Melancholia: Severe depression.

Mental mechanisms: Specific intrapsychic defensive processes that relieve a person from uncomfortable or intolerable situations; also called defense mechanisms.

Mental retardation: A deficit in intelligence that makes the individual's intellectual abilities lower than normal for his age and development.

Milieu: The people and factors within an environment with which a person interacts.

Molest: To annoy or disturb; to unjustifiably meddle with sexually.

Motivation: The force within the individual that impels him to act.

Mutism: The inability to speak.

Narcissism: A psychoanalytic term meaning self-love.

Narcolepsy: A condition in which the individual is overcome by an uncontrollable desire to sleep.

Negative feelings: Unfriendly, hostile feelings.

Negativism: Strong resistance to suggestions or advice.

Negotiate: A discussion whereby an agreement is reached.

Neologism: The formation or development of a new word from parts of existing words.

Nervous breakdown: A nonmedical, nonspecific term for emotional illness.

Neurasthenia: A neurotic behavior in which the main pattern is motor and mental fatigue.

Neurosis: Maladaptive behavior patterns that produce psychic distress for the individual. Neuroses are classified as minor disorders although they can cause extreme suffering and may impair and weaken parts of the individual's coping ability. They are characterized by an inability of the individual to perform at his normal capability.

Nightmare: A frightening dream, often accompanied by a sensation of helplessness and impending doom.

Nosological: Classification or list of diseases.

Object: A psychoanalytic term meaning person.

Object relationship: The emotional bonds that exist between one individual and another.

Obsession: Persistent and uncontrollable thoughts.

Oedipus complex: A psychoanalytic phase of psychosexual development whereby the child (roughly age 4-7) has feelings of attachment for the parent of the opposite sex and also feelings of envy and aggression toward the parent of the same sex.

Operant conditioning: A technique of behavior therapy in which the desired behavior is rewarded and the undesired behavior is either ignored or acknowledged by punishment.

Oppositional behavior: Actions that go contrary to prescribed behavior.

Oral eroticism: Pleasurable sensations obtained from the mouth.

Oral stage: A psychosexual phase of development that refers to both the oral-erotic and oral-sadistic phases of the first year of life.

Organic mental illness: A mental illness caused by organic changes.

Orthopsychiatry: Psychiatry concerned with the study of children in which the emphasis is placed on preventive techniques to emphasize normal, healthy emotional development.

Overcompensation: A defense mechanism whereby a physical or psychological deficit produces exaggerated correction.

Panic: A term used in psychiatry to indicate acute, intense, and overwhelming anxiety.

Paranoid: A term used in psychiatry to indicate feelings of persecution, suspicion; may develop into delusions.

Personality: The sum total of the behavior style and patterns of the individual.

Perversion: A deviation from socially acceptable patterns of sexual gratification.

Phallic stage: A psychosexual phase of development (roughly ages 4-6) during which the child's interest centers around issues of potency and strength.

Phobia: An obsessive, persistent, and unrealistic fear of an external object or situation. Common phobias are: acrophobia (heights), agoraphobia (open spaces), aquaphobia (water), crudanophobia (crowds), claustrophobia (closed spaces), mysophobia (dirt), myctophobia (dark), pyrophobia (fire).

Pica: The abnormal ingestion of substances that have no nutritional value, such as paper, paint, soil.

Play therapy: A technique used in child psychiatry to establish interaction between the child and a therapist.

Pleasure principle: A basic psychoanalytic concept that man seeks to avoid pain and strives for gratification and pleasure.

Preconscious: That part of the psychic structure in which thoughts are not in immediate awareness but can be recalled by conscious effort.

Prevention, primary: The promotion of health and the prevention of illness.

Prevention, secondary: Early detection of illness and prompt treatment.

Prevention, tertiary: Rehabilitative efforts to minimize the effects of an illness.

Projection: A defense mechanism whereby thoughts, attitudes, and motivations are directed out into the environment and not to the person.

Psychiatric nursing: A specialty within the nursing profession in which efforts are directed by the nurse toward promotion of mental health, prevention of mental illness, early casefinding of and intervention in emotional problems, and follow-up care to minimize long-term effects of mental illness.

Psychiatrist: A doctor of medicine who deals with the origins, diagnosis, treatment, and prevention of mental illness.

Psychiatry: A specialty within medicine that deals with mental illness.

Psychoanalysis: A theory of human development, human behavior, and a form of psychotherapeutic treatment developed by Sigmund Freud and his followers.

Psychoanalyst: A psychiatrist or a lay therapist who has had additional training in psychoanalysis and who practices the techniques of psychoanalytic therapy.

Psychodynamics: The systematized knowledge and theory of human behavior, its motivation, and psychoanalytic principles.

Psychogenesis: The causation of symptoms by mental or emotional factors, as opposed to organic reasons.

Psychologist: A health professional who specializes in psychology and has earned a graduate degree (an M.A. or a Ph.D.).

Psychology: A science and a profession that deals with knowledge of the psyche in relation to problems of mind and behavior.

Psychoneurosis: A psychiatric term used interchangeably with neurosis.

Psychosexual development: A psychoanalytic term that distinguishes phases of development of the person from birth to adult life.

Psychosis: A severe disability: involving coping mechanisms of the individual that is commonly characterized by a loss of contact with reality, distortion of perception, regressive behavior, and abnormal mental content.

Psychotherapy: A form of treatment for psychiatric disorders characterized by a special relationship between the patient and a professional whose goal is to modify particular symptoms or patterns of behavior that are considered maladaptive by the patient.

Racism: A belief in the inherent superiority of a given race and its right to domination over others; a political or social system based on racism.

Rape (forcible): Unlawful sexual intercourse by force and against a person's will.

Rape trauma: The resulting symptomatology to the act of rape.

Rationalization: A defense mechanism whereby the individual substitutes one reason for his behavior for the real one motivating his behavior.

Reaction formation: A defense mechanism operating unconsciously, whereby an opposite attitude or behavior takes the place of the real attitudes, impulses, or behavior the individual harbors either consciously or unconsciously.

Reality: The character of being true to life.

Reality principle: A psychoanalytic concept whereby the individual's desires and wishes are regulated in accord with the demands of reality.

Requests: The wishes or hopes of a person for a desired service or item.

Regression: A defense mechanism whereby the individual reverts to earlier patterns of behavior.

Rejection: The state of refusing to accept.

Repression: A defense mechanism that keeps unpleasant experiences and thoughts from conscious awareness.

Resistance: A psychiatric term used to imply an individual's reluctance to bring repressed thoughts or impulses into awareness.

Role: A set of expectations which is associated with a position in a social system and which determines behavior within specified limits regardless of the personality of the incumbent.

Rorschach test: A psychological test designed to disclose conscious and unconscious traits and emotional conflicts. The person being tested tells what is suggested to him when viewing a series of standard inkblot patterns.

Sadism: Pleasure derived from inflicting physical or psychological pain on others.

Schizoid: Used as an adjective to describe traits of introversion, withdrawal, aloofness.

Schizophrenia: A psychiatric syndrome characterized by a thinking disorder, withdrawal from reality, regressive behavior, poor communication, and severely impaired interpersonal relationships.

Sex: All the characteristics which distinguish between the female and the male.

Sexual assault: An attack to an individual which has sexual connotations.

Sexuality: The quality or state of being sexual.

Sibling: A term for brother or sister.

Sociology: The scientific study of society, social institutions, and social relationships, especially the study of the development, structure, and function of human groups conceptualized as processes of interaction or as organized patterns of collective behavior.

Soma: The physical aspect of humans as distinguished from the psyche.

Somatic: Physical.

Stall: A loss in the amount of forward progress necessary to maintain the therapeutic process.

Stress: A physical, chemical, or emotional factor that can cause mental tension and ready the person to act.

Stressful situation: A situation that has a stressor in it.

Stressor: The incident or event that provokes stress.

Style: The distinctive and characteristic mode of one's behavior.

Subconscious: A lay term to imply that part of the mind not in awareness.

Sublimation: A defense mechanism in which libido energy is utilized in socially acceptable avenues.

Substitution: A defense mechanism by which one attitude or emotion is replaced by another.

Suburban: An outlying and adjacent part of a city.

Superego: A psychoanalytic term to represent that part of the psychic structure that is the individual's standard of values, ethics, and conscience.

Supervision: In psychiatric nursing a teaching or educative process by which therapy is managed.

Suppression: A defense mechanism in which conscious effort is made to overcome unpleasant thoughts or experiences.

Surrogate: One who takes the place of another; a substitute person.

Symbiosis: A term used in psychiatry to identify the relationship between two people who are totally dependent on each other.

Symbolization: A defense mechanism in which an abstract representation is made to an acutal object.

Testify: To give evidence under oath in court.

Therapeutic: Serving to cure or heal.

Tranquilizer: Medication prescribed to calm an individual.

Trauma: The result of an injury or wound violently produced; in psychiatry, the result of an emotional wound which is long-term in effect.

Transference: Feelings and attitudes of the patient toward a therapist that are displacements of the patient's feelings toward other people in his life.

Unconscious: A psychoanalytic concept describing thoughts, feelings, and behavior not in awareness. It also refers to a division of the mind.

Undoing: A defense mechanism by which something is verbalized or acted on in reverse in the hopes of "undoing" something which the ego finds intolerable.

Victim: Someone who is harmed, injured, killed, destroyed or sacrificed, whether it be by ruthless design or incidentally or accidentally.

Victimology: The study of the victim.

Withdrawn: A form of behavior that implies a retreat from reality.

INDEX